Obstetric Anesthesia Practice

Obstetric Anesthesia Practice

Edited by

Alan D. Kaye, MD, PhD

Vice-Chancellor of Academic Affairs, Chief Academic Officer, and Provost;
Professor, Departments of Anesthesiology and Pharmacology, Toxicology,
and Neurosciences Louisiana State University School of Medicine
Department of Anesthesiology
Louisiana State University School of Medicine
Shreveport, LA, USA

Richard D. Urman, MD, MBA, FASA

Associate Professor of Anesthesia
Harvard Medical School
Department of Anesthesiology, Perioperative and Pain Medicine
Brigham and Women's Hospital
Boston, MA, USA

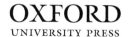

OXFORD
UNIVERSITY PRESS

OXFORD
UNIVERSITY PRESS

Oxford University Press is a department of the University of Oxford. It furthers
the University's objective of excellence in research, scholarship, and education
by publishing worldwide. Oxford is a registered trade mark of Oxford University
Press in the UK and certain other countries.

Published in the United States of America by Oxford University Press
198 Madison Avenue, New York, NY 10016, United States of America.

Library of Congress Cataloging-in-Publication Data
Names: Kaye, Alan D., editor. | Urman, Richard D., editor.
Title: Obstetric Anesthesia Practice / edited by
Alan D. Kaye and Richard D. Urman.
Description: New York, NY : Oxford University Press, [2021] |
Includes bibliographical references and index.
Identifiers: LCCN 2020041606 (print) | LCCN 2020041607 (ebook) |
ISBN 9780190099824 (paperback) | ISBN 9780190099848 (epub) |
ISBN 9780190099855 (online)
Subjects: MESH: Anesthesia, Obstetrical—methods |
Pregnancy Complications—surgery
Classification: LCC RG732 (print) | LCC RG732 (ebook) |
NLM WO 450 | DDC 617.9/682—dc23
LC record available at https://lccn.loc.gov/2020041606
LC ebook record available at https://lccn.loc.gov/2020041607

DOI: 10.1093/med/9780190099824.001.0001

1 3 5 7 9 8 6 4 2

Printed by Integrated Books International, United States of America

To my wife Dr. Kim Kaye and my children, Aaron and Rachel Kaye, for being the inspiration to work hard in my life;
To my mother Florence, sister Sheree, and brother Adam for sticking with me all of my life;
To all my colleagues at the LSU School of Medicine in Shreveport, including Dr. Ghali Ghali, Dr. Charles Fox, Dr. Chris Kevil, and Dr. David Lewis for their support and friendship.
—**Alan D. Kaye**

To all my mentors for all their advice and for being there when I need them;
To my wife Dr. Zina Matlyuk and my children, Abigail and Isabelle, for their love and support;
To my patients who ultimately will be the beneficiaries of this book;
To my colleagues who inspire me every day.
—**Richard D. Urman**

Contents

viii   Contents

Foreword

Obstetrics as a specialty continues to evolve. Here in the United States, preterm delivery rates are finally decreasing, while cesarean section rates have continued to increase in some locations. Recently, maternal mortality has become the major concern occupying the attention of physicians, hospitals, and beaurocrats. Despite all of these issues, one major change in the last forty-years, which has dramatically transformed the field of obstetrics, pain control.

Obstetric anesthesia as a specialty has been around for some time. The journey has gone from medication and specifically administered local anesthesia, such as pudendal blocks, to epidurals that remove the vast majority of pain during this otherwise painful process. As an obstetrician, it is quite common for my patients to think more highly of the anesthesiologists that they just met, than myself who has cared for them during the course of their pregnancy. Pain elimination has that effect on people.

Like most specialties, obstetrical anesthesia has evolved and become an art. Scientific evidence has shown us the best techniques, medications, and the best timing for their use. The current book by Kaye and Urman is a comprehensive evaluation of anesthesia's use in obstetrics. It includes all the current techniques and drugs.

As a health care provider, we are called to always practice our best. This includes keeping up with the latest techniques and information. This book provides the necessary foundation for the reader to accomplish this goal.

David F. Lewis, MD, MBA
Professor and Chair, Department of Obstetrics and Gynecology
Dean, School of Medicine, LSUHSC-S

Preface

The first edition of *Obstetrical Anesthesia* is intended to provide a timely update in the field of obstetrical anesthesia and continue the mission of providing a concise, up-to-date, evidence-based, and richly illustrated book for students, trainees, and practicing clinicians. The book comprehensively covers a robust list of topics focused to improve understanding in the field with emphasis on recent developments in clinical practices, technology, and procedures. We strived for a simple, accessible format that avoids encyclopedic language and lengthy discussions.

As the practice of obstetric anesthesia becomes increasingly recognized as a major sub-specialty of anesthesia, there is a growing interest from current practitioners to evolve their neuraxial, regional, and general anesthesia techniques and understanding of the latest evidence. This book contains all the essential topics that are required for the practitioner to quickly assess the obstetric patient and stratify her risk; decide on the type of analgesic and anesthetic plan that is most appropriate for the patient, including its feasibility and safety; provide expert consultation to the other members of the obstetric team; manage anesthesia care and complications; and arrange for advanced care if needed. We placed particular emphasis on clear, detailed anatomic color drawings; latest techniques and images; an easy-to-read outline format when appropriate; and clinically relevant, practical aspects of obstetric anesthesia. The chapter contributors are national and international experts in the field, and the book's compact size makes it easy to carry around in the labor and delivery suite.

There is nothing as miraculous as watching a healthy baby be born into this world full of opportunity. We as clinicians must consistently strive to improve ourselves to deliver the best care for newborns and mothers each day. We hope you enjoy our book!

Alan D. Kaye, MD, PhD
Shreveport, LA, USA

Richard D. Urman, MD, MBA, FASA
Boston, MA, USA

Contributors

Benjamin F. Aquino, MD
Attending Anesthesiologist
Department of Anesthesiology
Illinois Masonic Medical Center
Chicago, IL, USA

Elvera L. Baron, MD, PhD
Assistant Professor
Department of Anesthesiology, Perioperative
and Pain Medicine
Department of Medical Education
Icahn School of Medicine at Mount Sinai
New York, NY, USA

Gavin T. Best, MD
Department of Anesthesiology
Baylor College of Medicine
Houston, TX, USA

Shobana Bharadwaj, MBBS
Assistant Professor
Department of Anesthesiology
University of Maryland School of
Medicine
Baltimore, MD, USA

Darshna Bhatt, DO, MHA
Assistant Professor of Pediatrics, Division
of Neonatology
Department of Pediatrics
CHoR at VCU, Virginia COmmonwealth
University
Richmond, VA, USA

Michelle S. Burnette, MD
Department of Anesthesia and Critical Care
Medicine
The George Washington University
Washington, DC, USA

Paulina Cardenas, MD, FASA
Associate Professor
Department of Anesthesiology
UT Health San Antonio
San Antonio, TX, USA

Nayef Chahin, MD
Assistant Professor and Associate Program
Director
Department of Pediatrics
Children's Hospital of Richmond at VCU
Richmond, VA, USA

Everett Chu, MD
Resident Physician
Department of Anesthesiology and Critical
Care Medicine
Washington, DC, USA

Jacqueline Curbelo, DO
Assistant Professor
Department of Anesthesiology
Joe R. and Teresa Lozano Long School
of Medicine, University of Texas Health
Science Center
San Antonio, TX, USA

Marianne David, MD
Assistant Professor
Department of Anesthesiology and Critical
Care Medicine
The George Washington University
Washington, DC, USA

Aladino De Ranieri, MD, PhD
Attending Anesthesiologist
Advocate Illinois Masonic Hospital
Chicago, IL, USA

Yi Deng, MD
Assistant Professor
Department of Anesthesiology
Baylor College of Medicine
Houston, TX, USA

Thais Franklin dos Santos, MD
Obstetric Anesthesiologist
Neuroanesthesia Fellow
Department of Anesthesiology
University of Miami/Jackson Memorial Hospital
Miami, FL, USA

Michelle Eddins, MD
Anesthesiologist
Department of Anesthesiology and Pain Management
UT Southwestern Medical Center
Dallas, TX, USA

Beata Evans, MD
Assistant Professor
Department of Anesthesiology
VCU Health
Richmond, VA, USA

Fadi Farah, MD
Anesthesiologist, Pain Physician, Assistant Professor
Department of Anesthesiology and Pain Medicine
Montefiore Medical Center
Bronx, NY, USA

Daniel Fisher, MD
Resident Physician
Department of Anesthesia and Critical Care
The George Washington University Hospital
Washington, DC, USA

Jessica Galey, MD
Anesthesiologist
Department of Anesthesiology
University of Maryland School of Medicine
Baltimore, MD, USA

Kanchana Gattu, MD
Assistant Professor
Department of Anesthesiology, Division of Pain Medicine
University of Maryland School of Medicine
Baltimore, MD, USA

Arina Ghosh, MD
Resident Physician in Anesthesiology
Department of Anesthesiology, Perioperative Medicine, and Pain Management
University of Miami/Jackson Memorial Hospital
Miami, FL, USA

Sandra N. Gonzalez, MD
Assistant Professor of Anesthesiology
Department of Anesthesiology
University of Florida
Gainesville, FL, USA

David Gutman, MD, MBA
Assistant Professor
Department of Anesthesia and Perioperative Medicine
Medical University of South Carolina
Charleston, SC, USA

Leila Haghi, MD
Research Scholar
Department of Rheumatology
University of Chicago
Chicago, IL, USA

Afshin Heidari, MD
Department of Anesthesiology
Advocate Illinois Masonic
Chicago, IL, USA

Geoffrey Ho, MBBS
Research Assistant
Department of Anesthesiology and Critical Care
George Washington University School of Medicine and Health Sciences
Washington, DC, USA

Najmeh Izadpanah, MD, BS
Anesthesiologist
Department of Anesthesiology
University of Maryland Medical Center
Baltimore, MD, USA

Arunthevaraja Karuppiah, MBBS, MD
Obstetric Anesthesiology Clinical Fellow
Department of Anesthesiology and Critical Care
University of Maryland
College Park, MD, USA

Daniel Katz, MD
Associate Professor
Department of Anesthesiology, Perioperative and Pain Medicine
Department of Medical Education
Icahn School of Medicine at Mount Sinai
New York, NY, USA

Alan D. Kaye, MD, PhD
Vice-Chancellor of Academic Affairs, Chief Academic Officer, and Provost; Professor
Departments of Anesthesiology and Pharmacology, Toxicology, and Neurosciences
Louisiana State University School of Medicine
Department of Anesthesiology
Louisiana State University School of Medicine
Shreveport, LA, USA

Faiza A. Khan, MBBS, MD
Associate Professor
Department of Anesthesiology
University of Arkansas for Medical Sciences
Little Rock, AR, USA

Joseph Khoury, MD
Associate Professor
Department of Pediatrics
Children's Hospital of Richmond at VCU
Richmond, VA, USA

Fatoumata Kromah, MD, FASA
Associate Professor
Department of Anesthesiology
Virginia Commonwealth University
Health System
Richmond, VA, USA

Seung Lee, MD, MBA
Assistant Professor
Department of Anesthesiology, Division
of Pain Medicine
University of Maryland School of Medicine
Baltimore, MD, USA

Lucy Li, MD
Resident Physician
Department of Anesthesia, Critical Care
and Pain Medicine
Massachusetts General Hospital
Boston, MA, USA

Henry Liu, MD
Professor
Department of Anesthesiology and
Perioperative Medicine
Penn State College of Medicine
Hershey, PA, USA

Michael Marotta, MD
Assistant Professor
Department of Anesthesia and Perioperative
Medicine
Medical University of South Carolina
Charleston, SC, USA

Nora Martin, MD
Anesthesiologist
Department of Anesthesiology
Kaiser Permanente-MAPMG
Rockville, MD, USA

Patrick McConville, MD, FASA
Physician
Department of Anesthesiology
University of Tennessee
Knoxville, TN, USA

Robert Mester, MD
Assistant Professor
Department of Anesthesia and Perioperative
Medicine
Medical University of South Carolina
Charleston, SC, USA

Jill M. Mhyre, MD
Professor and Chair
Department of Anesthesiology
University of Arkansas for Medical
Sciences (UAMS)
Little Rock, AR, USA

Trevor Miller, MD
Anesthesiologist
Department of Anesthesiology
Integrated Anesthesia Associates LLC Fairfield
Division
East Hartford, CT, USA

Shairko Missouri, MD
NYU School of Medicine
Department of Anesthesiology, Pain Medicine
and Intensive Care
Clinical Assistant Professor
New York, NY, USA

Taylor Mueller, MD
Anesthesiologist
Department of Anesthesiology
New York University
New York, NY, USA

Melissa A. Nikolaidis, MD
Assistant Professor
Department of Anesthesiology
Baylor College of Medicine
Houston, TX, USA

Anvinh Nguyen, MD
Cardiothoracic Anesthesiologist
Department of Anesthesiology
Baylor College of Medicine
Houston, TX, USA

Samuel Onyewu, MBChB
Anesthesiologist/Clinical Fellow
Department of Anesthesiology
Yale University/Yale New Haven Hospital
New Haven, CT, USA

Easha Patel, MD
Resident Physician
Department of Obstetrics and Gynecology
Virginia Commonwealth University
Health System
Richmond, VA, USA

Rajanya S. Petersson, MD, MS, FACS
Associate Professor
Department of Otolaryngology—Head and Neck
Surgery
Virginia Commonwealth University
Health System
Richmond, VA, USA

Carrie Polin, MD
Assistant Professor
Department of Anesthesiology
University of Tennessee Medical Center
Knoxville, TN, USA

Kevin Quinn, MD
Resident
Department of Otolaryngology
Virginia Commonwealth University
Richmond, VA, USA

Shamantha Reddy, MD, FASA
Director, Obstetric Anesthesia
Department of Anesthesiology
Montefiore Medical Center
Bronx, NY, USA

Courtney Rhoades, DO, MBA
Medical Director of Labor and Delivery
Department of Obstetrics and Gynecology
University of Florida
Gainesville, FL, USA

Christa L. Riley, MD
Assistant Professor
Department of Anesthesiology
VCU School of Medicine
Richmond, VA, USA

Laura Roland, MD
Department of Anesthesia and CCM
The George Washington University
Washington, DC, USA

Joel Sirianni, MD
Assistant Professor
Department of Anesthesia and Perioperative
Medicine
Medical University of South Carolina
Charleston, SC, USA

Yelena Spitzer, MD
Anesthesiologist
Department of Anesthesiology
Montefiore Medical Center
Bronx, NY, USA

Lacey E. Straube, MD
Assistant Professor
Department of Anesthesiology
University of North Carolina School of Medicine
Chapel Hill, NC, USA

Agathe Streiff, MD
Assistant Professor
Department of Anesthesiology
Montefiore Medical Center
Bronx, NY, USA

Justin Swengel, MD
Anesthesiology Fellow
Department of Anesthesiology
University of North Carolina
Chapel Hill, NC, USA

Richard D. Urman, MD, MBA
Associate Professor of Anesthesia
Department of Anesthesiology, Perioperative
and Pain Medicine
Brigham and Women's Hospital
Boston, MA, USA

Kristen Vanderhoef, MD
Assistant Professor
Department of Anesthesiology
University of Florida
Gainesville, FL, USA

Jingping Wang, MD, PhD
Attending Physician
Department of Anesthesia, Critical Care and
Pain Medicine
Massachusetts General Hospital
Boston, MA, USA

Blake Watterworth, MD
Assistant Professor
Department of Anesthesiology, Division
of Pain Medicine
University of Maryland School of Medicine
Baltimore, MD, USA

Adam L. Wendling, MD
Associate Professor
Department of Anesthesiology
University of Florida
Gainesville, FL, USA

Timothy Wills, MD
Resident
Department of Anesthesiology
Virginia Commonwealth University
Richmond, VA, USA

Miheret Yitayew, MD, MPH
Neonatal-Perinatal Medicine Fellow
Department of Pediatrics
Children's Hospital of Richmond at Virginia
Commonwealth University
Richmond, VA, USA

Reine Zbeidy, MD
Assistant Professor, Clinical Anesthesiology
Program Director, Obstetric Anesthesia Fellowship
Division of Obstetric Anesthesiology
University of Miami Miller School of Medicine
Miami, FL, USA

Carole Zouki, MD
Physician
Department of Anesthesia
Illinois Masonic Medical Center
Chicago, IL, USA

1

Physiological Changes During Pregnancy

Shairko Missouri, Trevor Miller, and Taylor Mueller

The Cardiovascular System

A high-flow, low-resistance hyperdynamic circulation develops in pregnancy, at first driven by hormonally mediated peripheral vasodilation. This begins as early as 8 weeks of gestation. The heart rate steadily climbs before plateauing at 10–15 beats above baseline by 30-32 weeks gestation.[2] With the increase in heart rate, cardiac output also incrementally increases. Initially, the heart rate-mediated increases in cardiac output result in a slight decrease in mean arterial pressure (MAP) and widening pulse pressures. The decreased MAP activates renin-angiotensin autoregulation, resulting in improved salt and water retention and overall plasma volume expansion by up to 40–50%. The larger plasma volume increases preload, end-diastolic volumes, and thus stroke volume beginning around the middle of the first trimester. This is augmented by a 20% increase in blood volume.[4] The effects of peripheral vasodilation on systemic vascular resistance (SVR) and blood pressure (BP) are pronounced, resulting in an average decrease in SVR of 20% and decreased systolic and diastolic BP of 8% and 20%, respectively.[5] Despite the expansion in intravascular volume, the peripheral vasodilation and increased pulmonary vascular compliance cause the central venous pressure (CVP) and pulmonary capillary wedge pressures to remain relatively unchanged.[5] Additionally, the ejection fraction remains unchanged relative to baseline values.[6]

By 20 weeks of gestation, the enlarging uterus approaches the level of the umbilicus and begins compressing the inferior vena cava (IVC) and descending aorta in the supine position. The decrease in SVR also plateaus in the middle of the second trimester. The rise in cardiac output continues, but in a nonlinear[1] trajectory.

Cardiac output (CO) reaches its peak in the early third trimester, with heart rate (HR) peaking at 16 beats per minute above baseline.[1] There is also an average of 40 gram increase in left ventricular mass above baseline in the early third trimester.

By 38–40 weeks, cardiac output decreases by 25–30% when turning from lateral to supine position due to aortocaval compression. Because there is no autoregulation of uteroplacental blood flow, this can compromise flow to the fetus resulting in uteroplacental insufficiency and fetal heart rate decelerations. Maternal compensation includes an increase in sympathetic tone and diversion of blood flow through collateral circulation to reach the right heart through the azygous veins and vertebral plexus system.[1,2,3]

Electrocardiographic (EKG) changes occur late in pregnancy around gestational weeks 37 due to the cephalad displacement of the diaphragm, causing left-sided rotation of the heart. There will be widening of the lower chest wall by 5–7 cm associated with the 4 cm displacement of the diaphragm. Consequently, normal Q waves on the inferior leads and T wave inversion are not unexpected on the EKG during late pregnancy.[8]

Labor and Delivery

Epidural veins and venous plexus are engorged and during uterine contraction there is autotransfusion of 500 ml from the uterine vasculature as the muscular wall contracts. Increases in cardiac workload and autotransfusion pose a danger for pregnant patients with limited cardiac reserve, due to the risk of ventricular failure or development of pulmonary edema.

During early labor, CO increases 15% above baseline, and during active labor it increases by 25%. It rises by 50% during maternal pushes in the second stage of labor. These increases are tempered to varying degrees by the epidural anesthetic. Notably the increase in cardiac output with uterine contractions persists. In addition, the fact that positioning the patient in left lateral position significantly increases CO during labor relative to supine suggests CO during labor is preload dependent.[1] At the time of delivery, there is an 80% increase in CO as the uterus involutes following delivery of the fetus and placenta.

HR and BP return to baseline prepregnancy levels within 6–8 weeks[1] postdelivery. CO returns to normal over the course of a month. In as short as two weeks, there is a reduction in left ventricular size and contractility.[7]

Cardiovascular Parameters During Pregnancy

Parameters	Changes
Cardiac output	30–50% increase
Stroke volume	30% increase
Plasma volume	50% increase
Hear rate	15–25(bpm) increase
SVR	20% decrease
Systolic BP	slight decrease
Diastolic BP	20% decrease
CVP	unchanged
FVP	2–3 × increase

Pregnancy is a high-flow and low-resistance state.

SVR = systemic vascular resistance, BP = blood pressure, CVP = central venous pressure, FVP = femoral venous pressure

The Hematologic System

The pregnant patient prepares for hemorrhage during delivery through the development of physiologic anemia and a prothrombotic state. Overall there is an expanded plasma volume, mild neutrophilia, mild thrombocytopenia, increased procoagulant factors and decreased anticoagulants, and diminished fibrinolysis. There is an increase in plasma and red and white cell volumes during pregnancy. The increase in plasma volume is 40–50%, while the increase in red cell mass is only 15–20%.[9] The increase in red cell mass is 10–15% at 6–12 weeks and expands until 30–34 weeks before plateauing at near term.[9] This creates a physiologic anemia of pregnancy. The increase in red cell mass requires improved maternal stores of up to a two-fold increase in iron, a two-fold increase in B12, and a ten to twenty fold increase in folate.[15] This is driven by increased erythropoietin (EPO) levels, which climb to 50% above baseline. Corresponding with red cell mass expansion is an increase in 2,3—DPG (Diphosphoglycerides) which facilitates offloading of O_2 to the fetus.[16] As mentioned in the cardiovascular section, the plasma expansion is thought to be driven by an initial hormonally mediated (atrial naturietic peptide, estrogen, progesterone, and nitric oxide) vasodilation and transiently dropping blood pressure, and causes RAAS activation and compensatory fluid and salt retention.[10]

Pregnancy is associated with a mild leukocytosis, with mean values ranging from 10,000–16,000 with reported upper levels of 29,000. The leukocytosis is primarily neutrophilic-predominant and begins to develop in the second to third month of pregnancy, plateauing in third trimester.[17]

A gestational thrombocytopenia is common in pregnancy, with typical levels remaining in the normal range: 150,000–450,000. Levels less than 100,000 should be investigated, and differential diagnosis includes idiopathic thrombocytopenic purpura (ITP), severe pre-eclampsia, sepsis with disseminated intravascular coagulation (DIC), HELLP syndrome (Hemolysis, Elevated Liver enzymes, Low Platelets count), Thrombotic Thrombocytopenia Purpura (TTP, antiphospholipid syndrome, and drug-induced thrombocytopenia.

Overall, the coagulation profile demonstrates an increase in procoagulant factors, a reduction in anticoagulant factors, and a reduced state of fibrinolysis. Factor I, VII, VIII, IX, X, XII, and fibrinogen levels are elevated during pregnancy. Von Willebrand factors increases two- to fourfold during pregnancy and returns to baseline postpartum.[18] Factors XIII and antithrombin (AT) are decreased. AT levels may be slightly increased or stable during pregnancy with a noticeable fall in level by 30% below baseline following delivery. This is likely mediated by consumption. AT levels return to baseline 72 hours postpartum.[19] Thrombopoietin, platelet production, and destruction are all increased with a gradual decline in platelet counts as pregnancy progresses.[11] Resistance to activated protein C reaches a plateau in the second and third trimester.[12] Free protein S decreases.[13] Fibrinolytic inhibitor levels, including thrombin activated fibrinolytic inhibitor and plasminogen activator inhibitor 1 and 2, increase, thus leading to decreased fibrinolysis.[20] Hence, pregnancy is a hypercoagulable state and should return to normal 12 weeks postpartum.

Over the course of 6-8 weeks following delivery, the plasma volume, white blood cell count, red blood cell count, platelets, and coagulation fibrinolytic system return to baseline.[21]

Respiratory Changes

Most patients who have underlying lung pathologies, except for pulmonary hypertension or chronic respiratory insufficiency due to parenchymal or neuromuscular disease, can tolerate normal pregnancy.[22] Minute ventilation increases during pregnancy, due to higher respiratory center sensitivity and drive, compensated respiratory alkalosis, and reduced functional residual capacity (FRC). Vital capacity and forced expiration are preserved.

Anatomical Changes

The costochondral ligaments of ribcage become more relaxed, allowing for widening of the subcostal angle by approximately 68° to 103°. This causes an expansion in the lower rib cage circumference[25] by around 5 cm to accommodate for the enlarged uterus later in pregnancy.[23] Similar elastochondral relaxation takes place in the pelvic ligaments at the sacroiliac joints and the pubis. Such relaxation is mediated by the hormone relaxin.[24] It takes a few months after delivery for those changes to get back to normal.

There is also 4 cm elevation of the diaphragm, which compromises the chest wall compliance by 35–40%,[26] which progressively worsens as the gravid uterus increases intraabdominal pressure. This will also lead to a reduction in the end expiratory volume (EEV).

Despite the elevated diaphragm, tidal volume (TV) is increased during pregnancy as a result of the widening in the ribcage and strong respiratory stimulation from an increase in progesterone[30] which attenuate tidal volume dependency on diaphragmatic excursion. The inspiratory capacity (IC) will increase. The inspiratory reserve volume (IRV) is reduced early in pregnancy due to an increased TV (Figure 1.1). IRV increases in the third trimester due to reduced FRC.[27,28]

FRC will be reduced due to the reduction in chest wall compliance and this will be more noticeable at 12 weeks of gestation when the residual volume (RV) begins to decrease. This will maintain vital capacity (VC) at its normal pre-gravid level or cause a mild increase in VC.

The FRC will decline during the late stage of pregnancy with supine position and lead to closure of closing volume (CV) earlier in tidal volume, causing an increase in alveolar-arterial-gradient (PA-Pa).

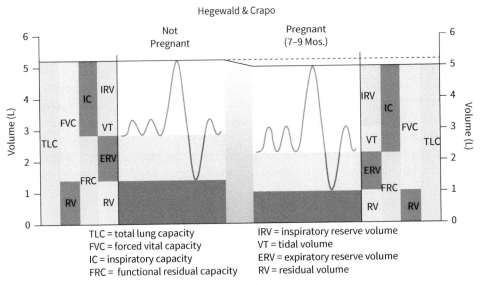

TLC = total lung capacity
FVC = forced vital capacity
IC = inspiratory capacity
FRC = functional residual capacity
IRV = inspiratory reserve volume
VT = tidal volume
ERV = expiratory reserve volume
RV = residual volume

Figure 1.1 Changes in lung volumes with pregnancy. The most significant changes are reductions in FRC and its subcomponents ERV and RV, and increases in IC and VT.

Reproduced with permission from Hegewald MJ, Respiratory physiology in pregnancy. *Clincal Chest Medicine.* 2001;32(1):1–13.

Minute volume (MV) will increase by 30% during pregnancy even at rest due to the increase in TV.[30]

Lung compliance will not change during a healthy pregnancy.

The CO_2 chemo-sensitivity and respiratory drive start early in pregnancy and return to normal soon after delivery.[31]

Pulmonary function test (PFT) values remain almost the same during pregnancy. The forced expiratory volume in 1 second (FEV1), peak expiratory flow rate (PEFR), and FEV1 to forced vital capacity (FVC) ratio are all normal during pregnancy.[27,28]

The volume compliance curve will stay the same as during nonpregnant women and dead space will be decreased in pregnancy due to the increase cardiac output and an improved physiological shunt at the apices.

Carbon dioxide production increases by up to 300 ml/min due to high metabolic production. However, a state of respiratory alkalosis with $PaCO_2$ during pregnancy between 30–34 mm Hg is normal. Pregnancy increases TV and MV, creating respiratory compensation.[29] Respiratory alkalosis will stimulate renal excretion of bicarbonate (HCO_3) to keep HCO^3 at the 15–20 mEq/L[30] level.

The alkalosis state will increase 2,3 diphosphoglycerate synthesis which will shift oxygen dissociation curve to the right, favoring oxygen delivery and extraction to fetus through the placenta.[30]

The hypoxic ventilatory drive doubles during pregnancy, despite the blood and cerebrospinal fluid alkalosis that inhibit hypoxic ventilatory response. The sensitivity of the drive is attributed to both estrogen and progesterone.

Due to hyperpnea in pregnancy, the partial pressure of oxygen (PaO_2) is mildly elevated, with ranges of 100–105 mm Hg, enhancing the diffusion gradient of oxygen across the placenta.[32,33]

The diffusing capacity of carbon monoxide (D_{CO}) is either unchanged in pregnancy or slightly reduced. The diffusion will increase with high cardiac output and the pulmonary capillary recruitments; however, this increase in diffusion is offset by the hemodilution of pregnancy.[34] Normally there is increase in D_{CO} in supine position which will be absent during pregnancy as a result of reduction in venous return.

Summary of the Respiratory Changes During Pregnancy

Parameters	Changes
Minute volume	increased
Tidal volume	increased
Respiratory rate	unchanged
TLC	unchanged/reduced
VC	unchanged/increased
LC	unchanged
Chest wall compliance	reduced
Inspiratory capacity	mild increase
FRC	reduced
RV	mild

Parameters	Changes
ERV	reduced
Thoracic diameter	increased 5–7 cm
Diaphragm	elevated 4 cm
FEV1	unchanged
FVC	unchanged
FEV1/FVC	unchanged
PH	7.44
PaO_2	107-105-103 mm Hg elevated 1st 2nd and 3rd trimesters consecutively
$PaCO_2$	30 mm Hg decreased
HCO_3^-	15–20 mEq/L decreased
D_{CO}	unchanged/mild reduction

TLC = total lung capacity, VC = vital capacity, LC = lung capacity, FRC = functional residual capacity, RV = residual volume, ERV = expiratory, residual volume, FEV1 = forced expiratory volume in 1 second, FVC = forced vital capacity, D_{CO} = diffusing capacity for carbon monoxide

High Altitude and Pregnancy

High altitude imposes certain changes and risk to pregnant women. D_{CO} is higher with pregnant women who reside at high altitudes compared to those who reside at sea level. The increase in D_{CO} supplements the increased MV and increased hemoglobin concentrations, thus increasing oxygen saturation.[37]

McAuliffe et al. demonstrated no significant differences in mean FVC, FEV1, FEV1/FVC, and PEFR of nonpregnant women at high altitude compared to nonpregnant women living at sea level. Pregnant women living at high altitude had larger mean TLC, IC, FRC ERV and RV than pregnant women living at sea level. Pregnant women living at high altitude compared with pregnant women living at sea level had higher mean FVC and FEV1, but their mean FEV1/FVC was lower. The mean PEFR of pregnant women living at high altitude did not differ significantly from that of pregnant women living at sea level.

TLC, RV, ERV, IC and FRC were elevated in pregnant women at high altitude.[37] Studies by Keyes et al. showing higher incidence of pre-eclampsia and stillbirth in pregnant women living at high altitude than dwellers pregnant living at sea level.[38]

Physiologic Dyspnea of Pregnancy

Shortness of breath at rest or on mild exertion during pregnancy is referred to as physiological dyspnea. By week 30 of pregnancy, 75% of women have exertional dyspnea.[39] The proposed cause is the increase in the work of breathing and minute volume in response to the enlarged uterus. Other factors contributing to the etiology of dyspnea include anemia, nasal congestion, and increased pulmonary blood flow.[40] Psychological studies suggest that dyspnea is due to the increased work of breathing rather than the increase in the sensitivity to mechanical loads.[40] Increasing endurance exercise didn't seem to show any evidence of improving the cardiovascular response compared to post-partum. Fetal response to short duration of exercise is moderate and returns to base-line after exercise. Furthermore, prenatal physical conditioning did affect fetal growth significantly.[41]

Clinicians need to differentiate the normal dyspnea of pregnancy from pathological ones referring to other clinical findings such as respiratory rate higher than 20 bpm, $PaCO_2$ less than 30 or greater than 35, hypoxemia, abnormal spirometry, and cardiac echocardiography.

The Renal System

Pregnancy induces significant functional, anatomical, and structural changes in the renal system. The high increase in progesterone plays a major mediator in many of those anatomical changes, namely reducing ureteral tone, peristalsis, and contraction pressure.

The importance of understanding those changes will not only help monitoring pre-natal progress but also distinguishing those changes from any pathological scenarios that may occur.

Changes in renal function during the menstrual cycle are similar to the changes happening at the early phase of pregnancy. Hormonal variations during the midluteal phase include lower mean arterial pressure and systemic vascular resistance, resulting in increased cardiac output, renal plasma flow (RPF), and glomerular filtration rate (GFR).[42]

The kidney size, volume, and length increase to approximately 30% of its original size 1–1.5 cm,[43] due to an increase in vascular and interstitial spaces, water retention, and hydronephrosis, even if the total number of nephrons remains constant. The kidneys start to shrink and return to normal size in up to six months postpartum.[44]

The renal pelvis, the calyces, and ureters are markedly dilated, which is often and mis-diagnosed as obstructive uropathy.[45,46] The dilation is due to smooth muscle relaxation from the increased secretions of progesterone.

There is also a slight reduction in cortical width without an ill effect.[46]

Physiological hydronephrosis and hydroureters will be experienced by 80% of preg-nant women. This ureteric dilatation develops during the second trimester and is more frequent and pronounced in primigravid women. It is prominent above the linea termi-nalis.[49] The right ureter is more affected because it crosses the iliac vessel and the ovary at its entrance to the pelvis.[46] Nonobstructive dilatation of the left ureter is often pre-sent.[47] The maximal incidence of hydronephrosis is reached at 28 weeks, with an inci-dence of 63% of overall hydronephrosis.[48] Au et al. found that hormonal balance during pregnancy is of less importance in causing hydroureter.[50]

Ureteric dilatation can be reduced clinically by placing the woman on the side least affected or in the knee-elbow position which will improve drainage while treating the commonly occurring ascending urinary tract infection during pregnancy.[51] There is a possible relationship with the development of pre-eclampsia as demonstrated by iso-topic Reno graphic studies.[52]

A worsening of an existing hydronephrosis or an acute hydronephrosis should be considered as a possible cause of uncertain abdominal pain during pregnancy.[53]

Renal plasma flow (RPF) increases by 80% during early pregnancy and falls to 40–65% during the third trimester. GFR remains at a level 50% above the nonpreg-nant throughout pregnancy.[54] The increase in GFR causes creatinine level and Blood Urea and Nitrogen (BUN) to decrease to below normal levels at term, and renal disease during pregnancy should be suspicious if serum creatinine level is greater than or equal 1.2 mg/dl.[55]

There is a study suggesting that hyperfiltration continues at levels 20% above normal at postpartum week two and resolves by one month postpartum.[56]

Those physiological and anatomic changes impose a few clinical implications:

- The dilated collecting system can hold 200 to 300 mL of urine, leading to urinary stasis and a 40% increased risk for asymptomatic bacteriuria and pyelonephritis.
- Elective radiologic examination of the urinary tract should be deferred until the an-atomical sizes of the renal system return to prepregnancy size. It should be consid-ered during radiological interpretation. Kidney size can take six months to return to prepregnant size.
- Rarely, massive ureteral and renal pelvis dilation might precipitate the "overdisten-sion syndrome."

Changes in Glomerular Filtration Rate (GFR) and Tubular Functions

The GFR and renal plasma flow RPF increase to levels about 50–60% above nonpregnant values. These increases occur shortly after conception and all increments are maximal in the second trimester. There is often a reduction in GFR of 15% during the final month of the third trimester and this must be taken into consideration, especially when assessing the course of pregnancy in a woman with known renal disease.

There are no substantial alterations in the production of creatinine and urea despite the increase in GFR. Creatinine levels fall from a nonpregnant level to 0.86 mg/dl in the first tri-mester, to 0.81 mg/dl in the second trimester, and to 0.87 mg/dl[57] in the third trimester. An increasing serum creatinine greater than 0.87 mg/dl in pregnancy could indicate an acute kidney injury.[57]

Serum urea is low in pregnancy due to a reduction in protein degradation and an in-crease in clearance. Average plasma urea levels of 7–12 mg/dl during first trimester, 3–13 mg/dl during the second and 3–11 mg/dl during the third trimester. In nonpregnant healthy woman, BUN is 7–20 mg/dl.

Glucose excretion is increased and tubular reabsorption of glucose is less efficient.

Proteinuria increases due to high RPF and should be considered abnormal when it is twice the normal limit. Normal proteinuria is 150–250 mg/24 hr in healthy women.

Changes in Water and Electrolytes Homeostasis

Arterial vasodilation in pregnancy stimulates the sympathetic nervous systems, baroreceptors and renin-angiotensinogen-aldosterone system (RAAS), leading to a release of arginine vasopressin peptide (AVP) from the posterior hypothalamus. These changes cause sodium and water retention, hypervolemia, and hypo-osmolar state.[58,59,60]

Maternal plasma volume increases by 30–50% with 40% of that volume composing the extracellular volume (ECV). Total plasma volume is expected to be 1600 to 2000 ml above nonpregnant level.[61] Plasma volume reaches a maximum of 50% during the second trimester. There is also fluid within fetal and maternal interstitial spaces, which is greatest at term. The thresholds for thirst and antidiuretic hormone secretion are depressed, resulting in lower osmolality and serum sodium levels 4–5 mEq/L lower than nonpregnant levels.[62]

Salt and water retention in the distal tubule and collecting duct takes place, due to high aldosterone secretions from the activation of the RAAS. The increase in aldosterone is responsible for the increase in plasma volume during pregnancy.[63]

Aldosterone has a high potency for sodium-retention; however, natriuresis is promoted by progesterone, which is an aldosterone antagonist. Renin synthesis increases during pregnancy as upregulation of RAAS. There is an extra renal production of inactive renin precursor which takes place in the ovaries and decidua during early pregnancy. The estrogen produced by the placenta will stimulate the synthesis of angiotensinogen by the liver. This will be converted into angiotensin II (ANG II). Though ANG II is a potent vasopressor, systolic blood pressure in known to be low during pregnancy. This is likely due to other factors that cause the vasodilatory state of pregnancy. This refractoriness to the ANG II can be due to other hormonal effect of progesterone and vascular endothelial growth factor mediated prostacyclin and/or the monomeric state of angiotensin 1 (AT_1) receptors.[64] This explains the reason for low systolic blood pressure despite high renin production. In patients with pre-eclampsia, there is a dysregulation of the RAAS and return of ANG II sensitivity.[64]

Potassium is kept constant during pregnancy despite the increase in total body level of potassium. This is due to a balance between excretion of potassium and increase in tubular reabsorption. Progesterone promotes antikaliuretic function.[65]

Hypothalamic AVP release increases early in pregnancy as a result of increased relaxin levels. AVP mediates an increase in water reabsorption via aquaporin 2 channels in the collecting duct. The threshold for hypothalamic secretion of AVP and the threshold for thirst is reset to a lower plasma osmolality level, creating the hypo-osmolar state characteristic of pregnancy. These changes are mediated by human chorionic gonadotropin (hCG) and relaxin.[66]

The production of aminopeptidase vasopressinase by the placenta increases fourfold in middle and late pregnancy. These changes enhance the metabolic clearance of vasopressin and regulate the levels of active AVP.

In pre-eclampsia or twin pregnancies, a transient diabetes insipidus may develop due to overproduction of vasopressinase, leading to high secretion of atrial natriuretic peptides. The levels of natriuretic peptides are higher in pregnant women with chronic hypertension and pre-eclampsia.[67]

Renal Changes During Pregnancy

Parameters	Changes	Causes / Comments
Kidney size	1–1.5 cm increase	Fluid retention, hydronephrosis, return to normal up to 12 weeks
GFR	Increases 20% at 4 weeks, 40% 9 weeks, 50% at term	Increase renal plasma flow, high progesterone. Normalizes 4–6 weeks postpartum
Blood pH	7.4–7.44 slight alkalosis	
Plasma osmolality	270 mOsm/kg	Increase plasma volume
BUN	9.0 mg/mL 25% decreased	Hyperfiltration high GFR
Serum Creatinine	0.5 mg/dL 25% decreased	Hyperfiltration high GFR
Uric acid	2–3 mg/dl 20–25% reduced	
Ureter diameter	increase	Return to normal 4–6 weeks post delivery
Serum HCO3-	18–20 mEq/L 20% decreased	
Serum Na+	135 mEq/L (4–5 mEq/L less than nonpregnant)	Normal or slightly low
Serum K+	3.8 mEq/L	Slightly low due antikaliuretic effect of progesterone
Urine Glucose	Increases	Reduced reabsorption

The Gastrointestinal System

Nausea and vomiting are common in pregnancy with incidence of 50–90%. The etiology is still unknown although it has been inferred to be related to the high production of estrogen and progesterone, hCG, and TSH hormones.[68]

As pregnancy reaches 20 weeks of gestation, the enlarging uterus will encroach into the intra-abdominal area, resulting in displacement of the digestive organs. The stomach is moved upward and to the left and is rotated 45 degrees to the right of its normal vertical position. This causes a displacement of the intra-abdominal portion of the esophagus into the thorax in many patients, resulting in decreased competency of the lower esophageal sphincter. Further, this reduces the ability of the lower esophageal tone to rise, which typically occurs under high intragastric pressure to prevent reflux. As pregnancy advances into the last trimester the continued cephalad movement of the abdominal contents results in up to 80% of women experiencing pyrosis. Growth of the fetus distends the abdomen stretching the peritoneum, leading to desensitization, which can make diagnosis of acute abdomen and peritonitis more difficult.

Hormonal changes during pregnancy affect GI transit time. Increasing levels of progesterone result in inhibition of GI contractility and a decrease in esophageal peristalsis and LES tone; however, overall gastric emptying is not affected. The placenta produces gastrin, which increases gastric hydrogen ion secretion, further lowering the gastric pH. These physiologic changes result in the incidence of pyrosis and reflux esophagitis symptoms in nearly 50–80% of parturient. Aspiration pneumonia is estimated to affect 0.1% of pregnant women.

The use of opioids, including epidural opioids, in the peripartum period contributes to the reduction of esophageal tone and impaired gastric emptying. Anticholinergics will also contribute to decreased smooth muscle motility and increased risk of aspiration. Due to the changes mentioned above, all pregnant women after 20 weeks gestation should be treated as if they have a full stomach, with a minimum of 6–8 hours fasting before any elective surgery. Rapid sequence intubation, cricoid pressure, and gastric suctioning should be performed for pregnant patients to minimize aspiration risk. Furthermore, the American Society of Anesthesiologists recommends "Timely administration of oral non-particulate antacids, intravenous IV H2-receptor antagonists, and/or metoclopramide for aspiration prophylaxis." Nonparticulate antacids, such as sodium citrate, work rapidly but can increase gastric volume, so administration should not be immediately prior to induction of anesthesia. Metoclopramide is a dopamine antagonist known to cause increased gastric emptying and a modest increase in LES tone. Within the first day of the postpartum period, gastric emptying and gastric volumes return to prepregnancy state.

Summary of Gastrointestinal Changes During Pregnancy

Parameters	Changes	Causes / comments
Gastric motility	Decrease	Increased progesterone
Gastric emptying time	Increase	
Hyperemesis gravidarum		Increased thyroid hormones, hCG, progesterone, estrogen
Gastroesophageal sphincter tone	Decrease	Anatomical displacement and increased gastrin
Bowel motility	Decrease	Increased gastrin
Bowel transit time	Increase	

The Hepatic System

While there is no change in liver size, morphology, and blood flow in the parturient, there are important changes in hepatic physiology. Plasma protein concentration is reduced secondary to hemodilution described earlier. Plasma albumin concentration decreases from 4.5 to 3.9 g/100 mL in the first trimester and continues to decline to 3.3 g/100 mL by the third trimester. Total protein decreases to 7.0 g/100 mL from 7.8 g/100 mL in the nonpregnant patient. Globulin levels will decrease 10% in the first trimester and then will rise to 10% above normal by the third trimester. Due to these changes the maternal colloid pressure declines 5% in the pregnant patient. There is a 25% decrease in plasma cholinesterase activity during pregnancy; however, this has limited clinical significance in anesthetic management.

The liver produces an assortment of proteins and clotting factors including Factors V, VII, IX, X, XI, antithrombin, Protein C and S, fibrinogen, and prothrombin. As highlighted previously in this chapter, the hepatic changes during pregnancy result in elevated production of coagulation factors I, VII, VIII, IX, X, and XII leading to increased fibrinolysis, clotting, and platelet turnover.

In the pregnant period, alanine and aspartate aminotransferase ALT, AST, LDH, and serum bilirubin will increase to the upper limits of normal. Alkaline phosphatases (ALP) increases to 2–4 times normal values in late pregnancy, attributed to the increased production of isoenzymes by the placenta, bones, liver, kidneys, and small intestine. Due to hormone mediated changes in smooth muscle tone, there is a slowing of gallbladder emptying, resulting in increases of fasting and residual gallbladder volumes, specifically in the second and third trimester. As the rate of gallbladder emptying slows, the bile concentrates and predisposes the pregnant patient to gallstone formation and further complications.

The Endocrine System

In the pregnant patient, the rapid increase of metabolic demands of both the mother and fetus requires the endocrine system to undergo many changes. The hypothalamic pituitary axis is critical in the coordination of these metabolic activities. The placenta releases increased amounts of corticotropin-releasing hormone (CRH) important for the initiation of labor, and Gonadotropin-releasing hormone (GnRH) which functions primarily to promote further growth of the placenta.

During pregnancy, in response to the increase in hypothalamic releasing hormones, the pituitary gland increases in size by three times. Growth hormone secretion is largely replaced by increased expression of placenta growth hormone. As progesterone and estradiol levels increase, there is decreased gonadotropin secretion.

The anterior lobe of the pituitary gland undergoes hypertrophy in order to produce lactotrophs. The anterior pituitary production of prolactin increases throughout pregnancy in preparation for breastfeeding. In nonbreastfeeding mothers, levels of prolactin will rapidly fall after delivery.

The anterior pituitary release of thyroid-stimulating hormone (TSH) decreases during the first trimester, before returning to normal by term. This initial decrease of TSH is due in large part by the rapid rise in human chorionic gonadotropin hormone (HCG) produced by the placenta. HCG has thyroid stimulating properties resulting in negative feedback suppression of TSH release. Due to the complex hormonal feedback loops mediating TSH levels, TSH should not be used for diagnosis of thyroid dysfunction during pregnancy. Instead, checking free-T4 levels is recommended. This rapid rise of HCG can result in hyperthyroid symptoms, which may contribute to the incidence of hyperemesis gravidarum. Increased levels of estrogen result in 200% increase in synthesis of thyroxine-binding globulin correlating to a resultant 50% increase in T4 and T3 levels. Due to high metabolic demands of the fetus, there is increased transport of iodine into the fetus, resulting in a state of iodine-deficiency in the mother.

The posterior pituitary gland releases antidiuretic hormone (ADH) and oxytocin. As the placenta enlarges, there is an increased clearance of ADH, which can be associated with increased risk for development of diabetes insipidus in some women. Oxytocin is increased during throughout pregnancy, and is involved in milk production and release.

The placenta produces both CRH and adrenocorticotropic hormone (ACTH), which overrides the typical negative feedback loop, resulting in a hypercortisol state. Corticosteroid binding globulin doubles during gestation due to estrogen induced hepatic synthesis, the elevated corticosteroid binding globulin results in a 100% increase of plasma cortisol concentration during first trimester, and 200% increase at term. Interestingly, and important for diagnosis of metabolic disorders, healthy pregnant women continue to maintain diurnal variation of cortisol and ACTH levels. Normal symptoms of pregnancy (weight gain, fatigue, insulin resistance, vomiting, etc.) can make diagnosis of cortisol-excess (Cushing disease) and adrenal insufficiency nearly impossible to recognize without meticulous analysis of ACTH and Cortisol levels. Untreated adrenal insufficiency is of specific concern to the anesthesiologist as labor and its associated stress response may culminate in adrenal crisis and ensuing profound hypotension response necessitating vasopressor infusion and intravenous hydrocortisone.

The metabolic demands of pregnancy and fetus maturation require changes in carbohydrate and fat metabolism. Hyperplasia of beta cells in the pancreas result in increased insulin secretion and a resultant 10–20% drop of fasting blood glucose levels, most significantly in third trimester. Placental lactogen results in diabetogenic effects. The relative hyperinsulinemia results in mild insulin resistance, this insulin resistance is noted by increase in postprandial glucose levels, especially after high carbohydrate loads. The effects of relative insulin resistance of pregnancy can be confounded in obese patients with pre-existing insulin resistance and patients with low pancreatic reserves resulting in gestational diabetes and higher insulin dose requirements, when compared of nonpregnant women.

Similar to carbohydrate metabolism, fat metabolism changes drastically leading to utilization of fatty acids and glycerol as maternal energy sources. Glycerol is vital for maternal gluconeogenesis, providing the glucose to cross the placenta for fetal consumption. In the second semester, there is marked increase in storage and accumulation of fat secondary to triglyceride and cholesterol synthesis. As women progress into the third trimester, the increased metabolic demands result in a shift from fat accumulation to consumption with an associated increase in lipolysis. This increase in lipolysis drives the release of fatty acids and glycerol. Fatty acids are involved in energy production during maternal fasting and are converted to ketones by the liver, ketones cross the placenta freely and are utilized by the fetus. Increase in fat cells is also associated with increase in Leptin and Adiponectin, which are important in energy homeostasis, these markers will be abnormal in gestational diabetes.

Summary of the Endocrine Changes During Pregnancy

Parameters	Changes	Causes / Comments
Progesterone	Increase	
Estrogen	Increases	
Pituitary gland size	100% increase	
CRH	Increased	Initiation of Labor
GnRH	Increased	Promote growth of placenta
Adrenal gland size	Unchanged	
Thyroid gland size	10 – 15% increase	
TTH	Increase	Due to high estrogen
TBG	increase	
TSH	Decreased	Suppressed by HCG
FTH	Unchanged	
HPL	Increase	

TTH = total thyroid hormone, TBG = thyroid binding globulins, CRH = corticotropin-releasing hormone, FTH = free thyroid hormone, HPL = human placental lactogen, GnRH = gonadotropin-releasing hormone, TSH = thyroid stimulating hormone, HCG = human gonadotropin hormone

The Central and Peripheral Nervous System

There is an increase in the sensitivity to both local and general anesthetics during pregnancy. The increase in sensitivity to local anesthetic was demonstrated by Datta et al. in isolated rabbit nerves. A, B, and C fiber types from pregnant and nonpregnant specimens were administered a standardized dose of bupivacaine and times to 50% blockade were recorded. Time to 50% blockade was significantly reduced in pregnant fibers relative to nonpregnant.[69] Butterworth et al demonstrated an analogous differential sensitivity in lidocaine-treated median nerves of pregnant vs. nonpregnant human women.[70]

Consistent with these findings, there is greater sensitivity to local anesthetics when injected in the epidural space. This results in wider dermatomal spread of sensory anesthesia during pregnancy relative to age matched controls.[71] Explanations for the increased sensitivity include the respiratory alkalosis of pregnancy, reduced plasma and CSF protein levels, and hormonal influences.[71]

Table 1.1 Risks of General Anesthesia for Cesarean Delivery

Risk	Reasons	Prevention
Awareness	Often emergent nature of surgery Immediate incision after induction Use of low concentration of volatile agent because of atony, hypotension, hemorrhage, or decreased requirements in pregnancy Avoidance of preoperative sedatives Use of NMBAs	Maintain adequate depth of anesthesia, utilizing IV agents and N_2O when decreasing volatile anesthetic Administer opioids & benzodiazepines after delivery Avoid long-acting NMBAs if possible Consider BIS monitor
Aspiration/ aspiration pneumonitis	Possible recent oral intake Decreased gastric transit time in labor Decreased LES tone	Avoid solid food in labor[1] Aspiration prophylaxis RSI OG suction before extubation Extubate awake
Hemorrhage	Impairment of uterine contractility by volatile anesthetics	Decrease volatile agent after delivery TIVA for persistent atony
Difficult/failed airway	Airway edema Increased breast mass Weight gain in pregnancy	Ramped, sniffing position Immediate availability of emergency airway supplies Consider awake intubation for anticipated difficult airway Know airway algorithm Call for help early
Rapid desaturation during apnea	Decreased FRC Increased oxygen consumption	Pre-oxygenate with 3 minutes of TV breaths or 8 deep breaths of 100% FiO_2[2]
Fetal exposure to anesthetic agents	Placental transfer	Facilitate efficient delivery Administer IV anesthetics after delivery if appropriate to wait
Postoperative pain	Absence of neuraxial opioids	Consider pre-emptive truncal block or wound infiltration Multimodal analgesia

The increase in sensitivity to general anesthesia during pregnancy is well documented. Palahniuk et al in 1974 observed a 25–40% decrease in minimum alveolar concentration (MAC).[72]

Progesterone may be responsible for increases in sensitivity to both general and local anesthesia. This is implicated in animal models. Injection of progesterone into oophorectomized rabbits resulted in decrease MAC.[73] Chronic exposure to progesterone in these animals resulted in increased sensitivity to local anesthetics as well.[74] It is not currently known when nervous system sensitivity reverts to prepregnancy levels (see Table 1.1).

References

1. Meah VL, Cockcroft JR, Backx K, Shave R, Stöhr EJ. Cardiac output and related haemodynamics during pregnancy: a series of meta-analyses *Heart*. 2016;102(7):518. Epub.
2. Mashini IS, Albazzaz SJ, Fadel HE, et al. Serial noninvasive evaluation of cardiovascular hemodynamics during pregnancy. *Am J Obstet Gynecol*. 1987;156(5):1208–1213.
3. Datta S, Kodali BS, Segal S. *Obstetric Anesthesia Handbook*. New York, NY: Springer; 2010. doi:10.1007/978-0-387-88602-2_1.
4. Clark SL, Cotton DB, Lee W, et al. Central hemodynamic assessment of normal term pregnancy. *Am J Obstet Gynecol*. 1989;161(6 Pt 1):1439–1442.
5. Robson SC, Hunter S, Moore M, Dunlop W. Haemodynamic changes during the puerperium: a Doppler and M-mode echocardiographic study. *Br J Obstet Gynaecol*. 1987;94(11):1028–1039.
6. Lang RM, Borow KM. Heart disease. In: Barron WM, Lindheimer MD, eds. *Medical Disorders During Pregnancy*. St. Louis, MO: Mosby Year Book, 1991: 184.
7. Robson SC, Dunlop W, Moore M, Hunter S. Combined Doppler and echocardiographic measurement of cardiac output: theory and application in pregnancy. *Br J Obstet Gynaecol*. 1987;94:1014.
8. Ash N, Chesnut MD. *Physiology of Normal Pregnancy*. Elsevier Inc.; 2004
9. Hytten FE, Lind T. Indices of cardiovascular function. In: Hytten FE, Lind T, eds. *Diagnostic Indices in Pregnancy*. Documenta Geigy: Basel; 1973.
10. Barron WM, Mujais SK, Zinaman M, Bravo EL, Lindheimer MD. Plasma catecholamine responses to physiologic stimuli in normal human pregnancy. *Am J Obstet Gynecol*. 1986;154(1):80–84.
11. Frolich MA, Datta S, Corn SB. Thrombopoietin in normal pregnancy and preeclampsia. *Am J Obstet Gynecol*. 1998;179(1): 100–104.
12. Walker MC, Garner PR, Keely EJ, et al. Changes in activated protein C resistance during normal pregnancy. *Am J Obstet Gynecol*. 1997;177:162.
13. Toglia MR, Weg JG. Venous thromboembolism during pregnancy. *N Engl J Med*. 1996;335:108.
14. Lund CJ, Donovan JC. Blood volume during pregnancy. Significance of plasma and red cell volumes. *Am J Obstet Gynecol*. 1967;98:394.
15. Whittaker PG, Macphail S, Lind T. Serial hematologic changes and pregnancy outcome. *Obstet Gynecol*. 1996;88:33.
16. Bille-Brahe NE, Rørth M. Red cell 2.3-diphosphoglycerate in pregnancy. *Acta Obstet Gynecol Scand*. 1979;58:19.
17. Kuvin SF, Brecher G. Differential neutrophil counts in pregnancy. *N Engl J Med*. 1962;266:877.

18. Sood SL, James AH, Ragni MV, et al. A prospective study of von Willebrand factor levels and bleeding in pregnant women with type 1 von Willebrand disease. *Haemophilia.* 2016;22:e562.

19. James AH, Rhee E, Thames B, Philipp CS. Characterization of antithrombin levels in pregnancy. *Thromb Res.* 2014;134:648.

20. Ku DH, Arkel YS, Paidas MP, Lockwood CJ. Circulating levels of inflammatory cytokines (IL-1 beta and TNF-alpha), resistance to activated protein C, thrombin and fibrin generation in uncomplicated pregnancies. *Thromb Haemost.* 2003;90:1074.

21. Saha P, Stott D, Atalla R. Haemostatic changes in the puerperium "6 weeks postpartum" (HIP Study)—implication for maternal thromboembolism. *BJOG.* 2009;116:1602.

22. Wise RA, Polito AJ, Krishnan V. Respiratory physiologic changes in pregnancy. *Immunol Allergy Clin North Am.* 2006;26(1):1–12.

23. Gilroy RJ, Mangura BT, Lavietes MH. Rib cage and abdominal volume displacements during breathing in pregnancy. *Am Rev Respir Dis.* 1988;137:668–672.

24. Goldsmith LT, Weiss G, Steinetz BG. Relaxin and its role in pregnancy. *Endocrinol Metab Clin North Am.* 1995;24:171–186.

25. Cohen ME, Thomson KJ. Studies on the circulation in pregnancy. The velocity of blood flow and related aspects of the circulation in normal pregnant women. *J Clin Invest.* 1936;15:607–625.

26. Marx GF, Murthy PK, Orkin LR. Static compliance before and after delivery. *Br J Anaesth.* 1970;42:1100–1104.

27. Blair E, Hickam JB. The effect of change in body position on lung volume and intrapulmonary gas mixing in normal subjects. *J Clin Invest.* 1955;34:383–389.

28. Schneider KT, Deckardt R. The implication of upright posture on pregnancy. *J Perinat Med.* 1991;19:121–131.

29. Prowse CM, Gaensler RA. Respiratory and acid-base changes during pregnancy. *Anesthesiology.* 1965;26:381–392.

30. Tsai CH, de Leeuw NK. Changes in 2,3 diphosphoglycerate during pregnancy and puerperium in normal women and in beta-thalassemia heterozygous women. *Am J Obstet Gynecol.* 1982;142:520–523.

31. Lyons HA, Antonio R. The sensitivity of respiratory center in pregnancy after the administration of progesterone. *Trans Assoc Am Phys.* 1959;72:173–180.

32. Bayliss DA, Gidlowski JA, Millhorn DE. The stimulation of respiration by progesterone in ovariectomized cat is mediated by an estrogen dependent hypothalamic mechanism requiring gene expression. *Endocrinology.* 1990;126:519–527.

33. Hannhart B, Pickett CK, Moore LG. Effect of estrogen and progesterone on carotid body neural output responsiveness to hypoxia. *J Appl Physiol.* 1990;68:1909–1916.

34. McAuliffe F, Kametas N, Rafferty GF, Greenough A, Nicolaides K. Pulmonary diffusing capacity in pregnancy at sea level and at high altitude. *Respir Physiol Neurobiol.* 2003;134:85–92.

35. Norregaard O, Schultz P, Ostergaard A, Dahl R. Lung function and postural changes during pregnancy. *Respir Med.* 1989;83:467–470.

36. McAuliffe F, Kametas N, Espinoza J, Greenough A, Nicolaides. Respiratory function in pregnancy at sea level and at high altitude. *BJOG.* 2004;111(14):311–315.

37. McAuliffe F, Kametas N, Espinoza J, Greenough A, Nicolaides. Pulmonary diffusing capacity in pregnancy at sea level and at high altitude. *Respir Physiol Neurobio.* 2003;34(2):85–92.

38. Keyes LE, Armaza JF, Niermeyer S, Vargas E, Young DA, Moore LG. Intrauterine growth restriction, preeclampsia and intrauterine mortality at high altitude in Bolivia. *Pediatr Res.* 2003;54(1):20–25.

39. Gilbert R, Auchincloss JH Jr. Dyspnea of pregnancy. Clinical and physiological observations. *Am J Med Sci.* 1966;252:270–276.

40. Field SK, Bell SG, Genaiko DF, Whitelaw WA. Relationship between inspiratory effort and breathlessness in pregnancy. *J Appl Physiol.* 1991;71:1897–1902.

41. Krampl E. Pregnancy at high altitude. *Ultrasound Obstet Gynecol.* 2002;19(6):535–539.

42. Chapman AB, Zamudio S, Woodmansee W, et al. Systemic and renal hemodynamic changes in the luteal phase of the menstrual cycle mimic early pregnancy. *Am J Physiol.* 1997;273(5):F777–F782.

43. Cietak KA, Newton J. Serial quantitative maternal nephrosonography in pregnancy. *Br J Radiol.* 1985;58(689):405–413.

44. Bailey RR, Rolleston GL. Kidney length and ureteric dilatation in the puerperium *J Obstet Gynaecol Br Commonw.* 1971;78(1):55–61.

45. Hussein W, Lafayette RA. Renal function in normal and disordered pregnancy. *Current Opinion Nephrology Hypertension.* 2014;23(1):46–53.

46. Schulman A, Herlinger H. Urinary tract dilatation in pregnancy. *Br J Radiol.* 1975;48:638–645.

47. Bailey RR, Rolleston GL. Kidney length and ureteric dilatation in the puerperium. *J Obstet Gynaecol Br Commonw.* 1971;78(1):55–61.

48. Cietak KA, Newton JR. Serial quantitative maternal nephrosonography in pregnancy. *Br J Radiol.* 1985;58:405–413.

49. Lin YJ, Ou YC, Tsang LC, Lin H. Diagnostic value of magnetic resonance imaging for successful management of a giant hydronephrosis during pregnancy. *J Obstet Gynaecol.* 2013;33(1):91–93.

50. Au KK, Woo JS, Tang LC, Liang S. Aetiological factors in the genesis of pregnancy hydronephrosis. *Aust N Z J Obstet Gynaecol.* 1985;25(4):248–251.

51. Rasmussen PE, Nielsen FR. Hydronephrosis during pregnancy: a literature survey. *European Journal of Obst & Gyne & Reproductive Biology.* 1988;27(3):249–259.

52. Satin AJ, Seiken GL, Cunningham FG. Reversible hypertension in pregnancy caused by obstructive uropathy. *Obstet Gynecol.* 1993;81(5 Pt 2):823–825.

53. Brown MA. Urinary dilatation in pregnancy. *American Journal of Obest & Gyne.* 1991;164(2):642–643.

54. Dunlop W. Serial changes in renal haemodynamics during normal human pregnancy. *An International Journal of Obst & Gynaecology.*1981;88(1).

55. Krane NK, Cucuzzella A. Acute renal insufficiency in pregnancy: a review of thirty cases. *Journal of Maternal-Fetal Medicine.* 1995;4(1).

56. Krutzén E, Olofsson P, Bäck SE, Nilsson-Ehle P. Glomerular filtration rate in pregnancy: a study in normal subjects and in patients with hypertension, preeclampsia and diabetes. *Scand J Clin Lab Invest.* 1992;52(5):387–392.

57. Wiles K, Bramham K, Seed PT, Nelson-Piercy C, Lightstone L, Chappell LC. Serum creatinine in pregnancy: a systematic review. *Kidney International report.* 4(3):408–419.

58. Chapman AB, Zamudio S, Woodmansee W, et al. Systemic and renal hemodynamic changes in the luteal phase of menstrual cycle mimic pregnancy. *Am J. Physiol.* 1997;273(5Pt2):F777–F782.

59. Lumbers ER, Pringle KG. Roles of the circulating renin-angiotensin-aldosterone system in human pregnancy. *Am J Physiol Regul Integr Comp Physiol.* 2014; 306(2):R91–R101.

60. Davison JM, Gilmore EA, Dürr J, Robertson GL, Lindheimer MD. Altered osmotic thresholds for vasopressin secretion and thirst in human pregnancy. *Am J Physiol.* 1984;246(1 Pt 2):F105–F109.

61. Chapman AB, Zamudio S, Woodmansee W, et al. Systemic and renal hemodynamic changes in the luteal phase of menstrual cycle mimic pregnancy. *Am J. Physiol.* 1997;273(5 Pt2):F777–F782.

62. Cheung KL, Lafayette RA. Renal physiology of pregnancy. *Adv Chronic Kidney Dis.* 2013;20(3):209–214.

63. Lumbers ER, Pringle K. Roles of the circulating renin-angiotensin-aldosterone system in human pregnancy. *Am J Physiol Regul Integr Comp Physiol.* 2014;306(2):R91–101.

64. Irani RA, Xia Y. Renin angiotensin signaling in normal pregnancy and preeclampsia. *Semin Nephrol.* 2011;31(1):47–58.

65. Tkachenko O, Shchekochikhin D, Schrier RW. Hormones and hemodynamics in pregnancy. *Int J Endocrinol Metab.* 2014;12(2):e14098.

66. Cheung KL, Lafayette RA. Renal physiology of pregnancy. *Adv Chronic Kidney Dis.* 2013;20(3):209–214.

67. Castro LC, Hobel CJ, Gornbein J. Plasma levels of atrial natriuretic peptide in normal and hypertensive pregnancies: a meta-analysis. *Am J Obstet Gynecol.* 1994;171(6):1642–1651.

68. American College of Obstetrics and Gynecology. American College of Obstetrics and Gynecology (ACOG) Practice Bulletin: Nausea and vomiting of pregnancy. *Obstet Gynecol.* 2004;103(4):803–814.

69. Datta S, Lambert DH, Gregus J, Gissen AJ, Covino BG. Differential sensitivities of mammalian nerve fibers during pregnancy. *Anesth Analg.* 1983;62(12):1070–1072.

70. Butterworth JFT, Walker FO, Lysak SZ. Pregnancy increases median nerve susceptibility to lidocaine. *Anesthesiology.* 1990;72(6):962–965.

71. Bromage PR. Continuous lumbar epidural analgesia for obstetrics. *Can Med Assoc J.* 1961;85:1136–1140.

72. Palahniuk RJ, Shnider SM, Eger EI, 2nd. Pregnancy decreases the requirement for inhaled anesthetic agents. *Anesthesiology.* 1974;41(1):82–83.

73. Datta S, Migliozzi RP, Flanagan HL, Krieger NR. Chronically administered progesterone decreases halothane requirements in rabbits. *Anesth Analg.* 1989;68(1):46–50.

74. Flanagan HL, Datta S, Lambert DH, Gissen AJ, Covino BG. Effect of pregnancy on bupivacaine-induced conduction blockade in the isolated rabbit vagus nerve. *Anesth Analg.* 1987;66(2):123–126.

75. Rosene-Montella K, Bourjeily G. Pulmonary problems in Pregnancy, 2009th edition, Humana Press.

2

The Placenta

Anatomy, Physiology, Uteroplacental Blood Flow, and Drug Transfer

Sandra N. Gonzalez, Easha Patel, and Christa L. Riley

Introduction

The placenta is a fetal–maternal organ critical to the normal implantation and development of the fetus that starts developing early in pregnancy and supports growth and development all the way to term, adjusting dynamically to successfully support fetal growth. Failure of the placenta to develop normally will result in adverse maternal–fetal outcomes such as preeclampsia/eclampsia, intrauterine growth retardation (IUGR), and even loss of the pregnancy. As the interface between the mother and the fetus, the placenta prevents rejection of the fetal allograft, regulates the transfer of nutrients and gases, and eliminates fetal waste products, and it has a pivotal role in regulating transfer of medications to the fetus. It also regulates fetal growth and maternal metabolism by synthesizing peptide and steroid hormones, glycogen, and proteins. Medications are commonly used in pregnancy for both pregnancy-related and nonpregnancy-related conditions.[1] One study states that in 2008 more than 93% of pregnant women took at least one over-the-counter or prescription medication during pregnancy.[2] Anesthetic medications are also commonly used in pregnancy, as surgery for nonpregnancy related conditions occurs in approximately 1–2% of all pregnancies and obstetric surgery occurs in approximately 20% of all pregnancies, with cesarean sections being the most common.[3] Given the prevalence of medication use, it is important to understand the role of the placenta in the transfer of drugs from the mother to the fetus, and the potential effects of these drugs on the developing fetus. Transport across the placenta takes place at the level of placental villous trees, which are the functional units through which the highly balanced and regulated transfer of nutrients, gases, hormones, antibodies, and medications occurs, involving multiple active and passive cellular transport mechanisms. This chapter will review the development, anatomy, and physiology of the placenta; mechanisms that control placental blood flow; and placental pharmacokinetics and pharmacodynamics.

Maternal Physiologic Changes in Pregnancy

There are multiple changes in maternal physiology that occur during pregnancy. These changes are related to hormonal changes that occur during pregnancy and to the enlarging uterus over the course of pregnancy.[4] These changes affect the metabolism and transport of medications as the pharmacokinetics of drugs can be altered.[5]

Cardiac

There is a 50% overall increase in maternal plasma volume during pregnancy.[6] With the increase in blood volume, there is decreased albumin concentration, which can affect drugs with high protein binding, leading to higher concentration of free drug in circulation. There is also increased maternal arterial pH, which can affect drug-protein binding.[5] The increased plasma volume allows pregnant patients to withstand effects of blood loss during delivery. Uterine blood flow increases as the fetus grows, and by term 20% of the cardiac output is seen by the uterus. This system is highly sensitive to exogenous agents such as catecholamines as well as to loss of maternal intravascular volume.[7]

Respiratory

The major respiratory change in pregnancy is the increase in tidal volume secondary to rising progesterone levels. This results in increased oxygen consumption as well as increased minute ventilation; however, the respiratory rate does not increase. This change[7] results in a compensated respiratory alkalosis with a pCO_2 of approximately 30 mm Hg and bicarbonate levels in the 19–20 mEq/L.

Gastrointestinal

Increased progesterone levels also decrease gastrointestinal motility along with a decrease in the resting tone of the lower esophageal sphincter. This predisposes pregnant patients to reflux. They are also at an increased risk from aspiration with general anesthesia.[7] Drug absorption can be decreased to due delayed gastric emptying and increase in gastric pH.[5]

Renal

There is an increase in renal blood flow and increased glomerular filtration rate in pregnancy. This can lead to increased clearance of many medications.[5] There is also reduced ureteral tone and peristalsis, which can result in a dilated ureter and hydronephrosis. Hydronephrosis can also be related to be compression from gravid uterus.[7]

Development of the Placenta

Placental development begins between the stages of the morula and blastocyst and progresses in multiple stages:

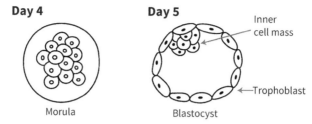

Figure 2.1 Pre-implantation stage.

Pre-Implantation Stage

Between the stages of morula and blastocyst (days 4 to 5 postfertilization), the trophoblast, from which the placenta originates, is the first cell lineage to differentiate.[8] The morula enters the uterus, and on day 5 the blastocyst forms as fluid accumulates and cells become polarized, forming the inner cell mass that will become the embryo and an outer layer of cells that becomes the trophoblast (Figure 2.1).[1]

Pre-Lacunar Stage

The portion of the trophoblast overlying the inner cell mass, the polar trophoblast, will lead to implantation of the blastocyst.[8] The trophoblast will give origin to the cytotrophoblast, which acts as a source of stem cells that differentiate into two pathways: the syncytiotrophoblast and the extravillous trophoblast (EVT). The syncytiotrophoblast, formed from fused cytotrophoblasts, will invade the uterine epithelium and implant the blastocyst into the uterine decidua at approximately 6 days postfertilization.[1] The syncytiotrophoblast completely surrounds the conceptus, preventing it from coming into contact with maternal tissues.[8] Once implanted, the blastocyst will have access to various substrates (e.g., glycogen) that are needed for continued growth (Figure 2.2).[1]

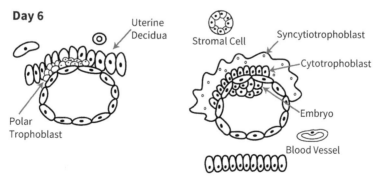

Figure 2.2 Pre-lacunar stage.

Lacunar Stage

Eight days after fertilization, vacuoles form within the syncytiotrophoblast and coalesce to form lacunae. The three fundamental zones of the placenta become more defined: the early chorionic plate facing the embryo, the lacunar system, and trabeculae develop into the intervillous space and villous trees, and the primitive basal plate comes into contact with the endometrium.[8] The EVT divides into the interstitial EVT, which invades the decidua, and the endovascular EVT, which invades and remodels the spiral arteries establishing the foundation for the uteroplacental circulation.[1]

Villous Stage

Approximately 13 days after fertilization, a layer of syncytiotrophoblast with a core of cytotrophoblast evaginates into the lacunar space to form primary villi, which acquire an inner core of embryonic mesoderm to become secondary villi. By day 21, the embryonic mesoderm will form blood vessels that connect to the vessels developing in the umbilical cord and embryo, forming the tertiary villi. Some villi anchor in the decidua, whereas others float free in the intervillous space. There is always a layer of trophoblasts separating the embryonic circulation from the maternal decidua (Figure 2.3).[1]

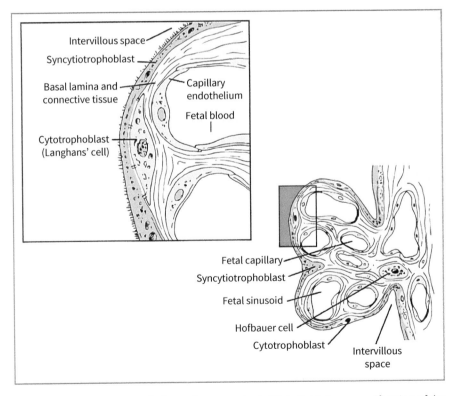

Figure 2.3 *Right:* Cellular morphology of two terminal villi. *Left:* Higher magnification of the boxed region exhibiting the placental barrier between fetal and maternal blood.

Reprinted with permission from *Chestnut's obstetric anesthesia: principles and practice*. 6th ed. Philadelphia, PA: Elsevier; 2019.

Anatomy of the Placenta

The placenta is a highly specialized organ that supports the growth and development of the fetus.[9] The main function of the placenta is to serve as an interface for gas exchange between the mother and the fetus, transfer of nutrients to the fetus and waste products from the fetus, and transfer of immunity via immunoglobulins. Additionally, the placenta secretes hormones that are necessary for the development of the fetus.[10] At term, the human placenta is a discoid organ with an approximate diameter of 22 cm, a central thickness of 2.5 cm, and an average weight[8] of 470 g. It has two surfaces: a fetal surface and a maternal surface.

Fetal Surface

The chorionic plate is covered by the amnion, which is a single-layer epithelium and amniotic mesenchyme. The chorionic vessels are continuous with the umbilical cord vessels and, deriving from the two umbilical arteries, the chorionic arteries will branch and their terminal branches will supply the villous trees. The chorionic veins are continuous with the veins of the villous trees and will give rise to the umbilical vein (Figure 2.4).[8]

Maternal Surface

The basal plate is the surface that emerges from the separation of the placenta from the uterine wall. It is divided into 10 to 40 lobes that correspond with the position of the villous trees arising from the chorionic plate. Each lobe is divided into one to four lobules (cotyledons), each one containing a villous tree.[8]

Physiology of the Placenta

Placental functions play a critical role in maintaining healthy maternal–fetal physiology. These functions include:

Implantation

Via invasion of the uterine decidua by the syncytiotrophoblast.

Synthesis of Energy Substrates and Hormone Precursors

- **Glycogen synthesis:** The placenta can synthesize significant amounts of glycogen, which is stored as an energy reserve. The uptake of glucose from the maternal circulation involves enzymes and regulators, and it is the rate-limiting step in this process.[1]
- **Cholesterol synthesis:** Placental cholesterol is a precursor for placental production of hormones (progesterone and estrogens).[1]

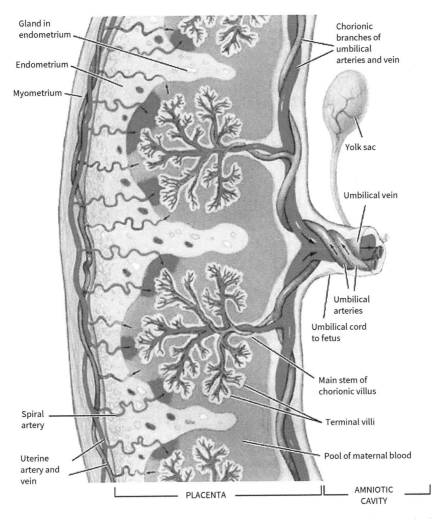

Figure 2.4 Placental vasculature. The terminal branches of the chorionic arteries supply the villous trees. There is continuity between villous trees veins and the chorionic veins. The latter will give rise to the umbilical vein.

Reproduced with permission from Vander AJ, Sherman JH, Luciano DS. *Human physiology: the mechanisms of body function.* 6th ed. Boston, MA: McGraw-Hill. 2001:679. Original figure 19-24.

- **Protein metabolism:** Placental synthesis of proteins is driven by the demands of growth, rising in production to 7.5 g per day by term.[1]
- **Lactate:** The placenta produces large amounts of lactate, which is removed efficiently by L-lactate transporters.[1]

Transport of Nutrients and Gas Exchange

These processes take place in the terminal villi. Maternal blood supplies nutrients, oxygen, water, and electrolytes that are exchanged for fetal carbon dioxide and other waste products. There are multiple mechanisms by which placental transfer occurs (Table 2.1):

Table 2.1 Mechanisms of Placental Transport

Mechanism	Description	Examples
Solvent drag	Bulk flow of water with dissolved solutes and nutrients. Driven by hydrostatic pressure	Water, ions
Simple diffusion	Passive transfer of solutes following concentration gradient	Respiratory gases
Transcellular transfer	Transport proteins	
	Channels (water filled pores in plasma membrane)	Aquaporins (transport of water and small molecules)
	Facilitated diffusion (saturable carrier proteins)	GLUT transporters (glucose)
	Carrier-mediated active transport (active transport, ATP dependent)	Na$^+$K$^+$ ATPase
Endocytosis and exocytosis	Endocytosis: engulfment of material within a fluid-filled vesicle	Immunoglobulin G, Liposomes, Nanoformulations
	Exocytosis: fusion of vesicles with cell membrane to release their contents	

- **Solvent drag** refers to the bulk flow of water that contains solutes and nutrients dissolved in response to hydrostatic pressure changes.[1]
- **Passive diffusion** is the passive transfer of solutes following concentration and electrical gradients. All solutes are transferred by diffusion to a degree determined by molecular properties. For example, respiratory gases and other lipophilic solutes are readily exchanged by simple diffusion.[1]
- **Transcellular transfer** is dependent on transport proteins in the microvilli or basal membrane of the syncytiotrophoblast. There are three different types:
  - *Channels:* Proteins that form water-filled pores in the plasma membrane. Ions and charged hydrophilic substances can be transported this way. Aquaporins are channels that exemplify this type of transport.
  - *Facilitated diffusion:* This occurs via saturable carrier proteins that are not dependent on metabolic energy. For example, GLUT transporters facilitate glucose transport.
  - *Active transport (carrier mediated):* Primary active transport requires ATP to move solutes against a gradient. Na-K ATPase is an example. Secondary active transport, such as Na-amino acid co-transport, uses concentration gradients.[1]
- **Endocytosis and exocytosis:** Endocytosis involves the formation of vesicles that engulf substances by invagination of the cell membrane; exocytosis is the opposite, whereby substances are released by vesicle fusion with the cell membrane. Specific solute–receptor interactions can mediate these processes.[1]
  - *Fatty acid transport:* Triglycerides are broken down to free fatty acids and glycerol, then re-esterified on the fetal side.[1]
  - *Immunoglobulin G (IgG) transfer:* IgG is readily transported across the placenta via the fragment crystallizable (FC) receptor. It confers immunity to the fetus. Immunoglobulin M cannot be transported across the syncytiotrophoblast.[1]

Placental Blood Flow

Maintenance of adequate placental blood flow is crucial for a successful pregnancy. The chorionic villi are the functional unit of the placenta, as the majority of the maternal–fetal exchange occurs in these units (see Figure 2.5). The villi are lined with syncytiotrophoblasts. Maternal blood enters the villi via the uterine spiral arteries, bathes the villi, and drains back into maternal circulation via endometrial veins.[9] Fetal capillaries take oxygenated blood from the villi to the umbilical vein, and deoxygenated fetal blood is brought back to the villi via umbilical arteries.[4] Nutrients, certain drugs, and various chemicals in the maternal blood pass from villi through the syncytiotrophoblasts, fetal connective tissues, and the endothelium of fetal capillaries into the fetal bloodstream.[10] See Figure 2.3 for detailed schematic of the placental transfer surface.

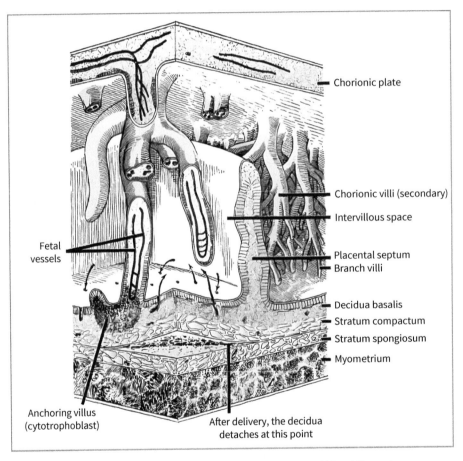

Figure 2.5 The relationship between the villous tree and maternal blood flow. The arrows indicate the maternal blood flow from the spiral arteries into the intervillous space and out through the spiral veins.

Reprinted with permission from *Chestnut's obstetric anesthesia: principles and practice.* 6th ed. Philadelphia, PA: Elsevier; 2019.

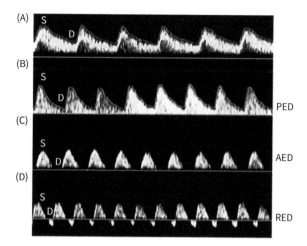

Figure 2.6 Umbilical artery FVW tracings obtained in normal and abnormal third trimester pregnancies. A) Normal: end diastolic velocities are high. B) End diastolic velocities are present, but clearly reduced (compare to A). This pattern is defined as PED. C) End diastolic velocities are absent. This pattern is defined as AED. D) During diastole flow velocities appear in the lower channel, indicating flow in the opposite direction relative to the systolic phase. This pattern is defined as RED. FVWs = flow velocity waveforms, PED = positive end diastole, AED = absent end diastole, RED = reverse end diastole, S = systole, D = diastole.

Reproduced with permission from *Placenta*. Vol 32, March 2011. T Todros, E Piccoli. *Review: Feto-placental vascularization: A multifaceted approach.* Elsevier, 2019.

The placental vasculature is low resistance; increased placental vascular resistance is frequently observed in pregnancies with IUGR, and it is a predictor of poor pregnancy outcomes. Umbilical blood flow rises as a pregnancy develops and can be estimated with Doppler waveform, which shows substantial placental blood flow in diastole. The absence or reversal of placental blood flow during diastole correlates strongly with poor pregnancy outcomes (Figure 2.6). The placenta has no neuronal input, and agents that are powerful constrictors of other vasculatures (e.g., catecholamines, angiotensin II, oxytocin, and vasopressin) are poor constrictors of fetal placental vessels.[11] Placental blood flow is entirely determined by humoral and structural factors:

Vasoactive Agents

- **Thromboxane:** Data from experimental studies consistently show thromboxane to be a potent vasoconstrictor of the fetal–placental circulation. Aggregating platelets are the most likely source of thromboxane in the placenta; indeed, disorders such as preeclampsia and systemic lupus erythematosus are associated with platelet aggregation and thromboxane release.[11]
- **Endothelin:** A potent constrictor of the fetal–placental vasculature. Elevated fetal serum concentrations of endothelin-1 have been reported at delivery in pregnancies associated with fetal hypoxia.[11]

- **Vasoactive prostanoids:** Prostaglandin E2 and prostaglandin F 2α constrict fetal–placental vessels, but they are far less potent than thromboxane or endothelin.[11]

Vasodilators

- **Nitric oxide (NO):** NO plays an important role in the control of fetal–placental vascular tone. NO is an inhibitor of platelet aggregation and reduces leukocyte adhesion. In pregnancies with IUGR and preeclampsia, NO synthetase levels are elevated, possibly as a compensatory response to poor placental blood flow.[11]
- **Atrial natriuretic peptide (ANP):** ANP may play a role in controlling placental blood flow as its receptors are found in human placenta. In addition, fetal ANP levels rise in response to volume expansion, suggesting an endocrine function.[11]
- **Prostacyclin:** Prostaglandin I2 has a dilator effect on umbilical vessels and may also play a role in controlling placental vascular tone; however, its half-life is very short and prostaglandin I2 is enzymatically inactivated by the placenta.[11]

Fetal–placental blood flow must be considered in conjunction with other events surrounding the pregnancy. The normal process of converting the spiral arteries into vessels of low resistance by the invasion of the trophoblast, if disrupted, will result in abnormally increased resistance within the placenta and abnormally decreased umbilical blood flow. Other pathological events such as the formation of microthrombus and areas of infarction in the placenta occur in pregnancies in women with preeclampsia, systemic lupus erythematosus, and antiphospholipid syndrome, in which placental blood flow is diminished.[11]

Mechanisms of Drug Transfer Across the Placenta

The mechanisms that regulate the passage of substances across the placenta are also involved in controlling the rate and extent of drug transfer across the placenta. Some medications accumulate at a higher concentration in the placenta itself, potentially altering its function. The evidence of placental permeability to drugs was reported earlier in the 20th century, even before the fetal malformations secondary to thalidomide intake during pregnancy were reported. Up until that point, the placenta was viewed as a perfect barrier, when in reality, most drugs cross the placenta to a certain extent.[12] Any drugs, nutrients, and other endogenous compounds that cross the placenta and enter the fetal circulation have to cross the syncytiotrophoblast, basement membrane, and fetal capillary endothelium.[5] The route of transport varies depends on the chemical and physical characteristics of the compound.[4] For example, in animal studies, silicon nanovectors of larger size have been found to not cross the placenta, remaining in the maternal circulation, potentially serving as carriers for harmful medications in order to prevent fetal exposure.[14] Substances in the maternal bloodstream are carried in free form dissolved in plasma, bound to carrier proteins, or bound to red blood cells.[13] Figure 2.7 illustrates the various mechanisms of transport across the human placental barrier, including passive diffusion, facilitated diffusion, active transport, and endocytosis.[5] Most drugs cross the placenta by passive diffusion and to a lesser extent through other mechanisms.

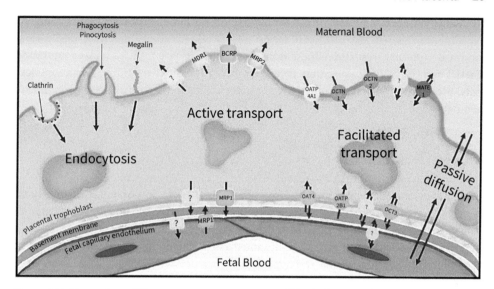

Figure 2.7 The various different transport processes within the human placental barrier.
Reprinted from Al-Enazy S, Ali S, Albekairi N, El-Tawil M, Rytting E. Placental control of drug delivery. *Advanced Drug Delivery Reviews*. 2017;116:63-72 with permission from Elsevier.

Passive Diffusion

This is the predominant route through which most drugs cross the placenta, and it applies mainly to hydrophobic molecules of less than 600 Da. Hydrophobic, lipophilic drugs, such as midazolam and paracetamol, cross the placenta by this mechanism.[5,10] Larger compounds, such as low molecular weight heparin, rarely cross the placenta.[15] Drugs with high plasma protein binding are unable to diffuse across the placenta. Compounds that move with this mechanism are more likely to move down a concentration gradient as this is not an energy-dependent process.[5] The concentration of drugs transferred by passive diffusion theoretically should be similar in maternal and fetal blood; however, lower fetal pH causes weakly basic drugs to accumulate in the fetus, more significantly during periods of fetal distress and acidosis, and fetal concentration of the drug may exceed maternal blood levels (e.g., local anesthetics). Drug binding to fetal proteins contributes to longer retention of the drug in the fetal compartment, with prolonged exposure to its effects in the fetus. The rate of transfer of solutes that diffuse rapidly across the placenta (e.g., inhalational anesthetics) is determined by the rate of placental blood flow, which increases as pregnancy progresses.[11]

Facilitated Diffusion

Various carrier proteins allow for uptake of hormones and nutrients from mother to fetus, as well as the removal of fetal metabolites and waste products to the maternal blood.[5] Energy is not needed for this mechanism, as substances move down a concentration gradient. Drugs such as cephalosporins and glucocorticoids are transported using this mechanism.[10] Carrier proteins have similar saturation kinetics and ability for competitive inhibition but are also distinct in terms of substrate selectivity, placental localization, and transcriptional regulation. These transport proteins share features such as saturation kinetics and the ability to be competitively inhibited but differ regarding substrate selectivity, placental localization, and transcriptional regulation. Most of these proteins are members of the adenosine triphosphate binding cassette and solute carrier transporters.[12]

Active Transport

Transport of substances across the placenta against a concentration or electrochemical gradient with use of energy, through carrier proteins that are present on both the maternal and fetal side. There are multiple different active transporters on the placenta that are involved in the transfer of drugs such as digoxin, dexamethasone, chemotherapeutic drugs, HIV protease inhibitors, norepinephrine, and dopamine.[10]

Endocytosis and Exocytosis

The syncytiotrophoblasts have the ability to use endocytosis as a mechanism of transport for both endogenous compounds as well as xenobiotics.[5] This occurs when the drugs are completely enveloped into the membrane and released on the other side.[10] There are multiple different mechanisms by which this process is carried out. Medications such as gentamicin and endogenous compounds such as albumin are transported with this mechanism.[5] Receptor-mediated endocytosis involves selective internalization of a specific extracellular ligand into cytoplasmic vesicles via interaction with specific receptors. In addition to IgG, biological agents such as infliximab and adalimumab (IgG1 antibodies), nanoparticles, and liposomes are transferred to the fetus this way.[12]

Drug Transfer to Fetus

Pharmacokinetic Factors

Most studies report fetal exposure in terms of fetal-to-maternal (F/M) drug concentrations. Maternal drug concentrations are measured in peripheral venous blood drawn at delivery. Umbilical vein blood is used to represent fetal blood concentrations. In addition to placental permeability, the pharmacokinetics of drugs determine the maternal metabolism of drugs, transfer of drugs across the placenta, and exposure of the fetus to maternal drugs. Most drugs are transferred across the placenta by passive diffusion. Lipid solubility, maternal and fetal protein and tissue binding, pKa, pH, and placental blood flow all affect fetal exposure to maternal medications.[16]

High lipid solubility facilitates diffusion across cell membranes but can trap drugs in placental tissue.[16,17] Fetal exposure to drugs that are highly protein bound is dependent on both maternal and fetal plasma protein concentrations, which vary by gestational age. The

Table 2.2 Drugs That Readily Cross the Placenta

Anticholinergic Agents	Atropine
	Scopolamine
Antihypertensive Agents	β-adrenergic receptor antagonists
	Nitroprusside
	Nitroglycerin
Benzodiazepines	Diazepam
	Midazolam
Induction Agents	Propofol
	Ketamine
	Etomidate
	Thiopental
	Dexmedetomidine
Inhalational Anesthetic Agents	Halothane
	Isoflurane
	Sevoflurane
	Desflurane (presumed)
	Nitrous oxide
Local Anesthetics	
Opioids	
Vasopressor	Ephedrine

(Reprinted with permission from *Chestnut's Obstetric Anesthesia: Principles and Practice*. Sixth Edition. Philadelphia, PA: Elsevier; 2019.)

primary binding proteins are albumin and α_1-acid glycoprotein (AAG), and fetal plasma concentrations of both proteins increase over the duration of gestation.[18] The pKa of a medication determines the fraction of ionized drug at physiologic pH. Drugs that are weak bases such as local anesthetics and opioids may be transferred more readily to the fetus in fetal acidemia.[19] Tables 2.2 and 2.3 summarize the placental transfer of medications commonly used in anesthesia.

Table 2.3 Drugs That Do Not Readily Cross the Placenta

Anticholinergic Agent	**Glycopyrrolate**
Anticoagulant	Heparin
Muscle Relaxants	Succinylcholine
	Non-depolarizing Agents
Non-depolarizing Agent Binder	Sugammadex
Vasopressor	Phenylephrine

Reprinted with permission from *Chestnut's Obstetric Anesthesia: Principles and Practice*. Sixth Edition. Philadelphia, PA: Elsevier; 2019.

Anesthetic Agents

- **Induction Agents:** The key feature that makes a drug useful for inducing anesthesia is high lipid solubility, which allows for passage across the blood brain barrier, so these medications also readily cross the placenta. Propofol studies showed an F/M ratio of 0.65 and 0.85, and that there may be sedative effects on the neonate when administered for the induction of anesthesia based on lower Apgar scores at 1 and 5 minutes compared to thiopental.[20–22] Propofol is highly protein-bound to albumin and therefore maternal alterations in albumin can affect the transfer of total concentration of propofol.[23] Ketamine readily crosses the placenta with an F/M ratio of 1.26 within 2 minutes of administration to the mother.[24] An induction dose of etomidate resulted[25] in an F/M ratio of 0.5. Dexmedetomidine has an F/M ratio of 0.12 and evidence of high placental tissue binding due to its high lipid solubility.[26] Benzodiazepines vary in their ionization and lipid solubility. Diazepam is the most lipophilic with an F/M ratio of 1 within a few minutes of administration to the mother, while midazolam is the most polar with an F/M ratio of only 0.76 that rapidly decreases.[27,28]

- **Opioids:** Opioid medications cross the placenta and therefore have the potential to cause neonatal respiratory depression. Intravenous (IV) dosing of morphine to the mother results in a lower biophysical profile score of the fetus at 20 minutes due to reduced fetal breathing and fewer heart rate accelerations.[29] Intrathecal morphine actually has an F/M ratio close to 1 but because the typical total intrathecal dose of morphine used is so small, the absolute fetal concentrations of morphine are well below the concentrations associated with neonatal respiratory depression.[30] Fentanyl is highly lipophilic and highly protein bound and rapidly transfers across the placenta.[31] In vitro perfusion of the human placenta shows bidirectional fentanyl transfer with collection of fentanyl in the placenta itself. Sufentanil has a higher F/M ratio than fentanyl but its increased lipid solubility results in rapid uptake by the central nervous system (CNS) when administered in the epidural space, resulting in less vascular absorption in the mother, reducing risk of fetal exposure.[32] Despite a low F/M ratio, alfentanil given at the induction of anesthesia has been shown to decrease Apgar scores at 1 minute.[33] Remifentanil administered by patient-controlled analgesia during labor is more likely to cause maternal respiratory depression than adverse fetal effects. Rapid metabolism by nonspecific esterases reduces the fetal exposure risk[34] despite an F/M ratio of 0.5. It is important to note that with opioid medications, pharmacokinetics of the specific medication and route of administration influence fetal and neonatal side effects more than a high F/M ratio.

- **Muscle Relaxants and Reversal Agents:** Muscle relaxants are large, ionized quaternary ammonium salts and do not readily cross the placenta. Although muscle relaxants have been detected in fetal blood as time from induction to delivery increases, a single dose of muscle relaxant administered to the mother for the induction of general anesthesia rarely affects muscle tone of the neonate.[35] Succinylcholine is not detectable in blood taken from the umbilical vein when the administered maternal dose[36] is less than 300 mg. Neonatal neuromuscular blockade can occur with a single induction dose of succinylcholine when mother and fetus are homozygous for atypical pseudocholinesterase deficiency.[37] Atropine and scopolamine both readily cross the placenta and may increase fetal heart rate.[38,39] Glycopyrrolate does not cross the placenta easily and does not affect fetal heart rate.[40] Anticholinesterase agents are ionized quaternary ammonium compounds in vivo and do not readily cross the placenta.[41] Sugammadex also does not easily cross the placenta due to its large molecular structure and high molecular weight.[42]

Medications Commonly Used in Pregnancy

Pregnant women often have many chronic medical conditions needing prescription medications.[5] This next section will describe some common classes of medications used in pregnancy.

- **Selective Serotonin Reuptake Inhibitors/Serotonin-norepinephrine Reuptake Inhibitors:** Depression is common in pregnancy with up to 20% of pregnant women affected.[43,44] Studies have shown that 7–13% of pregnancies have some exposure to antidepressant medications, with most being selective serotonin reuptake inhibitors (SSRIs).[43,45] Antidepressants cross the placenta primarily by passive diffusion and enter the intrauterine environment with varying degrees of bioavailability. The effect of antidepressants on the fetus is a syndrome called postnatal adaptation syndrome (PNAS), which is a constellation of behavioral symptoms.[43] This has been found in about 30% of infants exposed to SSRIs or selective norepinephrine reuptake inhibitors (SNRIs). Fluoxetine, paroxetine, and venlafaxine are all associated with PNAS more often than other antidepressants.[46]
- **Metformin:** Gestational diabetes is a common complication in pregnancy, affecting 5–13% of pregnancies in the United States. Metformin is an oral antiglycemic agent that is being used commonly for glucose control in gestational diabetes mellitus (GDM) patients.[47] Metformin readily crosses the placenta barrier.[48] There is a theoretical risk of development of lactic acidosis in a fetus exposed to metformin. Most data does not reflect an increase risk in miscarriage or congenital malformations with exposure to metformin.[49]
- **Antihypertensive Drugs:** Hypertensive disorders are a common medical complication in pregnancy including both pregestational hypertension and pregnancy-induced hypertensive disorders, especially in developing countries,[50] and it is a leading cause of maternal and perinatal morbidity and mortality worldwide.[49] Antihypertensive drugs are often used in pregnancy with the aim of reducing risk of cerebrovascular complications and avoiding progression of pregestational hypertension into superimposed preeclampsia. All antihypertensive medications cross the placental barrier and have varying effects on fetal metabolism. The two classes of medications that are largely avoided in pregnancy are ACE inhibitors and angiotensin II receptor blockers due to neonatal complications, such as renal failure and death.[51]
- **Anticoagulants:** Pregnancy is a hypercoagulable state with a 5-fold increase in the risk of venous thromboembolism (VTE) during pregnancy, a risk that remains until 12 weeks postpartum.[52] Vitamin K antagonists, such as warfarin, readily cross the

placenta with an increased risk of adverse outcomes, such as miscarriage and still-birth. In special populations, such as those with mechanical heart valves, the risk versus benefits has to be weighed before discontinuation of vitamin K antagonists. An alternative method of anticoagulation is the use of low molecular weight heparin, as it does not readily cross the placenta. It also has better bioavailability than unfractionated heparin.[53]

References

1. Roberts V, Myatt L. Placental development and physiology. UpToDate. Available at *https://www.uptodate.com/contents/placental-development-and-physiology*. Accessed July 12, 2019.
2. Mitchell AA, Gilboa SM, Werler MM, et al. Medication use during pregnancy, with particular focus on prescription drugs: 1976–2008. *Am J Obstet Gynecol.* 2011;205(1):51.e1–e8. doi:10.1016/j.ajog.2011.02.029
3. Rasmussen AS, Christiansen CF, Uldbjerg N, Nørgaard M. Obstetric and non-obstetric surgery during pregnancy: A 20-year Danish population-based prevalence study. *BMJ Open.* 2019;9(5):e028136. doi:10.1136/bmjopen-2018-028136
4. Juhasz-Böss I, Solomayer E, Strik M, Raspé C. Abdominal surgery in pregnancy. *Dtsch Aerzteblatt Online.* July 2014. doi:10.3238/arztebl.2014.0465
5. Al-Enazy S, Ali S, Albekairi N, El-Tawil M, Rytting E. Placental control of drug delivery. *Adv Drug Deliv Rev.* 2017;116:63–72. doi:10.1016/j.addr.2016.08.002
6. Yeomans ER, Gilstrap LC. Physiologic changes in pregnancy and their impact on critical care. *Crit Care Med.* 2005;33(10 Suppl):S256–258. doi:10.1097/01.ccm.0000183540.69405.90
7. Skubic JJ, Salim A. Emergency general surgery in pregnancy. *Trauma Surg Acute Care Open.* 2017;2(1):e000125. doi:10.1136/tsaco-2017-000125
8. Huppertz B. The anatomy of the normal placenta. *J Clin Pathol.* 2008;61(12):1296–1302. doi:10.1136/jcp.2008.055277
9. Gude NM, Roberts CT, Kalionis B, King RG. Growth and function of the normal human placenta. *Thromb Res.* 2004;114(5-6):397–407. doi:10.1016/j.thromres.2004.06.038
10. Griffiths SK, Campbell JP. Placental structure, function and drug transfer. *Contin Educ Anaesth Crit Care Pain.* 2015;15(2):84–89. doi:10.1093/bjaceaccp/mku013
11. Poston L. The control of blood flow to the placenta. *Exp Physiol.* 1997;82:377–387.
12. Tetro N, Moushaev S, Rubinchik-Stern M, Eyal S. The placental barrier: the gate and the fate in drug distribution. *Pharm Res.* 2018;35(4):71. doi:10.1007/s11095-017-2286-0
13. Koren G, Ornoy A. The role of the placenta in drug transport and fetal drug exposure. *Expert Rev Clin Pharmacol.* 2018;11(4):373–385. doi:10.1080/17512433.2018.1425615
14. Refuerzo JS, Godin B, Bishop K, et al. Size of the nanovectors determines the transplacental passage in pregnancy: study in rats. *Am J Obstet Gynecol.* 2011;204(6):546.e5–546.e9. doi:10.1016/j.ajog.2011.02.033
15. Forestier F, Daffos F, Capella-Pavlovsky M. Low molecular weight heparin (PK 10169) does not cross the placenta during the second trimester of pregnancy study by direct fetal blood sampling under ultrasound. *Thromb Res.* 1984;34(6):557–560. doi:10.1016/0049-3848(84)90260-3

16. Dancis J. Why perfuse the human placenta. *Contrib Gynecol Obstet.* 1985;13:1–4.
17. Roy Krishna B, Zakowski M, Grant G. Sufentanil transfer in the human placenta during in vitro perfusion. *Can J Anaesth.* 1997;44(9):996–1001. doi:10.1007/BF03011972
18. Syme M, Paxton J, Keelan J. Drug transfer and metabolism by the human placenta. *Clin Pharmacokinet.* 2004;43(8):487–514. doi:10.2165/00003088-200443080-00001
19. Johnson RF, Herman NL, Johnson HV, Arney TL, Paschall RL, Downing JW. Effects of fetal pH on local anesthetic transfer across the human placenta. *Anesthesiology.* 1996;85(3): 608–615.
20. Dailland D, Cockshott D, Lirzin C, et al. Intravenous propofol during cesarean section: placental transfer, concentrations in breast milk, and neonatal effects. a preliminary study. *Anesthesiology.* 1989;71(6):827–834. doi:10.1097/00000542-198912000-00003
21. Valtonen M, Kanto J, Rosenberg P. Comparison of propofol and thiopentone for induction of anaesthesia for elective Caesarean section. *Anaesthesia.* 1989;44(9):758–762. doi:10.1111/j.1365-2044.1989.tb09264.x
22. Sánchez-Alcaraz A, Quintana MB, Laguarda M. Placental transfer and neonatal effects of propofol in caesarean section. *J Clin Pharm Ther.* 1998;23(1):19–23. doi:10.1046/j.1365-2710.1998.00124.x
23. He Y-L, Seno H, Tsujimoto S, Tashiro C. The effects of uterine and umbilical blood flows on the transfer of propofol across the human placenta during in vitro perfusion. *Anesth Analg.* 2001;93(1):151–156. doi:10.1097/00000539-200107000-00030
24. Ellingson A, Haram K, Sagen N, Solheim E. Transplacental passage of ketamine after intravenous administration. *Survey of Anesthesiology.* 1977;21(6):543–543. doi:10.1097/00132586-197712000-00043
25. Gregory MA, Davidson DG. Plasma etomidate levels in mother and fetus. *Anaesthesia.* 1991;46(9):716–718. doi:10.1111/j.1365-2044.1991.tb09762.x
26. Ala-Kokko TI, Pienimäki P, Lampela E, Hollmén AI, Pelkonen O, Vähäkangas K. Transfer of clonidine and dexmedetomidine across the isolated perfused human placenta. *Acta Anaesthesiol Scand.* 1997;41(2):313–319. doi:10.1111/j.1399-6576.1997.tb04685.x
27. Myllynen P, Vähäkangas K. An examination of whether human placental perfusion allows accurate prediction of placental drug transport: studies with diazepam. *J Pharmacol Toxicol Methods.* 2002;48(3):131–138. doi:10.1016/S1056-8719(03)00038-8
28. Wilson CM, Dundee JW, Moore J, Howard PJ, Collier PS. A comparison of the early pharmacokinetics of midazolam in pregnant and nonpregnant women. *Anaesthesia.* 1987;42(10):1057–1062. doi:10.1111/j.1365-2044.1987.tb05168.x
29. Kopecky EA, Ryan ML, Barrett JFR, et al. Fetal response to maternally administered morphine. *Am J Obstet Gynecol.* 2000;183(2):424–430. doi:10.1067/mob.2000.105746
30. Hée P, Sørensen SS, Bock JE, Fernandes A, Anni S. Intrathecal administration of morphine for the relief of pains in labour and estimation of maternal and fetal plasma concentration of morphine. *Eur J Obstet Gyneco.* 1987;25(3):195–201. doi:10.1016/0028-2243(87)90099-2
31. Bower S. Plasma protein binding of fentanyl. *J Pharm Pharmacol.* 1981;33(1):507–514. doi:10.1111/j.2042-7158.1981.tb13849.x
32. Loftus JR, Hill H, Cohen SE. Placental transfer and neonatal effects of epidural sufentanil and fentanyl administered with bupivacaine during labor. *Anesthesiology.* 1995;83(2):300–308. doi:10.1097/00000542-199508000-00010

33. Gin D Tony, Ngan-Kee K Warwick, Siu C Yuk, Stuart E Joyce, Tan K Perpetua, Lam K Kwok. Alfentanil Given Immediately Before the Induction of Anesthesia for Elective Cesarean Delivery. *Anesth Analg.* 2000;90(5):1167–1172. doi:10.1097/00000539-200005000-00031

34. Volikas I, Butwick A, Wilkinson C, Pleming A, Nicholson G. Maternal and neonatal side-effects of remifentanil patient-controlled analgesia in labour. *Br Anaesth.* 2005;95(4):504–509. doi:10.1093/bja/aei219

35. Iwama H, Kaneko T, Tobishima S, Komatsu T, Watanabe K, Akutsu H. Time dependency of the ratio of umbilical vein/maternal artery concentrations of vecuronium in caesarean section. *Acta Anaesthesiol Scand.* 1999;43(1):9–12. doi:10.1034/j.1399-6576.1999.430103.x

36. Kvisselgaard N, Moya F. Investigation of placental thresholds to succinylcholine. *Anesthesiology.* 1961;22(1):7–10. doi:10.1097/00000542-196101000-00002

37. Baraka A, Haroun S, Bassili M, Abu-Haider G. Response of the newborn to succinylcholine injection in homozygotic atypical mothers. *Anesthesiology.* 1975;43(1):115–116. doi:10.1097/00000542-197507000-00028

38. Kivalo I, Saarikoski S. Placental transmission of atropine at full-term pregnancy. *Br J Anaesth.* 1977;49(10):1017–1021. doi:10.1093/bja/49.10.1017

39. Kanto J, Kentala E, Kaila T, Pihlajamäki K. Pharmacokinetics of scopolamine during caesarean section: relationship between serum concentration and effect. *Obstetric Anesthesia Digest.* 1990;10(1):12–12. doi:10.1097/00132582-199004000-00016

40. Ali-Melkkilä T, Kaila T, Kanto J, Iisalo E. Pharmacokinetics of glycopyrronium in parturients. *Anaesthesia.* 1990;45(8):634–637. doi:10.1111/j.1365-2044.1990.tb14385.x

41. Briggs GG author. *Drugs in pregnancy and lactation: a reference guide to fetal and neonatal risk.* 10th ed. Philadelphia, PA: Lippincott Williams & Wilkins; 2015.

42. Palanca JM, Aguirre-Rueda D, Granell MV, et al. Sugammadex, a neuromuscular blockade reversal agent, causes neuronal apoptosis in primary cultures. *Int J Med Sci.* 2013;10(10):1278. doi:10.7150/ijms.6254

43. Ewing G, Tatarchuk Y, Appleby D, Schwartz N, Kim D. Placental transfer of antidepressant medications: implications for postnatal adaptation syndrome. *Clin Pharmacokinet.* 2015;54(4):359–370. doi:10.1007/s40262-014-0233-3

44. Bennett HA, Einarson A, Taddio A, Koren G, Einarson TR. Prevalence of depression during pregnancy: systematic review. *Obstet Gynecol.* 2004;103(4):698–709. doi:10.1097/01.AOG.0000116689.75396.5f

45. Cooper WO, Willy ME, Pont SJ, Ray WA. Increasing use of antidepressants in pregnancy. *Am J Obstet Gynecol.* 2007;196(6):544.e1–544.e5. doi:10.1016/j.ajog.2007.01.033

46. Byatt N, Deligiannidis KM, Freeman MP. Antidepressant use in pregnancy: a critical review focused on risks and controversies. *Acta Psychiatr Scand.* 2013;127(2):94–114. doi:10.1111/acps.12042

47. Lee N, Hebert MF, Wagner DJ, et al. Organic cation transporter 3 facilitates fetal exposure to metformin during pregnancy. *Mol Pharmacol.* 2018;94(4):1125–1131. doi:10.1124/mol.118.112482

48. Vanky E, Zahlsen K, Spigset O, Carlsen SM. Placental passage of metformin in women with polycystic ovary syndrome. *Fertil Steril.* 2005;83(5):1575–1578. doi:10.1016/j.fertnstert.2004.11.051

49. Lindsay RS, Loeken MR. Metformin use in pregnancy: promises and uncertainties. *Diabetologia.* 2017;60(9):1612–1619. doi:10.1007/s00125-017-4351-y

50. Singh S, Ahmed EB, Egondu SC, Ikechukwu NE. Hypertensive disorders in pregnancy among pregnant women in a Nigerian teaching hospital. *Niger Med J*. 2014;55(5):384–388. doi:10.4103/0300-1652.140377

51. Khedun SM, Maharaj B, Moodley J. Effects of antihypertensive drugs on the unborn child. *Paediatr Drugs*. 2000;2(6):419–436. doi:10.2165/00128072-200002060-00002

52. Heit JA, Kobbervig CE, James AH, Petterson TM, Bailey KR, Melton LJ III. Trends in the incidence of venous thromboembolism during pregnancy or postpartum: a 30-year population-based study. *Ann Intern Med*. 2005;143(10):697–706. doi:10.7326/0003-4819-143-10-200511150-00006

53. Alshawabkeh L, Economy KE, Valente AM. Anticoagulation during pregnancy: evolving strategies with a focus on mechanical valves. *J Am Coll Cardiol*. 2016;68(16):1804–1813. doi:10.1016/j.jacc.2016.06.076

3
Fetal Physiology and Antepartum Fetal Surveillance

Agathe Streiff and Yelena Spitzer

Fetal Physiology

In order to understand antepartum fetal surveillance, it is important to be familiar with normal fetal physiology, especially neurologic, respiratory, and cardiac physiology, which are commonly assessed in the third trimester of pregnancy. This section will discuss these topics, with a focus on late-term fetal stages.

Neurophysiology

The neural tube develops by the third to fourth week from conception. This neural tube gives rise to the brain and spinal cord, and errors in formation can lead to many fatal conditions including anencephaly, encephalocele, myeloschisis, and craniorachischisis totalis. Less severe conditions include spina bifida, which may nevertheless result in lifelong disability. The neural tube differentiates into the prosencephalon, mesencephalon, and rhombencephalon, which give rise to the cerebrum and thalamic structures, the midbrain, and the brainstem and cerebellum, respectively. This differentiation occurs during the second to third months of gestation.[1]

The remainder of in utero neurologic development consists of neuron and glial cell proliferation and migration. This portion is not insignificant, with cortical gray matter increasing volume four to five times in the third trimester. Premature birth has been shown to result in decreased cortical volume.[2,3] It is important to note that neurodevelopment does not conclude until the second decade of life, and fetal insults in the peripartum period can have significant impact. These insults include hypoxia, ischemia, sepsis, and malnutrition.[2] It is estimated that approximately 50% of low birth weight infants born in the United States annually have a degree of cerebral white matter injury.[4] Prematurity is associated with intraventricular hemorrhage, periventricular leukomalacia, hydrocephalus, cerebellar disease, encephalopathy of prematurity, and other neurologic conditions with lifelong implications.[5]

While cerebral blood flow (CBF) in infants, children, and adults is autoregulated across a range of normal blood pressures, CBF in the developing fetus and premature neonate is more pressure-passive. This immature autoregulation renders it vulnerable to sudden decreases in blood pressure that may result in ischemia, as well as sudden increases in blood pressure that may result in rupture of fragile blood vessels. The germinal matrix proliferates in the second and early third trimester and is the most common site of intraventricular hemorrhage.

Even small deviations in blood pressure from normal can result in the CBF becoming more pressure-passive.[5]

Fetal movement is often assessed as a measure of fetal well-being and neurologic function. The first fetal movements occur after 7 weeks gestational age (GA) and are typically head and trunk movements.[6] These develop prior to the completion of spinal reflex pathways at weeks 10 to 11. More general movements (GM) of all parts of the body are typically seen at week 10, and increased tone of each movement is appreciated. These GMs persist until 5 months post-term, when they are replaced by more sophisticated goal-directed movements.[6]

Respiratory Physiology

The lung is derived from an invagination of the foregut endoderm. Lung development occurs throughout fetal life, but terminal bronchioles capable of gas exchange do not start to develop until 17 weeks of gestation.[7] Terminal bronchiole development is not complete until after 27 weeks of gestation, thus severely limiting the chances of survival of neonates born before this period despite advances in technology and neonatal care (Table 3.1).[7] Preterm delivery is one of the most important determinants of fetal lung development.

In utero, respiratory functions include normal fetal breathing movements, as well as the production and clearance of fetal lung fluid. Fetal breathing movements are important in maintaining pressure within airways and in stimulating lung growth and differentiation (Figure 3.1, Box 3.1).[7] Fetal breathing movements may be increased by hypercapnia, hyperglycemia, acidosis, hyperthermia, caffeine, indomethacin, and theophyllines. Conversely, these breathing movements may be decreased by hypoxia, hypoglycemia, prostaglandin E2, maternal smoking, maternal alcohol, intrauterine infection, diazepam, and morphine.[7] When the amniotic fluid volume is inadequate, such as in preterm rupture of membranes and fetal renal disease, pulmonary hypoplasia is seen.[7] The chest cavity must be of adequate

Table 3.1 The Different Stages of Lung Development[a]

Stage	Weeks in utero	Lung structures
Embryonic	0–7	Trachea Main bronchus Bronchi
Pseudoglandular	7–17	Bronchioli Terminal bronchioli
Canalicular	17–27	Alveolar ducts Respiratory bronchioli
Saccular	28–36	Increased gas exchange surface area
Alveolar	36 weeks to 2 years postnatal	Secondary septa Definitive alveoli

[a]Kotecha S. Lung growth for beginners. *Paediatr Respir Rev.* 2000;1(4):308–13.

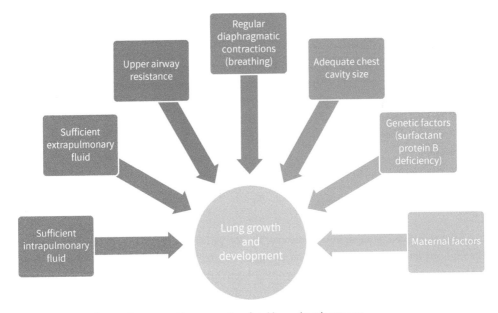

Figure 3.1 Key factors important in promoting fetal lung development.

size and unoccupied in order to achieve normal fetal lung development. Congenital diaphragmatic hernia is a failure of the diaphragm to close by weeks 10 to 12 of gestation. The presence of bowel in the chest cavity halts lung growth.[8]

The oxygen content formula is as follows:

$$(\text{hemoglobin})(1.34 \text{ mL O}_2 \text{ / g of hemoglobin})(\text{SaO}_2) + (0.03 \text{ mL O}_2)(\text{PaO}_2)$$

There are key differences in fetal physiology compared to that of adults.[8] The O_2 dissociation curve is left-shifted and the arterial P_{50} is 18 mm Hg in the fetus, compared to 26 in the adult, and the normal range of arterial oxygenation saturation is lower in the fetus. The lower P_{50} results in an offloading of oxygen from the maternal circulation to the fetal circulation down a concentration gradient. Oxygenated blood is supplied by the umbilical vein from the placenta, and the lungs do not engage in gas exchange in utero. The pulmonary vascular resistance (PVR) in late gestation is five times greater than that of newborns, and fetal pulmonary arterial blood flow is only 50% of that of newborns. These

---

Box 3.1 Maternal Factors Influencing Fetal Lung Development[a]

Maternal Factors
Nutrition
Endocrine factors
Smoking
Medical comorbidities
Concurrent intrauterine infection

[a]Kotecha S. Lung growth for beginners. *Paediatr Respir Rev.* 2000;1(4):308–13.

factors result in markedly different umbilical artery cord blood gas compared to adult arterial blood gases: pH 7.29, $PaCO_2$ 49, PaO_2 18, base deficit 2.7 mmol/L, bicarbonate 23 mmol/L.[9]

Cardiac Physiology

Three key differences exist in the fetal heart compared to the neonatal, infant, and adult heart—sarcomere and myofibril structure, myocardial cytoskeleton, and autonomic innervation. The myofibrils and sarcomeres in the fetus are arranged irregularly and in thinner layers, rendering force generation by the myocardium less efficient compared to later in development.[10] Additionally, the high collagen content of fetal and neonatal myocardium, with relatively high type I collagen compared to type II, results in a noncompliant neonatal and fetal heart.[11] Differences in extracellular matrix and cytoskeleton of the myocardium also are contributory. The neonatal and fetal heart is thus unable to respond as briskly to volume loading.[11] Lastly, sympathetic innervation is immature until the newborn period, leaving a predominance of the parasympathetic nervous system, and reflexive bradycardia is more frequent than tachycardia from the baseline. The maturation of the sympathetic system in term neonates contributes to increased heart rate variability, an indicator of fetal well-being and lack of stress.[12]

Similar to adults, fetal cardiac output is dependent on heart rate and stroke volume. The determinants of ventricular performance are preload, afterload, and myocardial contractility. Due to the relatively noncompliant myocardium, the stroke volume is fixed and the cardiac output is described as heart rate–dependent.[13]

Neonatal asphyxia has a profound effect on the fetus. After only a minute of umbilical cord occlusion, the PaO_2 of the fetus decreases sharply to less than 5 mm Hg, eventually resulting in a decreased cardiac output, hypotension, and further acidosis, including compromised neurological activity (Figure 3.2).[14] Continuous fetal heart rate tracings demonstrate such asphyxia from cord compression or fetal stress that occurs with contractions with periods of bradycardia and will be discussed subsequently.

Antepartum Fetal Surveillance

Fetal health is an important part of prenatal care. Antepartum fetal assessment is used to test for fetal well-being and to identify those fetuses that are at risk of hypoxic injury or death in pregnancies that are complicated by high risk maternal and fetal conditions (Box 3.2). The goal of fetal testing is to identify suspected fetal compromise and intervene before significant fetal neurologic injury or death occurs. In this chapter, we will discuss

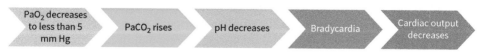

Figure 3.2 Systemic effects of hypoxia on the fetus.

Box 3.2 Antepartum Fetal Assessment Techniques in Clinical Use Currently[a]

Antepartum fetal assessment techniques
Maternal-fetal movement assessment
Nonstress test (NST)
Biophysical profile (BPP)
Modified BPP
Umbilical artery Doppler velocimetry
Contraction stress test

[a]ACOG Practice Bulletin No. 145: Antepartum Fetal Surveillance. *Obstet Gynecol.* 2014; 124(1):182–192.

---

antepartum fetal surveillance techniques, indications for testing, and management guidelines for intervention.[15]

Maternal-Fetal Movement Assessment

One of the most important tools for fetal surveillance is maternal perception of fetal movement.[15,16] This is an assessment that the mother can do daily in the form of "kick counts." A decrease in the perception of fetal movement may precede fetal death, even as much as by several days.[15,16]

There are several approaches to performing kick counts. In one approach, the woman is instructed to lie on her side and count distinct fetal movements. Feeling 10 distinct "kicks" in a period of up to 2 hours is reassuring.[15] In another approach, women are instructed to count fetal movements for 1 hour three times per week. If the count equals or exceeds her prior baseline count, it is considered reassuring. If the fetal kick count is not reassuring, the mother is advised to seek medical attention for further fetal assessment.

Nonstress Test

The nonstress test (NST) is a simple test that is performed by auscultation of the fetal heart rate using an electronic monitor. The NST is usually the initial assessment for fetal well-being. The NST is based on the premise that, in a healthy fetus, movement will result in an acceleration in the fetal heart rate (FHR).[15] The NST may be performed with the parturient in either the semi-Fowler (sitting with the head elevated 30 degrees) or lateral recumbent position. The FHR tracing is observed for accelerations that peak at least 15 beats per minute above the baseline and last 15 seconds.[15] The NST should be conducted for at least 20 minutes, but monitoring may be necessary for 40 minutes or longer to account for fetal sleep cycles. Nonstress tests are categorized as reactive or nonreactive. A reactive NST has 2 or more fetal accelerations in a 20 minute period.[15] A reactive NST is reassuring and is highly predictive of current fetal well-being (Figure 3.3). It is a short-term indicator of fetal acid-base status. A fetus with a reactive NST is not acidotic or neurologically

(A)   (B)

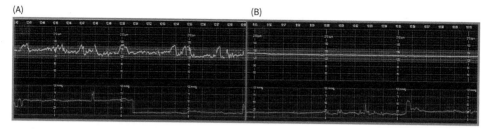

Figure 3.3 Nonstress test. Each small vertical square is 10 heart beats. Each small horizontal square represents 10 seconds. Each large horizontal square represents 1 minute. A) Reactive NST. Note the variability and accelerations. B) Nonreactive. Note the lack of accelerations.

depressed. A nonreactive NST lacks FHR accelerations over 40 minutes.[15] A nonreactive NST requires further fetal testing, usually with either a biophysical profile or modified biophysical profile.

Biophysical Profile

The biophysical profile (BPP) consists of an NST combined with four observations made by ultrasound (Figure 3.4, Table 3.2 and Box 3.3). It is usually performed if the NST was nonreactive.

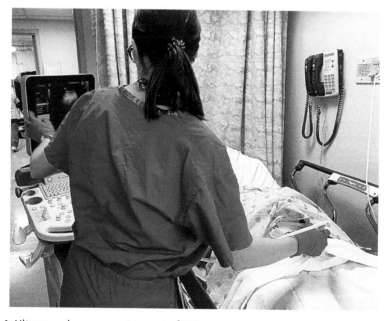

Figure 3.4 Ultrasound assessment as part of BPP.

Table 3.2 Components of the Biophysical Profile[a]

BPP component	Definition
Nonstress test	2 or more accelerations at least 15 bpm above baseline in a 20 minute period
Amniotic Fluid Volume	A single deepest vertical pocket greater than 2cm
Fetal Breathing Movements	At least one episode of rhythmic fetal breathing movements of 30 sec or more within 30 minutes
Fetal Movements	At least 3 discrete body or limb movements within 30 minutes
Fetal Tone	At least 1 episode of extension of a fetal extremity with return to flexion, or opening or closing of a hand

[a]Manning FA, Morrison I, Lange IR, Harman CR, Chamberlain PF. Fetal biophysical profile scoring: selective use of the nonstress test. *Am J Obstet Gynecol.* 1987;156:709–712.

Modified Biophysical Profile

The modified BPP combines the NST with amniotic fluid volume assessment (Figure 3.5).[15,16,17,18] It is easier to perform than the full BPP, but provides important information on fetal status.[19] As mentioned above, the NST is a short-term indicator of fetal acid-base status.[15] Amniotic fluid volume assessment, however, is a marker of long-term uteroplacental function.[15,20] During the late second trimester and third trimester, amniotic fluid volume is a reflection of fetal urine production. In the setting if uteroplacental insufficiency, decreased fetal renal perfusion may ultimately lead to oligohydramnios.[15,20]

The modified BPP may show one of the two following results:

- Normal: NST is reactive and the amniotic fluid volume is greater than 2 cm in the deepest pocket.
- Abnormal: NST is nonreactive or amniotic fluid volume in the deepest vertical pocket is 2 cm or less (oligohydramnios).

Box 3.3 Scoring the Biophysical Profile[a,b,c,d]

BPP scoring
Each of the 5 components is scored at either 2 (present) or 0 (not present)
A composite score of 8 to 10 is normal
Score of 6 is equivocal
Score of 4 or less is abnormal
Regardless of the composite score, oligohydramnios, defined as an amniotic fluid volume of 2cm or less in the deepest vertical pocket, should prompt further evaluation

[a]ACOG Practice Bulletin No. 145: Antepartum Fetal Surveillance. *Obstet Gynecol.* 2014;124(1):182–192.
[b]Pearson JF, Weaver JB. Fetal activity and fetal wellbeing: an evaluation. *Br Med J.* 1976;1:1305–1307.
[c]Manning FA, Morrison I, Lange IR, Harman CR, Chamberlain PF. Fetal biophysical profile scoring: selective use of the nonstress test. *Am J Obstet Gynecol.* 1987;156:709–712.
[d]Magann EF, Doherty DA, Field K, Chauhan SP, Muffley PE, Morrison JC. Biophysical profile with amniotic fluid volume assessments. *Obstet Gynecol.* 2004;104:5–10.

(A)   (B)   (C)

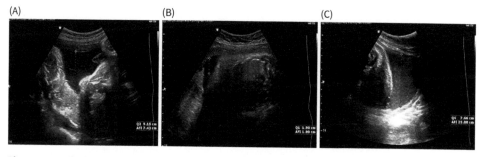

Figure 3.5 Ultrasound assessment of amniotic fluid volume. A) Normal amniotic fluid volume. B) Example of oligohydramnios. Amniotic fluid index (AFI) < 5 cm. Deepest vertical pocket is < 2 cm. C) Example of polyhydramnios. Single deepest pocket ≥ 8 cm or AFI ≥ 24 cm.

Umbilical Artery Velocimetry

Doppler ultrasonography is a noninvasive technique that is used to assess fetal status in pregnancies complicated by intrauterine growth restriction (IUGR; Figure 3.6). Flow velocity waveforms in the umbilical artery of normally growing fetuses differ from the waveforms of growth-restricted fetuses. In normally growing fetuses, the umbilical flow velocity waveform is characterized by high velocity diastolic flow.[15] In growth restricted fetuses, there is decreased umbilical artery diastolic flow.[15,21] In cases of severe growth restriction, diastolic flow may be absent or even reversed.[15,21] Umbilical artery Doppler velocimetry only provides information on fetal well-being for the growth-restricted fetus. There is no evidence that it can be applied to the fetus with normal growth.

Contraction Stress Test

Though the contraction stress test (CST) is technically a component of antepartum fetal surveillance, it is infrequently used for testing purposes. The contraction stress test necessitates that a mother has been admitted to the labor and delivery unit, intravenous access has been obtained, and oxytocin has been initiated.[15] The goal of the CST is to assess if the fetus will tolerate a temporary reduction in oxygenation associated with contractions. In a fetus with sufficient reserve, the contractions will not have an appreciable effect on the fetal heart rate (FHR) tracing. In the compromised fetus, however, the decrease in oxygenation with contractions will lead to a FHR pattern showing late decelerations.[15] CSTs are usually performed prior to an induction of labor to assess if the fetus will ultimately be able to tolerate labor. [15]

During a CST, a patient is positioned laterally, and FHR and uterine contractions are recorded simultaneously with an external fetal monitor. Contractions are observed over a 10-minute period and are deemed to be adequate when at least three contractions last for a minimum duration of 40 seconds (Figure 3.7).[15] Oxytocin administration is not indicated if the patient is spontaneously contracting. The CST is interpreted based on the presence or absence of late decelerations.[15,22] Contractions may also produce variable decelerations, which are usually caused by umbilical cord compression. CST can be categorized in Table 3.3.

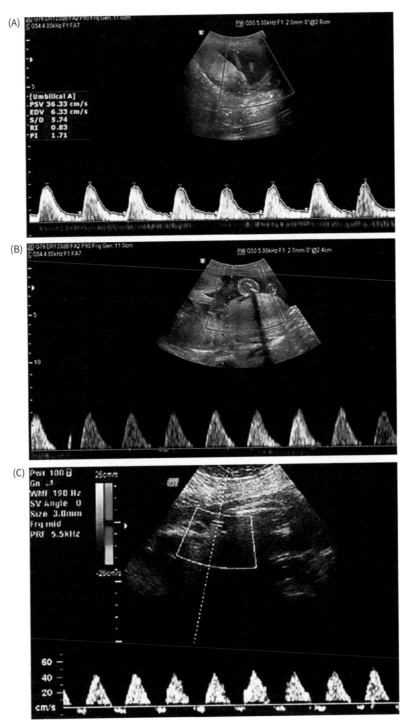

Figure 3.6 Examples of umbilical artery Doppler waveforms. A) Normal umbilical artery Doppler flow waveform. B) Absent end-diastolic Doppler flow in umbilical artery. C) Reversal of end-diastolic flow.

ACOG practice bulletin no. 145: antepartum fetal surveillance. *Obstet Gynecol*. 2014; 124(1):182–192.

(A)   (B)   (C)

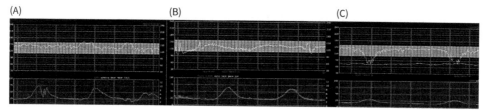

Figure 3.7 Contraction stress test. The yellow curve corresponds to the fetal heart rate. The green curve represents contractions. A) Negative contraction stress test. No decelerations noted with contractions. B) Variable decelerations. Abrupt decrease in FHR of > 15 beats per minute. The onset of deceleration to nadir is less than 30 seconds. The deceleration lasts > 15 seconds and less than 2 minutes. C) Example of late deceleration. A late deceleration is a visually apparent gradual decrease in FHR, with the timing of onset of the deceleration to its nadir being 30 second or longer. The nadir of the deceleration occurs after the peak of the contraction.
ACOG practice bulletin no. 145: antepartum fetal surveillance. *Obstet Gynecol.* 2014;124(1):182–192.

A negative CST is reassuring and suggests that the fetus has enough reserve to tolerate labor. With a positive CST, a discussion regarding mode of delivery should take place as the fetus has demonstrated diminished reserve.[15]

Indications for Antepartum Fetal Surveillance

Antepartum fetal testing is recommended for pregnancies in which the risk of fetal demise is increased. Risk factors can be separated into maternal and pregnancy-related. Some of the conditions for which testing may be indicated are listed in Table 3.4.[15]

Initiation of Fetal Surveillance

Antepartum fetal testing should be initiated at 32–34 weeks of gestation for most high-risk pregnancies.[23] In pregnancies with particularly concerning high-risk conditions, however, such as chronic hypertension with suspected intrauterine growth restriction, testing may

Table 3.3 Categorization of Contraction Stress Test[a]

Test Result	Criteria
Negative	No late decelerations or significant variable decelerations
Equivocal-suspicious	Intermittent late decelerations or significant variable decelerations
Equivocal	FHR decelerations that occur when contractions are ≥ 2 minutes or duration ≥ 90 seconds
Unsatisfactory	< 3 contractions in 10 minutes

[a]ACOG Practice Bulletin No. 145: Antepartum Fetal Surveillance. *Obstet Gynecol.* 2014;124(1):182–192.

Table 3.4 Maternal and Pregnancy Related Indications for Antepartum Fetal Testing[a]

Maternal conditions	Pregnancy-related conditions
Pre-existing diabetes mellitus	Gestational diabetes mellitus
Chronic hypertension / cardiovascular disease	Gestational hypertension / Preeclampsia
Autoimmune disease—systemic lupus erythematosus, antiphospholipid antibody syndrome	Decreased fetal movement
Chronic renal disease	Oligohydramnios / Polyhydramnios
Hyperthyroidism, poorly controlled	Fetal growth restriction
Hemoglobinopathies—sickle cell disease	Late term pregnancy
Thrombophilia	Multiple gestation (with significant discordance)
	Previous fetal demise
	Isoimmunization (moderate or severe)

[a]ACOG Practice Bulletin No. 145: Antepartum Fetal Surveillance. *Obstet Gynecol.* 2014;124(1):182–192.

begin at an earlier gestational age when delivery would be considered for fetal benefit, such as 26–28 weeks.[15]

Frequency of Fetal Testing

The frequency of antepartum fetal surveillance should be individualized to the patient. If the maternal and fetal condition that prompted testing remains stable and the tests are reassuring, weekly testing can be performed until delivery.[15] However, in certain high-risk conditions, more frequent testing can be performed. [15] Examples of such high-risk conditions include late-term pregnancy, gestational hypertension, diabetes, and intrauterine growth restriction.[15] The optimal frequency has not been established, but testing can occur 2-3 times per week or daily, depending on the condition.

Management of Abnormal Fetal Test Results

An abnormal fetal test result should be viewed in the context of the overall clinical scenario. It is important to understand that maternal conditions can adversely affect fetal status.[15] These conditions include maternal infection, poorly controlled diabetes, or a flare-up of an autoimmune disease. Optimizing the maternal status can improve the fetal status, and therefore repeat testing may be warranted in such situations. If there is no evidence of a potentially reversible maternal condition contributing to abnormal fetal testing, there should be a stepwise approach to fetal assessment (Figure 3.8).

Antepartum fetal testing has a high false-positive rate and low positive predictive values. Therefore, abnormal (positive) test results are usually followed by another test or delivery

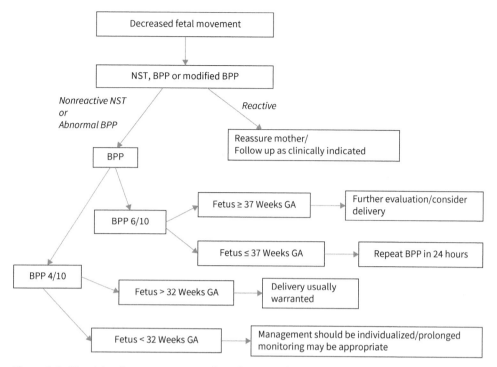

Figure 3.8 Algorithm for management of an abnormal fetal assessment in the presence of decreased fetal movement.

ACOG practice bulletin no. 145: antepartum fetal surveillance. *Obstet Gynecol*. 2014;124(1):182–192.

based on consideration of the test results, overall maternal and fetal status, and gestational age of the fetus.[15]

Management of Intrauterine Growth Restriction

There are currently no definitive guidelines for timing of delivery of the growth-restricted fetus on the basis of umbilical artery Doppler velocimetry (Figure 3.9). The Society for Maternal Fetal Medicine (SMFM) suggests that delivery should be considered based on gestational age of the fetus and umbilical artery Doppler findings.[24]

Management of Oligohydramnios

Oligohydramnios, as defined earlier, is a single deepest vertical pocket of amniotic fluid of 2 cm or less and an amniotic fluid index (AFI) of 5 cm or less. Available data has shown that using the deepest vertical pocket rather than AFI to diagnose oligohydramnios is associated with a decrease in unnecessary intervention without an increase in fetal morbidity.[25] Several factors must be assessed in the decision to intervene in cases of newly diagnosed

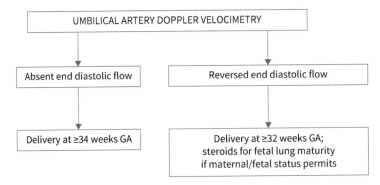

Figure 3.9 Example of an algorithm for delivery timing based on SMFM recommendations (Doppler assessment of the fetus with intrauterine growth restriction. Society for Maternal-Fetal Medicine).
Am J Obstet Gynecol. 2012;206:300–308. Published erratum appears in *Am J Obstet Gynecol.* 2012;206:508.

oligohydramnios. It is prudent to rule out the rupture of membranes as a potential cause of oligohydramnios.[15] If rupture of membranes is the etiology of oligohydramnios, it can no longer be considered an adequate predictor of placental status. According to the American College of Gynecology (ACOG), delivery is recommended at 36–37 weeks gestational age in the setting of persistent oligohydramnios without evidence of rupture of membranes.[26] At less than 36 weeks gestational age, oligohydramnios with intact membranes may be expectantly managed based on an individualized assessment of gestational age, and maternal and fetal status.[15]

Mode of Delivery

Delivery of the fetus is recommended in the setting of nonreassuring fetal testing. Management algorithms are shown in Figures 3.8 and 3.9. The mode of delivery of a potentially compromised fetus ought to be addressed by members of a multidisciplinary team. As per ACOG, in the absence of obstetric contraindications, vaginal delivery may be attempted via induction of labor.[15] If there is a concern that the fetus will not tolerate labor, a contraction stress test may be performed as described above. Continuous intrapartum monitoring of the FHR and uterine contractions is necessary.

Anesthetic Considerations

Patients with nonreactive fetal testing are at increased risk of undergoing cesarean delivery. These fetuses may have diminished reserve and may not tolerate induction of labor. It is important to perform a thorough preanesthetic assessment on these parturients should a cesarean delivery become necessary. Early neuraxial placement in these patients should be discussed to facilitate anesthetic care in case of emergent cesarean delivery. Close communication about fetal status is necessary with the obstetrics team to ensure safe and effective care.

References

1. Gregory GA, Bret CM. Neonatology for anesthesiologists. In: Davis P and Cladis FP, eds. *Smith's Anesthesia for Infants and Children.* 9th ed. Philadelphia, PA: Elsevier; 2016:513–570.
2. Allin M, Matsumoto H, Santhouse AM, et al. Cognitive and motor function and the size of the cerebellum in adolescents born very pre-term. *Brain.* 2001;124(Pt 1):60–66.
3. Limperopoulos C, Soul JS, Haidar H, et al. Impaired trophic interactions between the cerebellum and the cerebrum among preterm infants. *Pediatrics.* 2005;116(4):844–850.
4. Volpe JJ. Cerebral white matter injury of the premature infant—more common than you think. *Pediatrics.* 2003;112:176–179.
5. Khwaja O, Volpe JJ. Pathogenesis of cerebral white matter injury of prematurity. *Arch Dis Child Fetal Neonatal Ed.* 2008;93(2):F153–F161.
6. Hadders-Algra M. Early human motor development: From variation to the ability to vary and adapt. *Neurosci Biobehav Rev.* 2018;90:411–427.
7. Kotecha S. Lung growth for beginners. Paediatr Respir Rev. 2000 Dec;1(4):308–313.
8. Gao Y, Raj JU. Regulation of the pulmonary circulation in the fetus and newborn. *Physiol Rev.* 2010;90(4):1291–1335.
9. Dudenhausen JW, Luhr C, Dimer JS. Umbilical artery blood gases in healthy term newborn infants. *Int J Gynaecol Obstet.* 1997;57(3):251–258.
10. Nassar R, Reedy MC, Anderson PA. Developmental changes in the ultrastructure and sarcomere shortening of the isolated rabbit ventricular myocyte. *Circ Res.* 1987;61(3):465–483.
11. Klopfenstein HS, Rudolph AM. Postnatal changes in the circulation and responses to volume loading in sheep. *Circ Res.* 1978;52(6):839–845.
12. Cardoso S, Silva MJ, Guimaraes H. Autonomic nervous system in newborns: a review based on heart rate variability. *Childs Nerv Syst.* 2017;33(7):1053–1063.
13. Van Hare GF, Hawkins JA, Schmidt KG, Rudolph AM. The effects of increasing mean arterial pressure on left ventricular output in newborn lambs. *Circ Res.* 1990;67(1):78–83.
14. Rudolph AM, Heymann MA. Cardiac output in the fetal lamb: the effects of spontaneous and induced changes of heart rate on right and left ventricular output. *Am J Obstet Gynecol.* 1976;124(2):183–192.
15. ACOG Practice Bulletin No. 145: Antepartum Fetal Surveillance. *Obstet Gynecol.* 2014; 124(1):182–192.
16. Pearson JF, Weaver JB. Fetal activity and fetal wellbeing: an evaluation. *Br Med J.* 1976;1:1305–1307.
17. Manning FA, Morrison I, Lange IR, Harman CR, Chamberlain PF. Fetal biophysical profile scoring: selective use of the nonstress test. *Am J Obstet Gynecol.* 1987;156:709–712.
18. Magann EF, Doherty DA, Field K, Chauhan SP, Muffley PE, Morrison JC. Biophysical profile with amniotic fluid volume assessments. *Obstet Gynecol.* 2004;104:5–10.
19. Nageotte MP, Towers CV, Asrat T, Freeman RK. Perinatal outcome with the modified biophysical profile. *Am J Obstet Gynecol.* 1994; 170:1672–1676.
20. Clark SL, Sabey P, Jolley K. Nonstress testing with acoustic stimulation and amniotic fluid volume assessment: 5973 tests without unexpected fetal death. *Am J Obstet Gynecol.* 1989;160:694–697.
21. Gudmundsson S, Marsal K. Umbilical and uteroplacental blood flow velocity waveforms in pregnancies with fetal growth retardation. *Eur J Obstet Gynecol Reprod Biol.* 1988;27:187–196.

22. Freeman RK, Anderson G, Dorchester W. A prospective multi-institutional study of antepartum fetal heart rate monitoring. I. Risk of perinatal mortality and morbidity according to antepartum fetal heart rate test results. *Am J Obstet Gynecol.* 1982;143:771–777.

23. Rouse DJ, Owen J, Goldenberg RL, Cliver SP. Determinants of the optimal time in gestation to initiate antenatal fetal testing: a decision-analytic approach. *Am J Obstet Gynecol.* 1995;173:1357–1363.

24. Doppler assessment of the fetus with intrauterine growth restriction. Society for Maternal-Fetal Medicine [published erratum appears in Am J Obstet Gynecol 2012;206: 508]. *Am J Obstet Gynecol.* 2012;206:300–308.

25. Nabhan AF, Abdelmoula YA. Amniotic fluid index versus single deepest vertical pocket as a screening test for preventing adverse pregnancy outcome. Cochrane Database of Systematic Reviews 2008, Issue 3. Art. No.: CD006593.

26. Spong CY, Mercer BM, D'Alton M, Kilpatrick S, Blackwell S, Saade G. Timing of indicated late-preterm and early-term birth. *Obstet Gynecol.* 2011;118:323–333.

4

Coexisting Disease and the Parturient: Part One

Cardiovascular, Respiratory, Renal, Gastrointestinal Systems

Carole Zouki and Aladino De Ranieri

Introduction

Anesthesiologists play an important role in the care of a pregnant patient. Oftentimes, the first encounter they have with the parturient is in the perioperative period or while the patient is in labor. The ideal goal is to provide analgesia and render the mother's experience comfortable. Being aware of her comorbidities ahead of time, and preparing to anesthetize accordingly, is essential. Anesthesiologist and obstetricians need to work closely together in order to implement an individualized plan for the mother and deliver her baby in the most memorable and positive experience possible.

The pregnancy-related mortality ratio is defined as the number of pregnancy-related death per 100,000 live births.[1] Despite improvements in anesthesia and sterile techniques, the discovery of antibiotics, the rise in hospital births, and improvement in blood transfusions, the mortality ratio in the United States has more than doubled, rising from 7.2 deaths per 100,000 births in 1987 to 17.3 deaths in 100,000 births in 2013.[2] Pregnancy-related death is declining around the world but the pregnancy-related death continues to rise in the United States, and from 2003 to 2013 it was one of only eight countries with increasing maternal mortality.[3] Along with that, Americans continue to face an increase in hypertension, diabetes, chronic heart disease, and obesity.[1] Understanding maternal morbidity and implementing changes can guide physicians into reducing pregnancy-related events. The present chapter will discuss maternal physiology and associated maternal comorbidities.

Cardiovascular Disease

Cardiovascular disease is the leading cause of maternal mortality in the United States.[4,5] Approximately 0.4 to 4% of pregnancies are complicated by cardiovascular disease.[6] The severity of the cardiac disease before pregnancy can predict the outcome during pregnancy. This explains why some cardiac lesions are more dangerous than others.[7] It is important to understand the normal physiologic changes of pregnancy and the impact they have on the cardiovascular system in order to treat cardiovascular diseases of pregnancy. Maternal hemodynamics change tremendously during pregnancy and some important changes are an increase in cardiac output, an increase in intravascular volume, and a decrease in systemic vascular resistance. At term, plasma volume increases about 50% above the nonpregnant

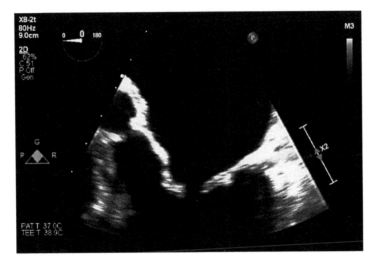

Figure 4.1 Mitral valve stenosis. TEE: mid-esophageal 5 chamber view.

state, and immediately after delivery of baby, cardiac output increases up to 80% above pre-term value. These physiologic changes of pregnancy can be challenging in women with cardiovascular disease, and some defects will tolerate these changes better than others. For example, in women with mitral stenosis (MS), the increase in heart rate and left ventricular volume can lead to atrial fibrillation or heart failure (Figure 4.1). On the contrary, women with mitral regurgitation will benefit from the decreased afterload and the increased left ventricular volume. The hemodynamic changes mentioned previously are what may lead a parturient to consult a cardiac specialist for the very first time. Many women remain asymptomatic and live with these heart defects silently up until pregnancy. They have no pre-existing diagnosis, but the cardiovascular changes and associated symptoms lead to seeking medical help.

Myocardial Infarction

Hemodynamic changes during labor and delivery secondary to anxiety, pain, and uterine contractions can result in a threefold increase in cardiac oxygen consumption.[8] A myocardial infarction occurs when there is an imbalance between oxygen demand and oxygen supply. Pregnancy in itself increases the risk of myocardial ischemia threefold to fourfold in women of reproductive age.[9,10] During labor, it is important to choose the delivery option with the least hemodynamic burden.[10] In women with atherosclerosis, the increase in cardiac output immediately postpartum might exacerbate underlying coronary artery disease.[10] The risk of myocardial infarction may occur anytime throughout pregnancy but it occurs more in the third trimester and commonly affects the anterior wall.[9] Medical management for a pregnant patient with ischemic heart disease consists of salicylates, beta blockers, calcium channel blockers, and heparin.[10,11] Fetal considerations may affect the choice of therapy, but survival is the primary concern and, if needed, revascularization should not be withheld.[10]

Aortic Dissection

Aortic complications are uncommon but, when they occur, they can lead to life-threatening complications.[12] Aortic complications can occur in women with no risk factors though they tend to occur mostly in women with connective tissue disease such as Marfan's or Ehlers-Danlos or in women with a family history of aortic disease.[12-15] The cardiovascular changes of pregnancy mentioned previously, such as increase in blood volume and cardiac output, pose a significant stress on the wall of the aorta.[12,16] Aortic dissection occurs when blood moves through a tear in the intima causing a shear stress and separating the intimal layer from adventitia.[16] Some risk factors associated with aortic dissection are hypertension, gender, age, family history, and connective tissue disease.[16] The common presenting symptom of a dissecting aorta is abrupt onset of severe pain described as sharp.[16] The treatment goal depends on the type of dissection. For Stanford Type A, treatment consists of surgical management, whereas in Stanford Type B, treatment involves medical management.[17]

Valvular Heart Disease

Valvular heart disease consists of one quarter of the cardiac diseases complicating pregnancy.[18] Valvular lesions can be separated into two types: stenotic or regurgitant. MS is the most commonly encountered valvular lesion in women of childbearing age.[19] The prevalence of mitral stenosis in developed countries is around 1% (Figure 4.2). However, the prevalence of MS in developing countries can be as high as 50% secondary to high incidence of MS.[18,19] Treatment goals aim to control the heart rate, limit volume expansion, and treat the atrial fibrillation or atrial flutter with a rate control medication or prompt cardioversion.[18,20] Aortic stenosis is most commonly caused by congenital bicuspid aortic valve and not by rheumatic fever.[18] Pregnancy is usually well tolerated and some favorable outcome during pregnancy are absent

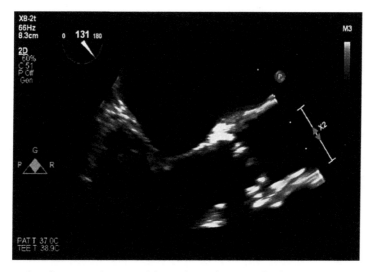

Figure 4.2 Aortic valve stenosis. TEE: mid-esophageal aortic valve long axis view.

symptoms, normal electrocardiogram (EKG), normal exertional blood pressure rise, aortic valve >1cm, and a normal left ventricular function.[21] These women have a fixed stroke volume and cannot handle the increase in plasma volume. Women with aortic stenosis who become symptomatic need to be treated with beta blockade and diuretics. If medical therapy fails, then and only then would valve replacement, after early delivery by cesarean, is necessary.[18,22]

Mitral regurgitation is a lesion that is favored early in pregnancy secondary to the increase in plasma volume and the decrease in systemic vascular resistance.[18] Nevertheless, the regurgitation may worsen in the third trimester secondary to volume overload and increase systemic vascular resistance.[18] When this occurs, medical management with diuretics usually suffices.[18] Aortic regurgitation is usually caused by a bicuspid aortic valve, and the presentation and management is similar to that of mitral regurgitation.[18]

Peripartum Cardiomyopathy

Peripartum cardiomyopathy is a rare form of heart failure, which by definition either occurs in late pregnancy or in the early postpartum period.[23,24] The etiology of peripartum cardiomyopathy is unknown but viral myocarditis has been suggested.[5] Presenting symptoms of women with peripartum cardiomyopathy are dyspnea on exertion, symptoms of congestion, orthopnea, paroxysmal nocturnal dyspnea, and edema of the lower extremities.[25] These symptoms may not always be obvious as they overlap with normal symptoms of pregnancy. Treatment of cardiomyopathy in pregnancy is similar to the management of heart failure with reduced ejection fraction.[5] Sodium restriction is the mainstay of volume management and loop diuretic may be added for symptoms of pulmonary edema.[26]

Respiratory Disease

Respiratory conditions encountered in pregnancy are a common cause of mortality.[27] Respiratory parameters start changing as early as the fourth week of gestation.[28] There is an increase in minute ventilation mainly due to a 30–50% increase in tidal volume.[28] This increase in minute ventilation leads to an increase in PaO_2 in the maternal circulation and a reduction in $PaCO_2$.[29,30] This decrease in $PaCO_2$ in pregnancy leads to a respiratory alkalosis, compensated by chronic metabolic acidosis.[31] The normal CO_2 in a pregnant woman should be below the nonpregnant level, and a finding of a "normal" $PaCO_2$ may be worrisome and indicative of respiratory failure.[32] Many of the respiratory hemodynamic changes in pregnancy are attributed to the increase in the hormone progesterone, a hormone directly causing an increase in respiration.[28,33] Some respiratory changes encountered in a pregnant woman are enlargement in the thoracic cage by 5–7cm and a vertical decrease in the chest by 4cm as a result of an elevated diaphragm.[34,35] Nasal congestion is common and it is often perceived as shortness of breath.[36]

Asthma

Asthma is a common comorbidity in pregnancy and its prevalence has increased in recent decades.[37] Asthma exacerbation are worrisome in pregnancy, and up to 45% of women need to seek medical help.[38] Some complications associated with asthma are a low birth weight, preeclampsia, preterm delivery, and an increase in perinatal mortality.[39–42] Some parturients with asthma are suboptimally medicated, as they fear the impact that asthma medication may have on the baby. Mothers need to understand that an asthma attack can decrease the oxygen level to the fetus, and this is more harmful to the fetus than the asthma medications.[43] Medications used in asthma such as short-acting inhaled beta agonists or inhaled corticosteroids have been shown to be safe in pregnancy and during lactation.[30,44] Current recommendations are to treat pregnant women with asthma in the same manner as we would the nonpregnant patient.[39]

Other Pulmonary Diseases of Pregnancy

Pulmonary edema may be cardiogenic or noncardiogenic in nature.[27] Pregnancy is associated with volume overload, as there is a progressive increase in blood volume. Women with congenital or rheumatic cardiac disorders may not tolerate this hemodynamic burden, eventually leading to pulmonary edema.[27] An iatrogenic cause of cardiogenic pulmonary edema in pregnancy is the use of tocolytic therapy, including beta-adrenergic agents such as ritodrine or terbutaline.[27] The cause of the pulmonary edema secondary to these agents is multifactorial and beyond the scope of this chapter. On the other hand, the cause of noncardiogenic pulmonary edema is due to acute lung injuries leading to an increased permeability in pulmonary vasculature.[45–47]

Women with pulmonary hypertension who become pregnant carry a poor prognosis with a mortality rate as high as 50%.[48] The combination of increased blood volume and an inability to increase cardiac output leads to right-sided heart failure and sudden death.[26] Pulmonary hypertension is a contraindication for pregnancy.[22,49–52] Respiratory failure in pregnancy is caused by a variety of diseases ranging from obstructive lung disease to restrictive lung disease, infection, and pulmonary edema.[53] Women will present with dyspnea and tachypnea.[27] Clues such as tachypnea, an inability to complete full sentences, and abnormal arterial blood gas should prompt intervention with either supplemental oxygen or temporary endotracheal intubation.[27]

Smoking

Cigarette smoking in pregnancy can have an impact on maternal and fetal health.[54] Pregnant women smokers tend to be younger, with a low socio-economic status, and a low level of education.[55] Smoking leads to an increase in blood concentration of carbon monoxide.[54] Consequentially, there is a left shift of the oxyhemoglobin curve leading to a decreased oxygen level.[53] Nicotine crosses the placenta and cigarette smoke impacts the fetus by restricting oxygen supply and nutrients.[56,57] Prenatal smoking may have adverse effects on child neurodevelopment such as language development and cognitive function.[58] Despite the known complications associated with smoking in pregnancy, up to 23% of women in the United States who smoked at conception time continued to smoke throughout pregnancy.[26] However, the cessation rate is higher in pregnancy than in the general population.[59]

Renal Disease

Pregnancy leads to an increase in cardiac output and a decrease in vascular resistance that can cause up to an 80% increase in renal blood flow and an almost 50% increase in glomerular filtration rate (GFR).[60,61] Along with those changes, pregnant women have a serum concentration of urea and creatinine that is slightly lower than in the nonpregnant state. Pregnancy in a woman with kidney disease can lead to negative sequelae. Fetal and maternal prognosis depends on the degree of renal function at conception.[62] There is a wide range of different kidney conditions and monitoring during pregnancy should be tailored to the severity of the disease.[60] The exact mechanism by which pregnancy exacerbates renal disease is unknown and common obstetric complications associated with chronic renal disease include intrauterine growth restriction (IUGR), preterm delivery, hypertension, preeclampsia, and an increased rate of cesarean delivery.[63] Depending on the degree of kidney function, chronic kidney disease is divided into five categories.[60] Stage one and two have a normal or mild renal impairment and the GFR is slightly reduced. This type of kidney disease is more common in pregnancy, as it doesn't affect renal prognosis and 3% of women of childbearing age are affected.[62] Women with more advanced kidney disease such as chronic kidney disease stage 3 to 5 have a very low GFR (< 60 ml/min). Pregnancy is less common, as there is an increase in infertility and miscarriage and 1 in 150 women of childbearing age are affected.[60] The goal in managing a patient with chronic renal disease is to further avoid kidney damage. Hypertension and proteinuria will further decrease GFR, a tool that can be used as a prognostic value for the progression of the disease.[62,64]

Treatment goals aim to involve a specialist early in the pregnancy. Some values need to be monitored regularly, such as blood urea, nitrogen, and creatinine; blood pressure; proteinuria midstream urine for infection; and sometimes even an ultrasound is needed to detect urological obstruction.[60] Medical treatment options will depend on the extent of the disease ranging from steroids to immunosuppressive agents.[65] Women with diabetic nephropathy should be taken off ACE inhibitors (ACEI) or angiotensin receptor blockers (ARB), and strict blood pressure control should ensure 110–129/65–79 mm Hg.[66] Patients with Lupus nephritis should be tested for anticardiolipin antibodies and lupus anticoagulants, and if positive should receive low-dose aspirin or subcutaneous heparin.[67] Lupus nephritis flares should be controlled with immunosuppressive therapy such as high-dose corticosteroids or azathioprine.[62]

End Stage Renal Disease

Fertility is rare in women with end-stage renal failure primarily secondary to hormone imbalance.[68] Despite a trend toward improvement in women and infant survival in patients with end-stage renal failure, hypotension and major fluid shift changes can cause uteroplacental insufficiency and lead to fetal compromise.[69] One can avoid the hemodynamic consequences of dialysis by more frequent and shorter dialysis runs. Goals of dialysis are to maintain blood urea levels in order to decrease the risk of developing polyhydramnios and subsequently preterm labor.[64]

Gastrointestinal System

Pregnant patients have multiple gastrointestinal (GI) complaints during labor and most of these are mild and managed conservatively.[70] Some changes seen in the GI tract are a delay in gastric emptying secondary to elevation in progesterone, which decreases lower esophageal tone (Figure 4.3). Further there is an increase in gastric acidity due to elevation in hormonal gastrin, a hormone secreted by the placenta.[30,70] Nausea and vomiting are the most common medical complaint in pregnancy, affecting 50–80% of women.[70,71] The exact mechanism of nausea vomiting is unknown, and these symptoms usually subside by the 20th week of pregnancy.[71] After excluding other causes of nausea and vomiting, the parturient is treated with dietary restrictions.[72] Pharmaceutical treatment, such as an antihistamine, is given for those who have failed conservative management.[70,71] Consequently, the concept that pregnant women are "full stomach" is not a myth. The increased intra-abdominal pressure, delayed gastric emptying, and reduced gastric-esophageal sphincter tone, all combined with increased gastric volume, are contributing factors that can increase the risk of aspiration.[73] Anesthesiologists should be cautious especially for anesthetic induction and keep in mind the aforementioned physiologic and anatomic changes.

Common Gastrointestinal Complaints

Gastroesophageal reflux disease (GERD) is reported to be present in 40–85% of pregnant women.[74] Symptoms usually begin in the end of the first trimester and last up until delivery of the baby.[70] Mild symptoms are treated conservatively, and if symptoms persist then pharmacological treatment with antacids containing calcium or magnesium is recommended.[74] A second-line agent is a type 2 antihistamine such as ranitidine or cimetidine.[71,74] Finally, if the patient does not respond to the last two mentioned treatment regimens, then a proton pump inhibitor (PPI) may be used.[75] PPI are reserved for women with GERD complications, as they can diminish iron reabsorption.[70] Hyperemesis gravidarum (HG) is a severe form of nausea and vomiting usually associated with 5% weight loss, dehydration, and electrolyte imbalances.[70] HG is a diagnosis of exclusion and hospital admission is often necessary. When patients are hospitalized, treatment goals aim to prevent dehydration with intravenous fluid therapy and the correction of electrolyte disturbances.[70] Constipation is another GI complaint affecting around 40% of pregnant patients and some factors leading to

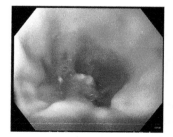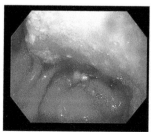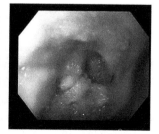

Figure 4.3 Delayed gastric emptying (endoscopic view left to right): undigested food in the esophagus, proximal, and distal stomach.

constipation in pregnancy are a higher level of serum progesterone or an increase in iron intake.[76,77] Constipation is usually managed with a high-fiber diet or fiber containing bulking agents such as Metamucil.[76]

References

1. Creanga, AA. Pregnancy-related mortality in the United States, 2006–2010. *Obstet Gynecol.* 2015;125(1):5–12.

2. Creanga, AA. Pregnancy-related mortality in the United States, 2011–2013. *Obstet Gynecol.* 2017;130(2):366–373.

3. Hirshberg, A. Epidemiology of maternal morbidity and mortality. *Semin Perinatol.* 2017;41(6):332–337.

4. Abir, G. Maternal mortality and the role of the obstetric anesthesiologist. *Best Pract Res Clin Anaesthesiol.* 2017;31(1):91–105.

5. Honigberg, MC. Peripartum cardiomyopathy. *BMJ.* 2019;364.

6. Burlew, BS. Managing the pregnant patient with heart disease. *Clin Cardiol.* 1990;13(11):757–762.

7. Chestnut, DH. *Chestnut's Obstetric Anesthesia: Principles and Practice* (4th edition). Elsevier Health Sciences; 2014.

8. Elkayam, U. High-risk cardiac disease in pregnancy: Part I. *J Am Coll Cardiol.* 2016;68(4):396–410.

9. James, AH. Acute myocardial infarction in pregnancy: a United States population-based study. *Circulation.* 2006;113(12):1564–1571.

10. Kealey, AJ. Coronary artery disease and myocardial infarction in pregnancy: A review of epidemiology, diagnosis, and medical and surgical management. *Can J Cardiol.* 2010;26(6):185–189.

11. Collins, JS. Asymptomatic coronary artery disease in a pregnant patient. A case report and review of literature. *Herz.* 2002;27(6):548–554.

12. Kamel, H. Pregnancy and the risk of aortic dissection or rupture: a cohort-crossover analysis. *Circulation.* 2016;134(7):527–533.

13. Gelpi, G. Should pregnancy be considered a risk factor for aortic dissection? Two cases of acute aortic dissection following cesarean section in non-Marfan nor bicuspid aortic valve patients. *J Cardiovasc Surg.* 2008;49(3):389–391.

14. Weissmann-Brenner, A. Aortic dissection in pregnancy. *Obstet Gynecol.* 2004;103(5 Pt 2):1110–1113.

15. Snir, E. Dissecting aortic aneurysm in pregnant women without Marfan disease. *Surg Gynecol Obstet.* 1988;167(6):463–465.

16. Immer, FF. Aortic dissection in pregnancy: analysis of risk factors and outcome. *Ann Thorac Surg.* 2003;76(1):309–314.

17. Patel, PV. Aortic dissection in a pregnant patient without other risk factors. *Case Rep Obstet Gynecol.* 2019;2019:1583509.

18. Anthony, J. Valvular heart disease in pregnancy. *Cardiovasc J Afr.* 2016;27(2):111–118.

19. Tsiaras, S. Mitral valve disease in pregnancy: outcomes and management. *Obstet Med.* 2009;2(1):6–10.

20. Windram, JD. Valvular heart disease in pregnancy. *Best Pract Res Clin Obstet Gynaecol.* 2014;28(4):507–518.

21. Myerson, SG. What is the role of balloon dilatation for severe aortic stenosis during pregnancy? *J Heart Valve Dis.* 2005;14(2):147–150.

22. European Society of Gynecology (ESG); Association for European Paediatric Cardiology (AEPC); German Society for Gender Medicine (DGesGM); Regitz-Zagrosek, V, Blomstrom Lundqvist, C, Borghi, C, Cifkova, R, Ferreira, R, Foidart, JM, Gibbs, JS, Gohlke-Baerwolf, C, Gorenek, B, Iung, B, Kirby, M, Maas, AH, Morais, J, Nihoyannopoulos, P, Pieper, PG, Presbitero, P, Roos-Hesselink, JW, Schaufelberger, M, Seeland, U, Torracca, L; ESC Committee for Practice Guidelines. ESC Guidelines on the management of cardiovascular diseases during pregnancy: the Task Force on the Management of Cardiovascular Diseases during Pregnancy of the European Society of Cardiology (ESC). *Eur Heart J.* 2011;32(24):3147–3197. doi:10.1093/eurheartj/ehr218. Epub 2011 Aug 26. PMID: 21873418.

23. Pearson, GD. Peripartum cardiomyopathy: National Heart, Lung, and Blood Institute and Office of Rare Diseases (National Institutes of Health) workshop recommendations and review. *JAMA.* 2000;283(9):1183–1188.

24. Hibbard, JU. A modified definition for peripartum cardiomyopathy and prognosis based on echocardiography. *Obstet Gynecol.* 1999;94(2):311–316.

25. Elkayam, U. Clinical characteristics of peripartum cardiomyopathy in the United States: diagnosis, prognosis, and management. *J Am Coll Cardiol.* 2011;58(7):659–670.

26. Kim, SY. The contribution of clinic-based interventions to reduce prenatal smoking prevalence among US women. *Am J of Public Health.* 2009;99(5):893–898.

27. Bhatia, P, Bhatia K. Pregnancy and the lungs. *Postgrad Med J.* 2000;76(901):683–689.

28. Datta, S. Maternal physiological changes during pregnancy, labor, and the postpartum period. In: *Obstetric Anesthesia Handbook* (5th edition). New York, NY: Springer New York; 2010:1–14.

29. Torgersen, CKL. A systematic approach to the physiologic adaptations of pregnancy. *Crit Care Nurs Q.* 2006;29(1):2.

30. Mehta, N. Respiratory disease in pregnancy. *Best Pract Res Clin Obstet Gynaecol.* 2015;29(5):598–611.

31. Tan, EK. Alterations in physiology and anatomy during pregnancy. *Best Pract Res Clin Obstet Gynaecol.* 2013;27(6):791–802.

32. Omo-Aghoja, L. Maternal and fetal acid-base chemistry: a major determinant of perinatal outcome. *Ann Med Health Sci Res.* 2014;4(1):8–17.

33. Bayliss, DA. Central neural mechanisms of progesterone action: application to the respiratory system. *J Appl Physiol (1985).* 1992;73(2):393–404.

34. Leontic, EA. Respiratory disease in pregnancy. *Med Clin North Am.* 1977;61(1):111–128.

35. Cohen, ME. Studies on the circulation in pregnancy. *J Am Med Assoc.* 1939;112(16):1556–1562.

36. Wise, RA. Respiratory and physiologic changes in pregnancy. *Immunol Allergy Clin North Am.* 2006;26(1):1–12.

37. Kwon, HL. Asthma prevalence among pregnant and childbearing-aged women in the United States: estimates from national health surveys. *Ann Epidemiol.* 2003;13(5):317–324.

38. Murphy, VE. Managing asthma in pregnancy. *Breathe.* 2015;11(4):258–267.

39. Murphy, VE. Asthma during pregnancy: mechanisms and treatment implications. *Eur Respir J.* 2005;25(4):731–750.

40. Triche, EW. Association of asthma diagnosis, severity, symptoms, and treatment with risk of preeclampsia. *Obstet Gynecol.* 2004;104(3):585–593.

41. Dombrowski, MP. Asthma during pregnancy. *Obstet Gynecol.* 2004;103(1):5–12.

42. Gordon, M. Fetal morbidity following potentially anoxigenic obstetric conditions. VII. Bronchial asthma. *Am J Obstet Gynecol.* 1970;106(3):421–429.

43. McDonald, CF. Asthma in pregnancy and lactation. A position paper for the Thoracic Society of Australia and New Zealand. *Med J Aust.* 1996;165(9):485–488.

44. National Heart, Lung, and Blood Institute, National Asthma Education and Prevention Program Asthma and Pregnancy Working Group. NAEPP expert panel report. Managing asthma during pregnancy: recommendations for pharmacologic treatment-2004 update. *J Allergy Clin Immunol.* 2005;115(1):34–46.

45. Russi, EW. High permeability pulmonary edema (ARDS) during tocolytic therapy—a case report. J Perinat Med. 1988;16(1):45–49.

46. Pisani, RJ. Pulmonary edema associated with tocolytic therapy. *Ann Intern Med.* 1989;110(9):714–718.

47. Phelan, JP. Pulmonary edema in obstetrics. *Obstet Gynecol Clin North Am.* 1991;18(2):319–331.

48. Dawkins, KD. Primary pulmonary hypertension and pregnancy. *Chest.* 1986;89(3):383–388.

49. Galiè, N. Guidelines for the diagnosis and treatment of pulmonary hypertension: the Task Force for the Diagnosis and Treatment of Pulmonary Hypertension of the European Society of Cardiology (ESC) and the European Respiratory Society (ERS), endorsed by the International Society of Heart and Lung Transplantation (ISHLT). *Eur Heart J.* 2009;30(20):2493–2537.

50. Thorne, S. Risks of contraception and pregnancy in heart disease. *Heart Br Card Soc.* 2006;92(10):1520–1525.

51. Pieper, PG. Pre-pregnancy risk assessment and counselling of the cardiac patient. *Neth Heart J Mon J Neth Soc Cardiol Neth Heart Found.* 2011;19(11):477–481.

52. Madden, BP. Pulmonary hypertension and pregnancy. *Int J Obstet Anesth.* 2009;18(2):156–164.

53. Noble, PW. Respiratory diseases in pregnancy. *Obstet Gynecol Clin North Am.* 1988;15(2): 391–428.

54. Wehby, GL. The impact of maternal smoking during pregnancy on early child neurodevelopment. *J Hum Cap.* 2011;5(2):207–254.

55. Chamberlain, C. Psychosocial interventions for supporting women to stop smoking in pregnancy. *Cochrane Database Syst Rev.* 2013;10(10):CD001055. Published 2013 Oct 23. doi:10.1002/14651858.CD001055pub4

56. Lambers, DS, Clark, KE. The maternal and fetal physiologic effects of nicotine. *Semin Perinatol.* 1996;20(2):115–126.

57. Berlin, I. Cigarette smoking during pregnancy: do complete abstinence and low level cigarette smoking have similar impact on birth weight. *Nicotine Tob Res.* 2017;19(5): 518–524.

58. Key, APF. Smoking during pregnancy affects speech-processing ability in newborn infants. *Environ Health Perspect.* 2007;115(4):623–629.

59. Schneider, S. Smoking cessation during pregnancy: a systematic literature review. *Drug Alcohol Rev.* 2010;29(1):81–90.

60. Williams, D. Chronic kidney disease in pregnancy. *BMJ.* 2008;336(7637):211–215.

61. Blom, K. Pregnancy and glomerular disease: a systematic review of the literature with management guidelines. *Clin J Am Soc Nephrol.* 2017;12(11):1862–1872.

62. Bili, E. Pregnancy management and outcome in women with chronic kidney disease. *Hippokratia.* 2013;17(2):163–168.

63. Reddy, SS. Management of the pregnant chronic dialysis patient. *Adv Chronic Kidney Dis.* 2007;14(2):146–155.

64. Imbasciati, E. Pregnancy and renal disease: predictors for fetal and maternal outcome. *Am J Nephrol.* 1991;11(5):353–362.

65. Lateef, A. Managing lupus patients during pregnancy. *Best Pract Res Clin Rheumatol.* 2013;27(3):435–447. doi:10.1016/j.berh.2013.07.005

66. Hod, M. Diabetic nephropathy and pregnancy: the effect of ACE inhibitors prior to pregnancy on fetomaternal outcome. *Nephrol Dial Transplant.* 1995;10(12):2328–2333.

67. Witter, FR. Management of the high-risk lupus pregnant patient. *Rheum Dis Clin North Am.* 2007;33(2):253–265.

68. Lim, VS. Reproductive function in patients with renal insufficiency. *Am J Kidney Dis Off J Natl Kidney Found.* 1987;9(4):363–367.

69. Krakow, D. Effect of hemodialysis on uterine and umbilical artery Doppler flow velocity waveforms. *Am J Obstet Gynecol.* 1994;170(5):1386–1388.

70. Gomes, CF. Gastrointestinal diseases during pregnancy: what does the gastroenterologist need to know? *Ann Gastroenterol.* 2018;31(4):385–394.

71. Body, C. Gastrointestinal diseases in pregnancy: nausea, vomiting, hyperemesis gravidarum, gastroesophageal reflux disease, constipation, and diarrhea. *Gastroenterol Clin North Am.* 2016;45(2):267–283.

72. van der Woude, CJ. Management of gastrointestinal and liver diseases during pregnancy. *Gut.* 2014;63(6):1014–1023.

73. Gal, O. Estimation of gastric volume before anesthesia in term-pregnant women undergoing elective cesarean section, compared with non-pregnant or first-trimester women undergoing minor gynecological surgical procedures. *Clin Med Insights Womens Health.* 2019;12:1179562X19828372. Published 2019 Mar 14. doi:10.1177/1179562X19828372

74. Ali, RAR. Gastroesophageal reflux disease in pregnancy. *Best Pract Res Clin Gastroenterol.* 2007;21(5):793–806.

75. Richter, JE. Review article: the management of heartburn in pregnancy. *Aliment Pharmacol Ther.* 2005;22(9):749–757.

76. Cullen, G. Constipation and pregnancy. *Best Pract Res Clin Gastroenterol.* 2007;21(5):807–818.

77. Wald, A. Constipation, diarrhea, and symptomatic hemorrhoids during pregnancy. *Gastroenterol Clin North Am.* 2003;32(1):309–322.

5

Coexisting Disease and the Parturient: Part Two

Hematologic, Neurologic, Musculoskeletal and Immune Systems

Benjamin F. Aquino, Afshin Heidari, and Leila Haghi

Coagulation Disorders

More than 50% of parturients with venous thromboembolism (VTE) have some sort of congenital deficiency in anticoagulant activity.[1] The most common among these are Factor V Leiden deficiency, Protein C deficiency, Protein S deficiency, and antithrombin III (ATIII) deficiency. Often diagnosed during pregnancy, they represent only 0.1% of all pregnancies, but of those parturients with untreated VTE, 24% develop pulmonary embolus.[2]

The risk increases during pregnancy (the 3rd trimester risk is greater than the first) and the greatest VTE risk actually occurs during the first postpartum week. The biggest risk factors include personal history of VTE, known congenital thrombophilia (Factor V Leiden conferring the greatest risk), and modifiable issues such as obesity and maternal mobilization.[3] Peripartum and antepartum thromboembolic disorders are managed by therapeutic anticoagulation, and these can obviously complicate placement of neuraxial anesthesia (see Table 5.1).

Coagulopathies

Frank coagulopathy of any kind is an absolute contraindication to neuraxial anesthesia. These include platelet disorders such as idiopathic thrombocytopenic purpura (ITP). This is old nomenclature—it is found to be due to IgG platelet destruction, and now properly known as autoimmune thrombocytopenic purpura (ATP)[4] Thrombotic thrombocytopenic purpura, or TTP, is from a defect of ADAMTS13 enzyme, which causes platelet aggregates and microemboli. Symptoms are signs from a classic pentad, but only the first two (low platelets, microangiopathic hemolytic anemia) are needed for diagnosis. The other three are fever, neurologic signs, and renal failure. Proper diagnosis is essential as the treatments are different. For ATP, conservative management is usually sufficient, but steroids can be given if platelets are < 30K before labor or < 50K before delivery.[5] For TTP, plasma exchange is the first line treatment, where 1 to 1.5 the predicted plasma volume is given.[6] Of the congenital coagulopathies, Von Willebrand's disease is

Table 5.1 Anticoagulation and Regional Anesthesia

MEDICATION	HOLD before Procedure	RESTART after Procedure	HOLD before Catheter Removal	RESTART after Catheter Removal	Additional Information	Half Life
Heparin						
IV Heparin	Wait until PTT < 40 (4–6 hours)	1 hour	4–6 hours after last dose (PTT < 40)	1 hour	Frequent Neuro check after removing catheter	1–2 hours
SC Heparin	Wait until PTT < 40 (4–6 hours)	Immediately	4–6 hours	Immediately		
LMWH (Low Molecular Weight Heparin)						
Enoxaparin (Lovenox®): Therapeutic Dose	• 24 hours; (anti-factor X_a activity in renal insufficiency)	• 24 hours after non-high bleeding risk procedure • 48–72 hours: after high bleeding risk procedure	Remove catheter before initiation of LMWH	• At least 24 hours after neuraxial procedure (4 hours prior to the first postoperative dose)	If bloody tap: wait >24 hours to restart medication	4–7 hours
Enoxaparin (Lovenox®): Prophylactic Dose	At least 12 hours	12 hours	Avoid	• 4 hours • At least 12 hours after neuraxial procedure	In OB patients: • In non-traumatic tap: and if catheter has been out >4 hours: restart in 6–12 hours • In traumatic tap: wait for 24 hours	
Warfarin						
Warfarin (Coumadin®)	INR ≤ 1.2	Immediately	• INR < 1.5: remove catheter • INR < 1.5 and > 3:Neuro check • INR > 3:hold warfarin	Immediately	• Frequent Neuro check after removing catheter for 24 hours. • Vitamin K, PCC, FFP for reversal if necessary	20–60 hours

(continued)

Table 5.1 Continued

MEDICATION	HOLD before Procedure	RESTART after Procedure	HOLD before Catheter Removal	RESTART after Catheter Removal	Additional Information	Half Life
Anti-Platelet Agents						
Aspirin			No restrictions			6 hours
Clopidogrel (Plavix®)	• 5–7 days	• Immediately: loading dose (–) • 6 hours*	• 1–2 days* • 24 hours: postop • No need: post-neuraxial procedure	• Immediately • 6 hours: loading dose (+)		
Factor Xa Inhibitors						
Rivaroxaban (Xarelto®)	72 hours	• At least 6 hours • Should be avoided while catheter is inside	22–26 hours	• 6 hours • Risks Vs. benefits	• CrCl < 30–50 ml/min: hold longer • CrCl < 15 ml/min: contraindicated	5–9 hours
Apixaban (Eliquis®)	72 hours	• At least 6 hours • Avoid while catheter is inside	26–30 hours	• 6 hours • Risks Vs. benefits	• CrCl < 30–50 ml/min: hold longer • CrCl < 15 ml/min: contraindicated	6–12 hours

From: Toledo P, Malinow AM. Embolic disorders. In: Chestnut D, Wong C, eds. *Obstetric anesthesia: principles and practice.* 5th ed. Philadelphia, PA: Elsevier; 2014:923–926.

the most common. It is a defect of the prothrombotic von Willebrand's factor (vWF) that binds factor VIII, which in turn binds platelets and collagen. There are three subtypes, but Type I, the most common subtype, may have a prevalence as high as 1% of the general population. The treatment is desmopressin (DDAVP), given 0.3 mcg/kg IV at the onset of labor.

Disseminated Intravascular Coagulation

Disseminated intravascular coagulation (DIC) is brought on by an inciting event that causes inappropriate activation of the coagulation cascade. Microvascular thrombi formation, resulting in end-organ failure, occurs alongside consumption of coagulation factors, which causes uncontrolled bleeding. Most common causes in pregnancy include pre-eclampsia, abruption, sepsis, retained products of conception, postpartum hemorrhage, fatty liver of pregnancy, and amniotic fluid embolism.[7]

For diagnostic criteria, lab findings, and treatment, see Table 5.2.

Table 5.2 DIC Diagnosis and Treatment in the Parturient

Diagnosis	• Prolonged PT/PTT ($\geq$ 1.5 times normal value) • Thrombocytopenia ($\leq$ 50,000) • Low fibrinogen (< 150 mg/dL) • Elevated fibrin degradation products (FDPs, also known as D-dimer) (> 0.5 mcg/mL fibrinogen equivalent units (FEU)) • Bleeding/oozing from mucosal surfaces, IV sites
Differential diagnosis	• Massive blood loss • HIT (Heparin-induced thrombocytopenia) • Vitamin K deficiency • Thrombotic microangiopathy • Liver insufficiency

Treatment and management[1]	• Treat the original cause of DIC—usually entails evacuation of uterine contents
	• Replacing coagulation factors:
	  1. If active bleeding: FFP, Cryoprecipitate or Fibrinogen concentrate and platelets to maintain PT and PTT in 1.5 time their normal value, fibrinogen concentration above 150–200 mg/dL and platelet count above 50,000, respectively.
	  2. Therapeutic doses of heparin either unfractionated or LMWH (assuming adequate maternal AT III levels) if DIC is complicated with thromboembolism or fibrin deposition.
	• Multisystem support:
	  1. Admission in ICU and mechanical ventilation
	  2. Thromboembolism prophylaxis with either heparin or mechanical ways or combination of both
	General anesthesia for patients with DIC requiring c-section

Adapted from: Wada H, Thachil J, Di Nisio M, et al. Guidance for diagnosis and treatment of DIC from harmonization of the recommendations from three guidelines. *J Thromb Haemost.* 2013;11:761–767.

Neurologic Disorders

Multiple Sclerosis

Multiple sclerosis (MS) is an autoimmune demyelinating disease, of which there are two types—exacerbating remitting (85%) and chronic progressive.[8] Symptoms include weakness, ataxia, vision changes, bladder dysfunction, and respiratory difficulty. There are several treatment options. IFN—Beta can reduce relapse and delay disability, but it has fetal side effects. IV immunoglobulin (IVIG) can reduce relapse, and it has the benefit of much less effect on pregnancy outcome.[9] Relapses during pregnancy are usually treated with IV steroids.

The effects on pregnancy on the course of the disease vary. Pregnancy can be protective, but the risk of relapse is higher in the postpartum period.[10] Of note, fetal effects, such as meconium aspiration and IUGR, are more common in mothers with MS. For a list of pertinent anesthesia concerns, see Table 5.3.

Myasthenia Gravis

Myasthenia gravis (MG) is an autoimmune neuromuscular disorder, which is caused by production of antibodies against nicotinic acetylcholine receptors on motor end plate in skeletal muscle. This destruction of the motor end plate causes symptoms such as muscle weakness that worsen with activity, as well ocular involvement. Severe generalized respiratory weakness can occur later in the course of the disease. The pharmacologic mainstay of treatment[11] is anticholinesterase medications, which inhibit acetylcholine breakdown and help maintain

Table 5.3 Anesthesia Considerations for Multiple Sclerosis

Global	• In general, active warming should be avoided—demyelinated nerves more susceptible to damage if body temperature is higher

Neuraxial anesthesia	• What effect does local anesthetic have on already abnormal, demyelinated neurons?
	• Complete and documented neurologic exam before block
	• Minimize dose of anesthetic with neuraxial block—
	  • Less motor block, and total amount of drug exposed to nerves is less
	  • Lower the concentration (< 0.25% bupivacaine)[a]
	  • Mix local anesthetic with opioids, either in infusion or with bolus
	• Epidural anesthesia associated with lower perioperative relapse rate[b]

General anesthesia	• Unpredictable response to muscle relaxants—train of four needs to be closely monitored

[a]Bader AM, Hunt CO, Datta S, et al. Anesthesia for the obstetric patient with multiple sclerosis. *J Clin Anesth.* 1988;1:21–24.

[b]Confavreux C, Hutchinson M, Hours MM, et al. Rate of pregnancy-related relapse in multiple sclerosis. Pregnancy in Multiple Sclerosis Group. *N Engl J Med.* 1998;339:285–291.

motor end plate integrity. Plasmapheresis has been tried, but for pregnant patients, thymectomy has been shown to have better outcomes, as well as less maternal and perinatal morbidity, than other modalities.[12] For affected parturients, the highest exacerbation rates are during the first trimester and postpartum.[13]

Key anesthetic considerations for such patients include awareness of risk factors for myasthenic crisis, which include bulbar symptoms, high intraoperative blood loss (>1000 ml), and serum anti-Ach receptor antibodies >100 nmol/mL. Neuraxial anesthesia may be best for patients with respiratory symptoms. They are known to be more susceptible to opioid induced respiratory depression, and neuraxial anesthesia can give them the benefit of opioid-free analgesia. General anesthesia is preferred if the patient has bulbar symptoms and/or respiratory compromise. Issues with muscle relaxants, however, confound general anesthesia in a patient with MG. These patients can have an unpredictable response to succinylcholine, and they are exquisitely sensitive to nondepolarizing NMBs. Sensitivity to NMBs correlates with severity of disease. In most cases, 50% of standard dose may be adequate, but anesthetics on MG patients can be done without NMBs altogether.

Connective Tissue Disorders

Ehlers-Danlos Syndrome

Ehlers-Danlos Syndrome (EDS) is an inherited connective tissue disorder, mainly affecting joints, skin, and blood vessels. Incidence thought to be about 1:5000. There are now 13 different recognized subtypes[14]—types I, II, and III are the most common (30% each), with type IV being the most severe (10%). Most subtypes have common features of general joint hypermobility, hyperextensibility of skin, and atrophic scarring. Of note, Type IV (vascular EDS in new nomenclature) patients are prone to organ rupture. They also tend to have thin, translucent skin that tears easily. Type VIIC (cardiac-valvular EDS) is associated with progressive cardiac and valvular problems, in addition to classic hypermobility problems. Fortunately, the incidence of adverse pregnancy outcomes have not been shown to be increased in parturients with EDS[15] but concerns remain.

As far as anesthesia, both general and regional anesthesia can be given in women with EDS. Subtype specific concerns include issues such as uterine rupture risk in Type IV patients, even ones without a prior c-section. Patients with cardiac-valvular EDS can have hemodynamically significant cardiac lesions like aortic insufficiency or mitral regurgitation (MR), as well as arrhythmias due to MR or atrial enlargement. If any of these issues are present, the patient may need invasive cardiac monitoring. Patients of all subtypes may have hypermobility of the cervical spine, which can cause instability and predispose to difficult intubation. They may also be more prone to vascular problems, such as difficult access and spontaneous arterial rupture. Their vascular fragility, a direct result of their connective tissue defect, puts them at risk of excessive peripartum bleeding, as well as epidural hematoma. Even in such patients, labs are often normal, with the most prominent problem being abnormal platelet aggregation. See Table 5.4 for other concerns in patients with EDS.

Table 5.4 Anesthetic Planning for Parturient With Ehlers-Danlos Syndrome (EDS)

	Associated Anesthetic Concerns and Actions
Patient history and counseling	Know patient's subtype and personal history of their disease course Assess bleeding risk Assess airway and potential difficulty
coordination	Discuss case with obstetrician Neonatal ICU—most subtypes autosomal dominant—50% chance infant also has EDS
c-section intraoperative concerns	Airway difficulty and necessary equipment Patient positioning Peripartum bleeding
Bleeding	Patient's personal history— prior surgeries, easy bruising Coordinate with blood bank DDAVP—useful in patient with positive bleeding history

Adapted from: Wiesmann T, Castori M, Malfait F, Wulf H. Recommendations for anesthesia and perioperative management in patients with Ehlers-Danlos syndrome. *Orphanet J Rare Dis.* 2014;9:109.

Autoimmune Disorders

Systemic Lupus Erythematosus

Systemic Lupus Erythematosus (SLE) is an autoimmune, multisystem disease, caused by antibodies against cellular antigens. Damage is from both the buildup of immune complexes, as well as the secondary inflammatory response. The female:male ratio is 9:1; Asians and African-Americans are affected more than Caucasians.[16] During pregnancy, SLE is generally associated with a greater incidence of adverse events. It affects only 1 in 1200 pregnancies, but 20% of all total lupus cases present initially during pregnancy.[17] Patients may have no previous history of the disease. Two thirds of those with pre-existing lupus will have worsening of their disease during pregnancy, with flare-ups most often from the second trimester onwards. Lupus nephritis is troublesome in that it can look like pre-eclampsia—both have hypertension, edema, and proteinuria. However, pre-eclampsia also presents with increased liver enzymes, increased serum uric acid, and proteinuria without active urinary sediment. These factors distinguish it from SLE mediated lupus nephritis. Proper diagnosis is key, because treatments are different. Lupus nephritis is treated with immunosuppressive therapy, while pre-eclampsia is treated by delivery of the fetus. Cornerstones of obstetric assessment and management include measurement of maternal serologic markers. As examples, anti-phospholipid antibodies predict higher maternal and fetal risk, and SLE patients with anti-phospholipid syndrome are at higher risk of VTE. Vaginal delivery is preferred, but the c-section rate is as high as 40% in parturients with SLE.[18] For anesthetic concerns and management of parturients with SLE, see Table 5.5.

Table 5.5 Anesthesia Concerns in Systemic Lupus Erythematosus (SLE)

System	Concerns
Cardiac	• Pericarditis • Coronary vasculitis—myocardial ischemia • Valvular abnormalities in up to 60% of SLE patients[a]—prophylactic antibiotics not recommended unless history of endocarditis or implanted prosthetic devices
Pulmonary	• Pulmonary hypertension—in up to 43% of SLE patients[a] • Need to maintain sinus rhythm, minimize peripheral resistance, avoid big decreases in systemic vascular resistance (SVR)[b]
Neurologic	• Neuropathies—in up to 25% of SLE patients • Cerebral vasculitis, lupus cerebritis—on differential of postpartum headache
Hematologic	• Transfusion: patients may have unusual antibodies—difficult cross matching • Lupus anticoagulant—laboratory artifact only • Coagulation abnormalities—likely due to autoantibodies against clotting factors
Other	• Patients currently on steroids need perioperative stress dose

[a]Popham B, Reid RW. Autoimmune Disorders. In: Chestnut D, Wong C, eds. *Obstetric Anesthesia: Principles and Practice*. Philadelphia, Elsevier, 5th ed. 2014:950.

[b]Cuenco J, Tzeng G, Wittels B. Anesthetic Management of the Parturient with Systemic Lupus Erythematosus, Pulmonary Hypertension, and Pulmonary Edema. *Anesthesiology*. 1999;91:568–570.

Adapted from: Ben-Menachem E. Review article: systemic lupus erythematosus: A review for anesthesiologists. *Anesth Analg*. 2010;111(3):665–676.

Infectious Diseases

Human Immunodeficiency Virus

Human Immunodeficiency Virus (HIV) is a retrovirus transmitted via infected bodily fluids. The virus affects CD4 cells and impairs immunity, causing susceptibility to opportunistic infections. Since the late 1990s, medical management has consisted of highly active anti-retroviral therapy (HAART) medications, which include nucleoside and non-nucleoside reverse transcriptase inhibitors, protease inhibitors, and integrase inhibitors. It is also necessary to treat opportunistic infections. Among the primary goals of obstetric management is preventing vertical transmission of the disease from mother to fetus.

To do this, maternal disease must of course be controlled. Transmission is greater in women with more severe HIV disease, such as those with active AIDS symptoms and higher viral loads.[19] Maternal drug therapies include zidovudine, which, when given to the mother throughout pregnancy and to the infant after delivery, decreases transmission rates to as low as 8.3%.[20] HAART is also used to treat aggressively, regardless of viral load. It has minimal fetal effects, with perinatal transmission as low as 1–2%.[21] Other aspects of obstetric management include minimizing time between rupture of membranes (ROM) and delivery, and avoiding other risk factors, such as chorioamnionitis, instrumentation (forceps, invasive monitoring, cerclage, etc.), and breast feeding.[22] Pertinent anesthesia concerns are enumerated in Table 5.6.

Table 5.6 Anesthesia Concerns in the HIV-Positive Parturient

Global	More likely to engage in high risk behaviors—need high index of suspicion for these and their associated problems C-section—best way to minimize time between ROM and delivery
Neuraxial anesthesia	Awareness and documentation of neurologic status—infections causing meningitis, cerebral edema, or increased ICP, may be contraindications to neuraxial anesthesia No evidence that neuraxial anesthesia increases neurologic complications, viral load, or speeds disease progression Epidural blood patch, in old and limited study, appears safe in HIV+ patients[a] Strict asepsis—be wary of infecting immunocompromised patient
General anesthesia	Provider precautions: strict universal precautions to avoid contracting infection or transmitting to others—gloves, eyewear, avoid recapping needles, etc. Postoperatively, clean anesthesia work space thoroughly and replace all equipment Possible negative effect on immune function—not significant in healthy patients,[b] but what about HIV positive parturients with active infection? Without active infection? Possibility of hastening or causing pulmonary issues in patient with underlying lung disease?

[a]Tom DJ, Gulevich SJ, Shapiro HM, et al. Epidural blood patch in the HIV-positive patient: review of clinical experience. San Diego HIV Neurobehavioral Research Center. *Anesthesiology.* 1992;76:943–947.

[b]Schneemilch CE, Schilling T, Bank U. *Best Pract Res Clin Anaesthesiol.* 2004;18(3):493–507.

Herpes Simplex Virus II

Herpes simplex virus II (HSV) is acquired by sexual contact and can cause genital infection, fever, lymphadenopathy, meningitis, encephalitis, and hepatitis, among other things. Long latent periods between symptomatic episodes are possible. Treatment is with antiviral meds, the mainstay of these being acyclovir. The prime obstetric concern is avoiding fetal transmission, as neonatal HSV infection has high morbidity and mortality. It is critical to avoid direct contact with active lesions. Vaginal delivery was once indicated, with elective c-section only if active lesions or prodromal symptoms are present. But more recent ACOG recommendations are for c-section even if mother is latent, because asymptomatic shedding of virus can occur, and preventing the fetal sequelae of HSV is worth the risk of a c-section.[23]

Anesthetic concerns include the theoretical risk of transmission of the virus from neuraxial blocks to the CNS. This has, however, been shown to be unlikely in a patient without active infection.[24] As such, asymptomatic latent infection is not a reason to deny neuraxial anesthesia.

On the other hand, the safety of neuraxial technique in patients with primary infection or signs of viremia is not known, and the anesthesia provider needs to weigh the risk and benefit of a neuraxial block.

Substance Use

Cocaine

Cocaine is a sympathomimetic vasoconstricting local anesthetic that inhibits the reuptake of NE, serotonin, and dopamine. An estimated 1.8 to 10% of pregnant women use

Table 5.7 Anesthetic Considerations: The Parturient and Cocaine

Global	Urine positive screen NOT an absolute contraindication to GA if patient without signs of acute cocaine intoxication—such patients show no increased hemodynamic extremes or worsened short term outcomes compared to cocaine negative controls[1] Increases abruption risk—need high index of suspicion BP responses to anesthesia may be exaggerated • Often relatively resistant to pressor effects • Ephedrine unpredictable due in part to indirect effects on catecholamine release—response depends on circulating catecholamine levels • Phenylephrine best BP choice—direct alpha-1 agonism
Neuraxial	Neuraxial anesthesia as soon as possible—decreases circulating catecholamine levels Need to be wary of unpredictable pressor response If clinical situation allows, can be beneficial to dose epidural slowly if concerned about pressor response
General	Best avoided in acute intoxication—significant hypertension and tachycardia can occur in response to laryngoscopy Avoid etomidate or ketamine—both can increase CNS stimulant effects of cocaine Increased aspiration risk—increased sympathetic tone delays gastric emptying even more than usual Chronic cocaine users may have prolonged response to succinylcholine

[1] From: Moon TS, Gonzales MX, Jun JJ, et al. Recent cocaine use and the incidence of hemodynamic events during general anesthesia: A retrospective cohort study. *J Clin Anesth* 2019;55:146–150.

the drug, and do so across socioeconomic, racial, and ethnic lines.[25] Notably, up to 90% of these patients abuse other substances.[26] Cocaine has multiple physiologic effects pertinent to both the parturient and the anesthesia provider. Its most obvious cardiovascular effect is hypertension, but it can also increase the risk of coronary vasoconstriction, chest pain, myocardial infarction, and tachyarrhythmias. Neurologic issues include increased risk of TIA, CVA, and seizures. Pulmonary effects include peripartum wheezing. Issues related specifically to pregnancy include the fact that cocaine crosses the placenta and decreases uterine blood flow. During pregnancy, there are also increased levels of active metabolite norcocaine, which means the duration and potency of drugs may increase[27] and physiologic effects can be accentuated. Cocaine use is associated with worse fetal outcomes, like preterm labor, preterm birth, and low birth weight infants. For anesthesia concerns see Table 5.7.

Marijuana/Cannabis

Marijuana is the most commonly used dependent substance in pregnancy. It too crosses the placenta, and cannabinoid receptors are present in the fetal brain;[28] its effects on development are unknown. Its use is even more prevalent now that legalization is becoming more common in the United States. Cannabidiol (CBD), a phytocannabinoid that accounts for 40% of the cannabis plant's extract, is putatively responsible for many of cannabis' therapeutic effects. It contains no THC (the cannabinoid with the most psychoactive effects), but often the exact mix of even commercially available CBD is varied and unknown; a recent study showed up to 62 different compounds in one commercially available extract.[29]

The anesthesia provider caring for a patient on cannabis needs to consider that such patients will often have a higher requirement of induction drugs[30] and increases of BIS

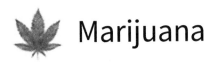

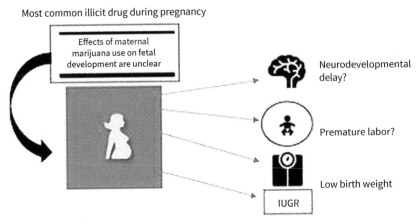

Anesthesia considerations:

- Some drugs (atropine, pancuronium, and ketamine) can exacerbate existing tachycardia associated with marijuana use.
- Sedative and volatile agents have effects, such as myocardial depression, that can be augmented in acute marijuana intoxication.
- Chronic marijuana smokers at risk for similar perioperative pulmonary complications as cigarette smokers.

Figure 5.1 Anesthesia considerations—marijuana and the parturient.

From: Jaques SC, Kingsbury A, Henshcke P, Chomchai C, et al. Cannabis, the pregnant woman and her child: weeding out the myths. *J Perinatol*. 2014;34(6):417–424.

Merlob P, Stahl B, Klinger G. For debate: does cannabis use by the pregnant mother affect the fetus and newborn? *Pediatr Endocrinol Rev*. 2017;15(1):4–7.

monitoring numbers are also possible.[31] Though cannabis is used for chronic pain, evidence is lacking for cannabis/CBD use in acute pain, although it is perceived by patients to be useful for such situations.[32] In addition, cannabis users have been shown to have higher pain scores and higher pain medicine requirements than noncannabis users in the postoperative period.[33] See Figure 5.1 for other anesthetic concerns in the cannabis-using patient.

References

1. Lockwood C, et al. Practice bulletin no. 124: Inherited thrombophilias in pregnancy. *Obstet Gynecol*. 2011;118(3):730–740.
2. James AH, Jamison MG, Brancazio LR, Myers ER. Venous thromboembolism during pregnancy and the postpartum period: incidence, risk factors, and mortality. *Am J Obstet Gynecol*. 2006;194(5):1311–1315.
3. Knight M. Antenatal pulmonary embolism: risk factors, management and outcomes. *BJOG*. 2008;194:1311–1315.

4. Sharma SK, Myhre JM. Hematologic and coagulation disorders. In: Chestnut D, Wong C, eds. *Obstetric Anesthesia: Principles and Practice*. Philadelphia, Elsevier, 5th ed., 2014, p. 1042.

5. Provan D, Stasi R, Newland AC, et al. International consensus report on the investigation and management of primary immune thrombocytopenia. *Blood.* 2010;115:168–186.

6. Rock GA, Shumak KH, Buskard NA, et al. Comparison of plasma exchange with plasma infusion in the treatment of thrombotic thrombocytopenic purpura. Canadian Apheresis Study Group. *N Engl J Med.* 1991;325(6): 393–397.

7. Thachil J, Toh CH. Disseminated intravascular coagulation in obstetric disorders and its acute haematological management. *Blood Rev.* 2009;23:167–769.

8. Kurtzke JF. Patterns of neurologic involvement in multiple sclerosis. *Neurology.* 1989;39(9): 1235–1238.

9. Achiron A, Kishner I, Dolev M, et al. Effect of intravenous immunoglobulin treatment on pregnancy and postpartum-related relapses in multiple sclerosis. *J Neurol.* 2006;251:1133–1137.

10. FInkelsztejn A, et al. What can we really tell women with multiple sclerosis regarding pregnancy? A systematic review and meta-analysis of the literature *BJOG.* 2011;118(7):790–797.

11. Bader AM. Neurologic and neuromuscular disease. In: Chestnut D, Wong C, eds. *Obstetric Anesthesia: Principles and Practice*. Philadelphia, Elsevier, 5th ed. 2014, p 1121.

12. Hoff JM, Daltveit AK, Gilhus NE. Myasthenia gravis in pregnancy and birth: identifying risk factors, optimising care. *Eur J Neurol.* 2007;14:38–43.

13. Ciafaloni E, Massey JM: The management of myasthenia gravis in pregnancy. *Semin Neurol.* 2004;24:95–100.

14. Malfait F, Francomano C, Byers P, et al. The 2017 international classification of the Ehlers-Danlos syndromes. *Am J Med Genet C Semin Med Genet.* 2017;175(1):8–26.

15. Sundelin HE, Stephansson O, Johansson K, Ludvigsson JF. Pregnancy outcome in joint hypermobility syndrome and Ehlers-Danlos syndrome. *Acta Obstet Gynecol Scand.* 2017;96(1): 114–119.

16. D'Cruz DP, et al. Systemic lupus erythematosus. *Lancet.* 2007;369:587–596.,

17. Gimovsky ML, Montoro M. Systemic lupus erythematosus and other connective tissue diseases in pregnancy. *Clin Obstet Gynecol.* 1991; 34:35–50.

18. Chakravarty EF, Nelson L, Krishnan E. Obstetric hospitalizations in the United States for women with systemic lupus erythematosus and rheumatoid arthritis. *Arthritis Rheum.* 2006;54:899–907.

19. Dickover RE, Garratty EM, Herman SA, et al. Identification of levels of maternal HIV-1 RNA associated with risk of perinatal transmission: effect of maternal zidovudine treatment on viral load. *JAMA.* 1996;275:599–605.

20. Connor EM, Sperling RS, Gelber R, et al. Reduction of maternal-infant transmission of human immunodeficiency virus type 1 with zidovudine treatment. Pediatric AIDS Clinical Trials Group Protocol 076 Study Group. *N Engl J Med.* 1994;331:1173–1180.

21. Cooper ER, Charurat M, Mofensen L, et al: Combination antiretroviral strategies for the treatment of pregnant HIV-1-infected women and prevention of perinatal HIV-1 transmission. *J Acquir Immune Defic Syndr.* 2002;29:484–494.

22. Dunn DT, Newell ML, Ades AE, Peckham CS. Risk of human immunodeficiency virus type 1 transmission through breastfeeding. *Lancet.* 1992:340:585–588.

23. American College of Obstetricians and Gynecologists: Management of herpes in pregnancy. ACOG Practice Bulletin No. 82. Washington, DC, June 2007 (Reaffirmed 2009). *Obstet Gynecol.* 2007;209:1489–1498.

24. Bader AM, Camaann WR, Datta S. Anesthesia for cesarean delivery in patients with herpes simplex virus typ-2 infections. *Reg Anesth.* 1990;15(5): 261–263.

25. Kuczkowski KM. Peripartum care of the cocaine-abusing parturient: Are we ready? *Acta Obstset Gynecol Scand.* 2005; 84(2):108–116.

26. Leffert L. Substance abuse. In: Chestnut DH, Wong CA, eds. *Obstetric Anesthesia—Principles and Practice.* Philadelphia, Elsevier, 2014:1204.

27. Fajemirokun-Odudeyi O, Lindow SW: Obstetric implications of cocaine use in pregnancy: a literature review. *Eur J Obstet Gynecol Reprod Biol.* 2004; 112:2–8.

28. Thompson R, DeJong K, Lo J. Marijuana use in pregnancy: A review. *Obstetric and Gynecological Survey.* 2019;74(7):415–428.

29. Lewis MM, Yang Y, Wasilewski E, et al. Chemical profiling of medical cannabis extracts. *ACS Omega.* 2017;2(9):6091–6103.

30. Flisberg, P, Paech MJ, et al. Induction dose of Propofol in patients using cannabis. *Eur J Anaesthesiol.* 2009;26(3):192–195.

31. Ibera C, Shalom B, Saifi F, et al. *Harefuah.* 2018;157(3):162–166.

32. Khelemsky Y, Goldberg AT, Hurd YL, et al. Perioperative beliefs regarding potential effectiveness of marijuana (cannabinoids) for treatment of pain: a prospective population study. *Reg Anesth Pain Med.* 2018:42:652–659.

33. Liu CW, Bhatia A, Buzon-Tan A, et al. Weeding out the problem: the impact of preoperative cannabinoid use on pain in the perioperative period. *Anesth. Analg.* 2019;129(3):874–881.

6

Parturient Pre-Anesthesia Assessment and Evaluation

Patrick McConville, Carrie Polin, and Justin Swengel

Current Status

Parturients that present for predelivery assessment and consultation with an anesthesiologist often have a different time course than one who arrives on a labor and delivery unit. A visit before the planned delivery date allows for complete medical record retrieval and additional testing or consultation if necessary. If the patient arrives at the delivery center, initial assessment begins with an understanding of why the patient is in the labor and delivery unit. Patients arriving in active labor or those sent from the obstetrical clinic for fetal or maternal distress carry a different urgency than those who are scheduled for induction of labor or for cesarean delivery. Many situations require a discussion with the admitting obstetrician and a review of the medical record for an understanding of the reason for arrival.

Parturients who are in active labor or who are admitted for either fetal distress or maternal complications require an initial focused physical exam with emphasis on vital signs, allergies, airway exam, and IV access (see Box 6.1). Additional information and assessment can be obtained through discussions and records review, but an evaluation for these critical pieces of information can prepare the anesthesiologist in the event that an arrival becomes an emergency. Obtaining the gestational age and the number of gravida and para can also aid in rapid patient assessment.

Delivery Plan

Once initial assessment and evaluation for emergent conditions are made, anesthesia providers should assess the plan for the patient. If a patient is being monitored, will she be delivered in the event of maternal or fetal decompensation? In the setting of decompensation, will she be induced or will she have a cesarean section? Patients in active labor may be augmented, allowed to proceed with passive labor, or they may receive tocolysis. In the scheduled induction patient, discussing pain control plans are necessary. In the setting of a scheduled cesarean section, is the patient amenable to a regional anesthetic? Depending on the current patient status and plan for delivery, assessing the need or presence for blood products may be required.

Box 6.1 Focused Exam of Parturient in Active Labor or for Emergent Cesarean Delivery

---

Focused Physical Exam for Parturient in Imminent Active Labor OR Emergent Cesarean Delivery
- Vital Signs
- Allergies
- Airway Exam
- IV access
- Medical History
- Obstetric History
- Anesthetic History
- Major Organ Systems

Past Medical History

A thorough medical history can be divided into less relevant medical conditions and those that are more significant. Important but less relevant medical conditions include diagnoses that are common, well controlled, and unlikely to be impactful on the parturient in the short term such as generalized mild anxiety, medication-controlled hypothyroidism, hypercholesterolemia, or insomnia. A particular emphasis on the current condition is necessary for parturients with chronic systemic disease.

Cardiac Disease

Patients with cardiac disease require an understanding of the diagnosis, surgical or medical treatments, and current status. The cardiac output requirements of parturients increase throughout pregnancy and are highest just after delivery. While these changes are generally well tolerated by a healthy heart, a parturient with cardiac disease may decompensate rapidly with increases in preload or heart rate (see Table 6.1).

Maternal functional status should be determined. Parturients who have minor limitations (New York Heart Association [NYHA] class I and II) will likely be able to tolerate labor and delivery without major complications. Women who are classified as NYHA class III and IV are at higher risk in the intrapartum and immediate postpartum phase and may require additional monitoring during delivery and the postpartum period. A recent echocardiogram can provide critical information regarding a parturient's current ejection fraction, valvular abnormalities, and pressure gradients.

Optimal management and monitoring of cardiac disease during pregnancy is necessary. In the delivery suite, the anesthesiologist or anesthetist can best manage the situation if they are equipped with an understanding of the physiological limitations of the disease.

Table 6.1 Organ-Specific Concerns in the Parturient

Cardiac	Pulmonary	Renal	Hepatic	Neurologic	Hematologic	Endocrine	Psychiatric	Substance Abuse
Those with congenital heart disease may not tolerate fluid shifts associated with delivery. Functional status is very important. NYHA class III and IV are at higher risk and require additional monitoring in the peripartum period.	Chronic respiratory disease is becoming more common. Examples include those with cystic fibrosis or other severe asthma. Know about their symptoms (wheezing/chest tightness) and predisposing factors. Always be vigilant and avoid Hemabate in asthmatic.	Be aware of renal status. Distinguish between chronic kidney disease and end-stage renal disease. Parturients with CKD are at risk for worsening renal function due to large fluid shifts. Be liberal with fluids. Those with ESRD require tight fluid control and are at risk for additional complications.	Important to know if acute inflammatory phase vs. fibrosis/cirrhosis phase. AST/ALT for acute inflammation. PT/PTT, platelet count, and albumin levels for chronic liver disease. Liver disease has many systemic effects including accumulation of toxins, altered metabolism of medications, malnutrition, and coagulopathy.	It is important to understand the nature of any neurologic disease state. Seizures can be associated with eclampsia, RPLS, or epilepsy. Be aware of patients with intracranial tumors, as this can change your anesthetic plan. Know of any peripheral neuropathies prior to labor, as patients can develop new or worsening symptoms due to physical changes with pregnancy.	Conditions of hypocoagulation and hypercoagulation can by unmasked in pregnancy. Be mindful of sickle cell crisis in the parturient and treat appropriately. DVT or PE may manifest in those with undiagnosed thrombophylic disorders. The use of recent anticoagulants can have an effect on the anesthetic plan.	Many hormones are elevated during pregnancy. Diabetic patients can have increased insulin requirements and may have issues with worsened peripheral neuropathy, autonomic dysfunction (including gastric emptying), and macrosomia increasing the chance of cesarean delivery. Patients requiring insulin in the peripartum period should be closely monitored for hypoglycemia. Restrictions of food and liquids during labor may result in maternal or fetal hypoglycemia which can result in distress. Glucose administration intravenously in fluids may be required.	It is important to have the patient optimized on any psych medications. Changing levels of hormones can lead to decompensation and lead to psychiatric admittance. Patients with eating disorders can have electrolyte disturbances, and evaluation prior to labor or cesarean delivery is warranted.	Chronic alcohol use can lead to hepatitis and other cardiovascular comorbidities. The use of IV drugs can cause many issues including difficult IV access, exposure to infectious disease, and difficulty with pain control in the postoperative period.

Pulmonary Disease

Pregnancy has become more common in women with chronic pulmonary disease with the advancement of medicine as well as fertility success rates. Cystic fibrosis once severely limited both fertility and pulmonary function, but due to assisted reproduction these patients are delivering more commonly.

Assessment of patients with pulmonary disease relies heavily on physical examination as well as patient history. The patients' medical history should include the frequency of wheezing and chest tightness, any precipitating factors, the last hospitalization for pulmonary symptoms, and history of mechanical ventilation. In the physical examination, the respiratory rate should be noted as well as use of any accessory muscles to breathe and wheezing present on auscultation of the chest.

It is important to note the severity of asthma in parturients as this may help to guide the administration or avoidance of Hemabate (15-methyl prostaglandin F2- alpha) in the event that additional oxytocic medications are needed during a postpartum hemorrhage (see Table 6.1).

Renal Disease

Patients with chronic renal disease, like others with systemic organ dysfunction, have been increasingly successful in carrying pregnancy to term. Improved detection, treatment of contributing factors, and management of renal insufficiency have enabled women to conceive in many cases. Chronic renal disease that results in end stage disease in particular has limited fertility in women of childbearing age. Limited menstruation or even anovulation occurs in women with renal failure. In-vitro or other assisted fertility treatments have enabled non-ovulatory patients to conceive in the setting of renal failure. Renal failure may also develop during pregnancy as a result of an obstetric disorder such as preeclampsia or acute fatty liver of pregnancy.

Parturients, as with any patients with renal disease, may have electrolyte disturbances or volume overload in the setting of acute renal failure. Patients with renal insufficiency in the peripartum period are at risk for worsening of renal function due to oral intake restrictions, blood loss, and volume shifts. Renal failure patients additionally are at risk for systemic hypertensive and hypotensive complications including hemorrhage, myocardial infarction, and stroke.

Initial assessment of renal function with an understanding of source of disease, trends in function, and treatments required are necessary in the parturient. The degree of renal dysfunction is critical to both assessment and fluid management in the perioperative period. Patients with chronic renal dysfunction in the absence of renal failure require generous hydration and sufficient renal perfusion to avoid the potential complications associated with end stage renal disease. Those already in renal failure, however, require careful hydration to avoid volume overload as well as regular assessments of electrolyte disturbances that may be present in renal failure.

Hepatic Disease

Hepatic disease in the parturient is largely dependent on either the degree of inflammation in the acute phase or the degree of fibrosis in chronic disease. Because of their commonly young age relative to surgical patients, most pregnant patients with a history of liver disease have not had long-standing disease. The liver is responsible for many homeostatic functions including toxin removal, drug metabolism, protein and cholesterol production, and glucose storage. Liver dysfunction therefore can result in accumulation of toxins resulting in altered mental status, prolonged effects of medications, malnutrition, and coagulopathy.

Evaluation of patients with known or suspected liver disease includes laboratory analysis of liver enzymes for degree of acute inflammation. ALT (alanine transaminase) and AST (aspartate transaminase) may be elevated due to cell lysis during acute liver inflammation or damage. Causes of acute liver inflammation in parturients are similar to those in the general population and include infections such as viral hepatitis or systemic sepsis, medications including acetaminophen and cholesterol medications, excessive alcohol consumption, and autoimmune disorders. Pregnant patients additionally may have acute hepatitis due to severe preeclampsia, intrahepatic cholestasis of pregnancy, or acute fatty liver of pregnancy.[1] Acute liver inflammation in the setting of abdominal surgery such as cesarean delivery is particularly high risk depending on the degree of inflammation present and can result in fulminant liver failure.

Patients with long-standing hepatic disease may undergo fibrosis and cirrhosis of the liver resulting in portal hypertension, hypocoagulation, and altered protein binding. Physical exam findings in cirrhotic patients may show elevated jugular venous distension, bruising, and signs of malnutrition. Laboratory analysis in patients suspected of having cirrhosis includes PT (Prothrombin Time), PTT (Partial Prothrombin Time), platelet counts, and albumin levels. Such patients may have contraindications to neuraxial anesthesia or may have exaggerated responses to drugs that bind to albumin or are metabolized by the liver, warranting careful titration of medications.

Neurologic Disease

Parturients may suffer from a variety of neurological disorders, including those that are pregnancy related as well as chronic conditions. Pregnancy-associated neurological disorders include eclampsia, reversible posterior leukoencephalopathy syndrome (RPLS), and stroke. Chronic conditions including epilepsy, neuropathies such as compression peripheral neuropathy and multiple sclerosis, cerebral aneurysms, myasthenia gravis, and brain tumors are also seen in parturients.

Blood pressure increases associated with preeclampsia may result in progression to eclampsia and seizures, leading to maternal or fetal morbidity. Pregnancy-associated RPLS can cause seizures, altered mental status, and visual disturbances. In this disorder, breakdown in normally autoregulated cerebral blood flow results in cerebral endothelial damage and vasogenic edema.

The presence of an intracranial tumor in a pregnant patient can significantly alter the delivery plan for the obstetrician and anesthesiologist. Parturients with a diagnosis of an intracranial tumor should be evaluated for any signs or symptoms of increased intracranial pressure (ICP) including headaches, nausea, vomiting, or seizures. Focal neurologic deficits should also be assessed and documented. Recent intracranial imaging should be obtained to evaluate the size and location of the tumor. The delivery plan may need to consider avoidance of any additional increases in ICP by either using a passive second stage or a cesarean delivery.

Stroke in a parturient can be devastating. Ischemic stroke is the most frequent type during pregnancy and is commonly due to preeclampsia. Less common etiologies of pregnancy-related ischemic stroke include amniotic fluid embolism and choriocarcinoma. Hemorrhagic stroke in pregnancy may occur due to vasculopathies, severe preeclampsia, or aneurysm rupture. A multitude of manifestations may occur including headache, focal neurological deficits, and altered consciousness. Parturients with neurological symptoms suggestive of possible stroke require emergent multidisciplinary care from obstetricians, anesthesiologists, neurologists, interventional radiologists, and neurosurgeons, preferably at a comprehensive care center proficient in both obstetrical and stroke care.

Hydrocephalus in parturients is typically due to conditions present prior to pregnancy. These women will commonly have shunts in place to correct the hydrocephalus. Parturients with a history of hydrocephalus should be questioned about headaches, visual changes, nausea, and other symptoms of increased ICP (see Table 6.1). If any of these symptoms are present, the need for neurosurgical consultation or radiologic studies should be considered.

Peripheral neuropathy in obstetrical patients, as in the general population, is a common condition and may be exacerbated late in pregnancy due to fetal or uterine nerve compression, weight gain, and peripheral edema (see Table 6.1). Multiple sclerosis (MS) may be exacerbated in parturients by a multitude of factors including hormonal changes, temperature alterations, or pain. Fetal and obstetrical complications such as spontaneous abortions, congenital malformations, and premature delivery have not been found to be increased in patients with MS. Cesarean delivery rates likewise may be increased in patients with MS.[2]

Myasthenia gravis is fortunately a rare disease in the general population as well as in parturients. Antibodies are formed which attach to the nicotinic acetylcholine receptor, resulting in muscle fatigue and weakness. Patients are treated with anticholinesterases and immunosuppressants to augment acetylcholine availability at the neuromuscular junction. Depletion or inadequate therapy puts parturients at increased risk for cesarean section[3] Management of patients with myasthenia gravis includes monitoring for myasthenic crisis and careful titration or avoidance of neuromuscular blockade.

Hematologic Disorders

A variety of hematological disorders can be manifest or exacerbated in the parturient. Conditions of hypocoagulation as well as thrombophylic disorders are commonly altered in the pregnant patient. Patients with sickle cell disease or sickle cell heterozygous traits may suffer from vaso-occlusive episodes during pregnancy resulting in maternal or fetal ischemia and resulting complications.

Expected hematological changes of pregnancy include an increase in erythropoietin in the setting of increased aldosterone, which results in a dilutional anemia. Normally, this physiological change may reduce the incidence of vaso-occlusion in patients at risk such as those with sickle cell disease or trait. Labor, however, may cause increased oxygen consumption or dehydration which can result in maternal vaso-occlusive crisis, end organ dysfunction, and placental ischemia. Severe muscle pain, stroke, renal failure, and hypoxemia in the mother can be life threatening. Placental ischemia can cause fetal distress and death in utero. Laboring patients with known sickle cell disease or heterozygous sickle cell traits therefore require careful monitoring for vaso-occlusion including pulse oximetry, fetal heart rate monitoring, and regular clinical assessments. Patients require pain control, sufficient hydration, and supplemental oxygen administration when vaso-occlusion is suspected or expected.

Pregnancy initiates increases in platelet production, aggregation, activation and consumption.[4–6] Clotting factors are typically increased during pregnancy. Preexisting or previously undiagnosed thrombophylic disorders such as antiphospholipid antibody syndrome, protein C or S deficiencies, or Factor V Leiden syndrome may manifest in parturients. Acute deep vein thrombosis (DVT) may result in severe leg cramping or embolism to the pulmonary vasculature resulting in hypoxemia from pulmonary embolism (PE). Cerebral or coronary artery thrombosis can result in ischemic stroke or cardiac arrest. Hypercoagulable parturients alternatively may be on anticoagulants or antiplatelet medications prior to delivery and therefore require consideration for bleeding from neuraxial anesthetics or cesarean section.

Patients with quantitative or qualitative platelet dysfunction such as Von Willebrand's disease typically improve their ability to function due to the physiological changes of pregnancy. Peripartum bleeding, however, may require administration of Von Willebrand's Factor (VWF), Desmopressin (DDAVP), Factor VIII, or tranexamic acid (TXA) depending on the type and severity of the deficient factors. Patients with either hypo- or hypercoagulopathies should be seen as often as needed by obstetricians and hematologists throughout the peripartum period (see Table 6.1).

Substance Abuse Disorders

In-utero exposure to smoking or alcohol has for decades been known to result in increases in fetal morbidity. The Surgeon General's reports since the 1960s have advised against smoking in parturients. The earliest reports included warnings on increased incidences of preterm birth and low birth weight. Additional evidence over the past 50 years has found that stillbirth, neonatal death, gastroschisis, and congenital heart defects may be increased due to maternal smoking.[7] Acutely the parturient who uses tobacco should be assessed for comorbidities associated with smoking common in all perioperative patients, including reactive airway disease, hypertension, and cardiovascular disease.

Maternal use of alcohol, as with tobacco, is known to increase the rate of birth defects and is most commonly associated with fetal alcohol syndrome. Physical defects, behavioral and cognitive dysfunction, and psychiatric disorders may manifest in children who suffer from fetal alcohol syndrome. Parturients with chronic alcohol exposure should be assessed for co-morbidities, including cardiovascular disease such as hypertension and cardiomyopathy. Excessive alcohol can result in acute hepatitis or cirrhosis, necessitating the need for laboratory analysis with emphasis on liver enzymes, protein and platelet counts, and evaluation for coagulopathy in the peripartum period. In the setting of acute alcohol intoxication, concerns for enhanced response to IV or general anesthetics are warranted. Patients with chronic alcohol abuse require monitoring for withdrawal, which can result in seizures and fetal compromise, necessitating emergent maternofetal intervention.

The drug epidemic in the United States has affected every patient population over the past decades, including parturients. Most recently, the opiate addiction that has exploded in frequency has been a public health crisis and has resulted in multiple maternal co-morbidities. Bacterial infections from contaminated intravenous injections of heroin, fentanyl, or pain pills may result in parturients with abscesses, valvular heart disease, and septic emboli, resulting in debilitating stroke or respiratory failure.

Many opiate-using pregnant patients are treated with opiate agonist-antagonist medications during pregnancy. Patients with a history of drug abuse that present for delivery may have difficult venous access, pose infectious risk to health care providers, and have labor or cesarean section pain that is difficult to control. Such patients should be extensively counseled on their risks of complications of anesthesia and delivery. Assessment for co-morbidities, obtaining IV access, and managing pain are vital to the successful care of such challenging patients. Opiate-using patients, like patients with chronic alcohol use, may have altered anesthetic requirements depending on whether they are acutely exposed to self-administered substances or are in withdrawal.

Psychiatric Disease

Psychiatric disease is prevalent in the general population and may present in the peripartum period. Depression and anxiety disorders affect up to 10% of the population and are more common in women than in men.[8] Bipolar disorder, schizophrenia, and eating disorders carry incidences of at least 1%. Changing levels of estrogen and progesterone, combined with the added challenges of caring for a new baby put women at their greatest risk of decompensation and result in psychiatric hospitalization.[9]

Pregnant patients should be assessed for proper treatment of psychiatric disease including a medication review that may include antidepressants, antipsychotics, or sedatives. Patients with eating disorders may have electrolyte disturbances that can impact their physical health and response to anesthetics and therefore require laboratory analysis of sodium, calcium, potassium and albumin.

Endocrine Disorders

Multiple hormones are increased during pregnancy including progesterone, estrogen, cortisol, human placental growth hormone, and human placental lactogen. Glucose elevation is met with increases in insulin secretion to maintain normal levels in the parturient. Fetal, uterine, and excessive tissue growth in the parturient, however, may result in insulin resistance and the development of gestational diabetes. Patients with previously diagnosed and well-managed diabetes may have increases in blood sugar that require increasing amounts of exogenous insulin.

Diabetic patients require a review of medications and an assessment for the degree of blood sugar control. Patients with poorly controlled diabetes are at increased risk of cesarean section due to both a higher incidence of induced labor and fetal macrosomia. Diabetic neuropathies may be present in patients and result in autonomic dysfunction. Slowed gastric emptying time should be expected in such patients. While neuraxial anesthetics are not contraindicated in patients with somatic neuropathies, parturients with such conditions should be examined and any motor or sensory deficits should be documented in the medical record.

Obstetrical History

Anesthesia providers should carefully review previous pregnancies including the number of previous deliveries. Prior anesthetics including regional or general administered to patients may assist in needle placement, expected response to spinal or epidural doses, or difficulties encountered in general anesthesia (see Box 6.2).

Previous obstetrical complications including fetal or maternal distress may indicate the need for early epidural placement. Peripartum hemorrhage in previous deliveries may recur, depending on the cause. Sources of peripartum bleeding from cervicitis or vasa previa that do not typically result in large blood loss may not require changes in management in future pregnancies. Uterine atony, placental accrete, placental previa, and uterine rupture, however,

---

Box 6.2 General Evaluation of the Parturient

- **Obstetrical History**
  - birth history—gravida/para, fetal presentation, twin pregnancy, pre-eclampsia, gestational DM, previous abruption, previous cesarean, placental accrete, cord prolapse, etc.
  - previous anesthetics—GA vs. epidural vs. spinal; any issues with placement?
- **General Medical History**
  - cardiovascular—hypertension, pulmonary hypertension, congenital heart disease (repaired or not)
  - pulmonary—asthma, COPD, smoking history
  - renal—CKD, ESRD, renal stones
  - gastrointestinal—hepatitis, cirrhosis, gallbladder disease
  - endocrine—diabetes, thyroid disease,
  - hematologic—anemia, sickle cell disease, Factor V leiden, antiphospholipid syndrome, use of anticoagulants, cancer diagnosis
  - neurologic—history of intracranial lesion, peripheral neuropathy, seizure history
  - psychiatric—eating disorders, depression, drug and alcohol use/abuse
  - allergies
- **Physical Exam**
  - airway—Mallampati, mylohyoid distance, dentition, cervical ROM, etc.
  - vital signs
  - IV access

are more likely to recur in subsequent pregnancies, and such histories necessitate sufficient IV access and blood product preparation.

History of Current Pregnancy

In addition to a review of the patient's past medical and obstetrical history, an assessment of current fetal condition is helpful in planning for optimal care during delivery. A review of recent ultrasound reports may indicate fetal position and size. Placental size and position may be pertinent for mode of delivery and be reported on ultrasound records. The labor nurse or obstetrician caring for the patient can summarize fetal status including heart rate and tolerance of labor, if present. Previous hospitalizations for nausea, bleeding, or fetal monitoring should be discussed in order to identify potential complications during delivery.

Finally, a review of recent obstetrical notes or discussion with the obstetrician is helpful to identify particular concerns with delivery of which the patient may not be aware.

References

1. Wakim-Fleming J. Liver disease in pregnancy. Cleveland Clinic Center for Continuing Education Web site. August 2010. http://www.clevelandclinicmeded.com/medicalpubs/diseasemanagement/hepatology/liver-disease-in-pregnancy

2. Armon C, Berman, SA. Neurologic disease and pregnancy. *Medscape.* November 2018. https://emedicine.medscape.com/article/1149405-overview

3. Shehata HA, Okosun H. Neurological disorders in pregnancy. *Curr Opin Obstet Gynecol.* 2004;16(2):117–122.

4. Gerbasi FR, Buttoms S, Farag A, Mammen E. Increased intravascular coagulation associated with pregnancy. *Obstet Gynecol.* 1990;75:385–389.

5. Tygart SG, McRoyan DK, Spinnato JA, et al. Longitudinal study of platelet indices during normal pregnancy. *Am J Obstet Gynecol.* 1986;154:833–837.

6. Fay RA, Hughes AO, Farron NT. Platelets in pregnancy: hyperdestruction in pregnancy. *Obstet Gynecol.* 1983;61:238–240.

7. National Center for Chronic Disease Prevention and Health Promotion (US) Office on Smoking and Health. The health consequences of smoking-50 years of progress: a report of the Surgeon General. Atlanta, GA: Centers for Disease Control and Prevention; 2014.

8. Waraich P, Goldner EM, Somers, JIM, et al. Prevalence and incidence studies of mood disorders: a systematic review of the literature. *Can J of Psychiatry.* 2004;49:124–138.

9. Cantwell R. (2016). Peripartum Psychiatric Disorders. In: Clark V, ed. *Oxford Textbook of Obstetric Anaesthesia.* Oxford University Press.

7

The High-Risk Obstetric Patient

Pregnancy-Induced Conditions

Jacqueline Curbelo

Gestational Diabetes Mellitus

Introduction

Gestational diabetes mellitus (GDM) is a hyperglycemic state in pregnancy secondary to insulin resistance, which was not existing prior to pregnancy.[1] The prevalence of GDM is 4.6–9.2%.[2] Risk factors include advanced maternal age, family history of diabetes mellitus (DM), history of GDM with previous pregnancies, obesity, and race (increased prevalence in Asian, Native American, and Hispanic).[3-5]

In the nonpregnant, nondiabetic state, an abundance of serum glucose triggers the pancreatic beta cells to release insulin, which then triggers peripheral tissues to uptake glucose, as illustrated in Figure 7.1. Normal pregnancy is associated with progressive insulin resistance, which enables shunting of nutrients across the placenta to a growing fetus. GDM is thought to develop when an individual's subclinical, pre-existing insulin resistance is then compounded with further insulin resistance associated with pregnancy.[1,6-8]

Diagnosis

The US Preventive Services Task Force recommends screening all pregnant women for GDM between 24–28 weeks of gestation.[9] The most widely accepted screening method for GDM is a nonfasting 50-gram oral glucose load test. The screen test is positive if plasma glucose levels are at or above 130 mg/dL one hour after the glucose load. GDM is subsequently diagnosed using a fasting 100-gram oral glucose tolerance test. The diagnosis is confirmed if at least two plasma glucose readings are elevated according to either the Carpenter-Coustan or National Diabetes Data Group criteria, which are shown in Table 7.1.[10-12]

The International Association of Diabetes and Pregnancy Study Group (IADPSG) recommended a one-step diagnostic test for GDM in 2010, which involved a fasting, 2-hour 75-gram oral glucose tolerance test.[13] However, there is insufficient evidence to support this approach, higher associated healthcare cost, and no clear maternal or neonatal benefit. Further studies are needed to determine a definite optimal screening strategy.[10,14-16] Therefore, the American College of Obstetricians and Gynecologists supports the 2-step approach utilizing the nonfasting 50-gram oral load screening followed by a confirmatory fasting 100-gram oral glucose tolerance test for diagnosis.[17]

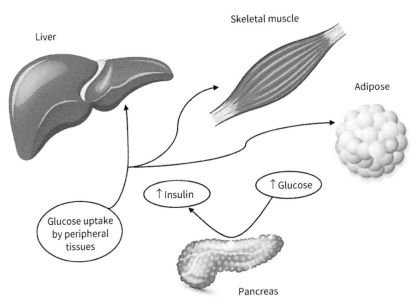

Figure 7.1 Normal physiologic response to a glucose load: abundant serum glucose triggers pancreatic release of insulin, which stimulates glucose uptake by peripheral tissues.

Management

Once GDM is diagnosed, the first-line recommendation for management is lifestyle modification, including diet and exercise recommendations.[18–21] Adequate treatment of hyperglycemia significantly reduces serious newborn complications and decreases rates of developing maternal preeclampsia.[22-24] Glycemic targets recommended by the American Diabetes Association include fasting blood glucose less than 95 mg/dL, and postprandial blood glucose less than 140 mg/dL after 1 hour and less than 120 mg/dL after 2 hours.[25] If diet and exercise inadequately controls blood glucose to target levels, then insulin therapy is

Table 7.1 Diagnostic Criteria for Gestational Diabetes Mellitus

Plasma glucose sample	Carpenter-Coustan	National Diabetes Data Group
Fasting	95 mg/dL (5.3 mmol/L)	105 mg/dL (5.8 mmol/L)
1 hour	180 mg/dL (10 mmol/L)	190 mg/dL (10.6 mmol/L)
2 hours	155 mg/dL (8.6 mmol/L)	165 mg/dL (9.2 mmol/L)
3 hours	140 mg/dL (7.8 mmol/L)	145 mg/dL (8.1 mmol/L)

Carpenter MW, Coustan DR. Criteria for screening tests for gestational diabetes. *Am J Obstet Gynecol.* 1982;144(7):769, Table II.[11]

National Diabetes Data Group. Classification and diagnosis of diabetes mellitus and other categories of glucose intolerance. *Diabetes.* 1979;28(12):1050, Table 5.[12]

recommended.[25] In spite of limited data on efficacy and safety, oral antidiabetic medications are being used increasingly in GDM when diet and exercise regimens fail.[26-31]

Maternal Complications

GDM typically resolves after pregnancy, but women who develop GDM are at increased risk of developing GDM in subsequent pregnancies (35–70%) and are at elevated risk of developing DM later in life (15–70%), particularly type 2 DM.[1,32-36] Women with pregnancies complicated by GDM should therefore be assessed for hyperglycemia in the postpartum period.[37]

Although diabetic ketoacidosis (DKA) is predominantly associated with pregestational DM, particularly type 1 DM, it can also complicate GDM.[38] Risk factors for DKA include emesis, infection, inadequate treatment/noncompliance, use of beta-adrenergic receptor agonists in preterm labor, and use of corticosteroids for fetal lung maturity.[38] Parturients with GDM are also at risk of developing gestational hypertension, preeclampsia, and polyhydramnios, and they have higher rates of cesarean delivery.[17,39-41] When a trial of labor after cesarean (TOLAC) is attempted, women with GDM have increased rates of operative delivery and repeat cesarean delivery.[42]

Fetal Complications

Fetal risks associated with GDM include fetal macrosomia and increased risk of shoulder dystocia and birth trauma with vaginal delivery.[43,44] Risk of major congenital anomalies is elevated, as well as intrauterine fetal demise (IUFD) and perinatal mortality.[45,46] Neonatal hypoglycemia is elevated to 5–7%, and results from fetal hyperinsulinemia secondary to chronic hyperglycemia in utero.[22,23,47] Neonatal hyperbilirubinemia is also associated with GDM.[48]

Obstetric Management

Obstetric management, and timing and mode of delivery, are determined in part by the degree of glycemic control. Due to an increased risk of antepartum fetal demise, the American College of Obstetricians and Gynecologists recommends antenatal fetal assessment for women with poorly controlled or medically controlled GDM beginning at 32 weeks of gestation or earlier if other risk factors for adverse outcome are present.[49] Women with abnormal antenatal testing may be considered for delivery, particularly if a strong likelihood of fetal lung maturity exists. With reassuring antenatal testing and good glycemic control, delivery is recommended between 39 to 39 6/7 weeks of gestation. If GDM is poorly controlled, then late-preterm or early-term delivery should be considered to avoid IUFD.[50,51]

There is no consensus regarding the necessity of antenatal surveillance for well-controlled GDM without medical management.[49] Generally, these patients can be managed expectantly up to 40 6/7 weeks of gestation, unless otherwise indicated. In general, vaginal delivery is recommended. However, the risks and benefits of cesarean delivery versus vaginal delivery should be considered in suspected fetal macrosomia and potential for birth trauma.[52]

Anesthetic Management

Anesthetic management of labor and delivery of the parturient with gestational diabetes is inadequately described in the literature, and recommendations are extended from those for nonpregnant diabetic patients or parturients with pregestational diabetes. In general, neuraxial analgesia is recommended for laboring women with DM, and may improve placental perfusion by reducing circulating catecholamines.[53] Additional benefits of neuraxial analgesia include reduced fetal acidosis, more effective and less depressive analgesia compared to systemic analgesia, and a useful means for providing emergency anesthesia when conversion to cesarean delivery is necessary.[54]

Parturients with gestational diabetes have an elevated risk for cesarean delivery, even in the absence of fetal macrosomia.[55] It is well known that normal physiologic changes of pregnancy place the parturient at high risk for aspiration, and diabetic parturients may have additional risk in the presence of gastroparesis and autonomic neuropathy. Aspiration prophylaxis should be administered prior to cesarean delivery, to include nonparticulate antacid, as well as consideration of histamine-2-receptor antagonist and metoclopramide.[54] Neuraxial anesthesia for cesarean delivery allows maintenance of the parturient's protective airway reflexes.[56] Epidural anesthesia may allow for slow titration of anesthesia compared to spinal anesthesia, and potentially less hemodynamic instability secondary to autonomic neuropathy associated with diabetes.[54] Vasopressors and crystalloids for volume expansion should be readily available to support maternal blood pressure and uteroplacental perfusion after neuraxial anesthesia.

When cesarean delivery is to proceed under general anesthesia, then the airway should be protected utilizing a rapid-sequence induction with cricoid pressure and intubation of the trachea.[56] Stiff joint syndrome associated with diabetes may affect the atlanto-occipital joint, making endotracheal intubation difficult.[54] Additional airway concerns such as high mallampati score or airway edema may contribute to potential difficult endotracheal intubation if obesity or preeclampsia are comorbid findings. Diabetic patients may have an exaggerated sympathetic response to laryngoscopy.[57]

Hypertensive Disorders of Pregnancy

Introduction

Hypertensive disorders of pregnancy are responsible for 13% of maternal deaths in developed countries.[58] In the United States, although the rate of pregnancy-related deaths has not significantly decreased in over 25 years, the cause of death related to hypertensive disorders of pregnancy has continued to decline from 17.6% in 1987–1990 to most recently 7.4% from 2011–2013.[59] Pregnancy-related mortality due to hypertensive disorders of pregnancy is illustrated in Figure 7.2. It remains a significant source of maternal and fetal morbidity and mortality.

The conventional threshold for hypertension in pregnancy is set at systolic blood pressure at or above 140 mm Hg or diastolic blood pressure at or above 90 mm Hg.[60] Hypertensive disorders of pregnancy are classified into the following four categories: (1)

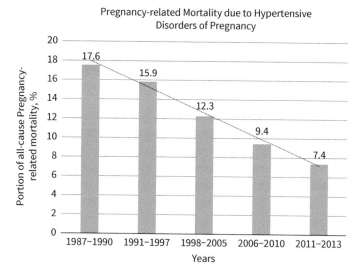

Figure 7.2 Maternal mortality due to hypertensive disorders of pregnancy.

Creanga AA, Syverson C, Seed K, Callaghan WM. Pregnancy-related mortality in the United States, 2011–2013. *Obstet Gynecol.* 2017;130(2): 366–373.

preeclampsia-eclampsia, (2) chronic hypertension, (3) chronic hypertension with superimposed preeclampsia, and (4) gestational hypertension.[61]

Gestational Hypertension

Gestational hypertension (GHTN) is defined as an elevated systolic blood pressure at or above 140 mm Hg or diastolic blood pressure at or above 90 mm Hg, occurring after 20 weeks of gestation, which resolves within 12 weeks postpartum.[62,63] It is not associated with proteinuria. It affects 5% of pregnancies, and 25–50% of parturients diagnosed with GHTN will develop preeclampsia.[64–68] When blood pressures elevate to severe range (systolic blood pressure $\geq$ 160 mm Hg or diastolic blood pressure $\geq$ 110 mm Hg), then management should proceed as that for preeclampsia with severe features.[69]

Preeclampsia

Preeclampsia presents as elevated systolic blood pressure at or above 140 mm Hg or diastolic blood pressure at or above 90 mm Hg, occurring after 20 weeks' gestation, but also with development of proteinuria or other end-organ findings.[61] The multisystemic involvement associated with preeclampsia distinguishes it from GHTN, and 3% to 4% of all pregnancies are affected.[65] Risk factors associated with the development of preeclampsia include the following: history of preeclampsia in a previous pregnancy; chronic medical conditions such as chronic hypertension, kidney disease, or pregestational DM; antiphospholipid antibody syndrome; and multiple pregnancy.[70]

Preeclampsia is associated with significant morbidity and mortality for both the mother and fetus. Maternal complications include progression to eclampsia, stroke, pulmonary edema, kidney failure, liver rupture or failure, and placental abruption. Fetal complications include intrauterine growth restriction, fetal demise, and preterm delivery and associated morbidities of prematurity.[71]

Diagnosis

Historically, a diagnosis of preeclampsia was established when hypertension developed after 20 weeks of gestation in the presence of proteinuria. However, concern arose regarding the accuracy of measuring proteinuria and minimizing the importance of other clinical and laboratory finding associated with preeclampsia in the absence of proteinuria.[72] Therefore, the International Society for the Study of Hypertension in Pregnancy introduced revisions to the diagnostic criteria in 2014 with the intent to reduce maternal and fetal adverse events and improve pregnancy outcome.[70] For hypertension with absent proteinuria, the diagnosis of preeclampsia can be made if there is evidence of thrombocytopenia, kidney dysfunction, liver dysfunction, pulmonary edema, or cerebral or visual disturbances. Diagnostic criteria as outlined by the American College of Obstetricians and Gynecologists (ACOG) are summarized in Table 7.2.[61]

Severe Features

The presence or development of more severe disease hastens the delivery process. Such ominous manifestations are labeled "severe features" and are illustrated in Figure 7.3. These findings include severe hypertension resistant to antihypertensives, worsening thrombocytopenia, evidence of liver dysfunction, worsening kidney function, pulmonary edema, and cerebral or visual changes. Severe features of preeclampsia as outlined by the ACOG are summarized in Box 7.1.[61]

Table 7.2 Diagnostic Criteria for Preeclampsia

Blood Pressure	SBP ≥ 140 mm Hg or DBP ≥ 90 mm Hg	
Proteinuria Status	A. Present	B. Absent
	1. ≥ 300 mg in 24-hour urine collection	1. Platelets < 100,000/mcL
	2. Spot protein/creatinine ≥ 0.3 (measured in mg/dL)	2. Serum creatinine > 1.1 mg/dL or doubling of creatinine in absence of kidney disease
	3. Dipstick 1+ protein if quantitative measurement capability unavailable	3. Elevated liver enzymes above twice normal
		4. Pulmonary edema
		5. Cerebral or visual symptoms

Preeclampsia is diagnosed when at least one criterion from column A or B exists in the presence of hypertension.

SBP = systolic blood pressure; DBP = diastolic blood pressure

American College of Obstetricians and Gynecologists. Hypertension in pregnancy: Report of the American College of Obstetricians and Gynecologists' Task Force on Hypertension in Pregnancy. *Obstet Gynecol.* 2013;122(5):1125, Table E-1.

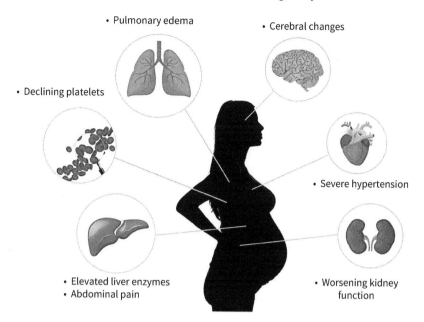

- Pulmonary edema
- Cerebral changes
- Declining platelets
- Severe hypertension
- Elevated liver enzymes
- Abdominal pain
- Worsening kidney function

Figure 7.3 Severe features of preeclampsia are manifestations of the systemic effects of the disease, including severe hypertension, declining platelets, elevated liver enzymes and abdominal pain, worsening kidney function, pulmonary edema, and cerebral changes.

Syndrome of Hemolysis, Elevated Liver Enzymes, and Low Platelets

The syndrome of hemolysis, elevated liver enzymes, and low platelets (HELLP) is thought to be a severe manifestation of preeclampsia, and is associated with increased morbidity and mortality.[73] The diagnostic criteria as outlined by the ACOG are listed in Box 7.2.[69]

Box 7.1 Severe Features of Preeclampsia

- SBP ≥ 160 mm Hg
- DBP ≥ 110 mm Hg
- Platelets < 100,000/μL
- Elevated liver enzymes above twice normal and/or RUQ or epigastric pain not relieved by medication
- Serum creatinine > 1.1 mg/dL or twice the baseline value in the absence of kidney disease
- Pulmonary edema
- New cerebral or visual changes

SBP = systolic blood pressure; DBP = diastolic blood pressure; RUQ = right upper quadrant

American College of Obstetricians and Gynecologists. Hypertension in pregnancy: Report of the American College of Obstetricians and Gynecologists' Task Force on Hypertension in Pregnancy. *Obstet Gynecol.* 2013;122(5):1124, Box E-1.[61]

Box 7.2 HELLP Syndrome Diagnostic Criteria

- LDH ≥ 600 IU/L
- AST and ALT above twice normal
- Platelets < 100,000/μL

HELLP = hemolysis, elevated liver enzymes, low platelets; LDH = lactate dehydrogenase; AST = aspartate aminotransferase; ALT = alanine aminotransferase

ACOG Practice Bulletin No. 202: Gestational Hypertension and Preeclampsia. *Obstet Gynecol.* 2019; 133(1): e3.[69]

Eclampsia

Eclampsia is the development of new-onset seizure activity during pregnancy, and is a severe manifestation of hypertensive disorders of pregnancy. It may occur during pregnancy or postpartum and lead to maternal hypoxia, aspiration pneumonia, stroke, and even death.[69,74] Administration of parenteral magnesium has been shown to reduce the incidence of eclampsia by about 50%.[75]

Obstetric Management of Hypertensive Disorders of Pregnancy

After an initial thorough evaluation, expectant management with continued observation is appropriate for women with GHTN and preeclampsia without severe features before 37 weeks of gestation. Frequent monitoring of blood pressure and for signs of severe features of preeclampsia is recommended, including ultrasonography of the fetus and laboratory testing. If maternal clinical condition progresses to preeclampsia with severe features, or if fetal testing becomes abnormal, then the decision to deliver or to continue with expectant management depends upon the availability of resources to monitor mother and fetus, maternal and fetal condition, and fetal gestational age. The decision to proceed with delivery requires balancing the risk of fetal prematurity with the maternal risk of complications from progressive disease. Additionally, expectant management of women with preeclampsia with severe features requires hospitalization and inpatient monitoring at a center with available maternal and neonatal intensive care. Mode of delivery may be by induction of labor with anticipated vaginal delivery, or by cesarean delivery, depending on routine obstetric considerations.[69]

Antihypertensive medications are recommended if blood pressure elevates to severe levels (systolic blood pressure of 160 mm Hg or higher, or diastolic blood pressure of 110 mm Hg or higher). Recommended agents include parenteral labetalol or hydralazine, or oral nifedipine for treatment of acute severe hypertension, which can then be transitioned to oral labetalol or calcium channel blockers for maintenance.[69]

Anesthetic Management of Hypertensive Disorders of Pregnancy

Anesthetic management of parturients with preeclampsia requires multidisciplinary coordination of care and careful preparation. Disease severity may rapidly progress without warning. A thorough history and physical examination should place particular emphasis on detection of signs and symptoms indicative of systemic involvement. All pertinent laboratory values should be reviewed and discussed with the obstetricians, including complete blood count, coagulation panel, liver function tests, and magnesium levels. These tests are typically ordered serially and require follow-up throughout labor, delivery, and postpartum.

Hypertension

The anesthesiologist may be consulted to help manage severe hypertension resistant to first-line antihypertensive therapy (parenteral labetalol and hydralazine, or oral nifedipine). The goal of reducing blood pressure to a range of 140–150/90–100 mm Hg is to avoid cerebral complications and heart failure.[76] Although invasive blood pressure monitoring is not universally recommended in preeclampsia, it can be considered for resistant severe hypertension, particularly if cesarean delivery is recommended or if general anesthesia is anticipated. It may have the additional benefit of allowing frequent blood draws for serial laboratory analysis.[77] Second-line antihypertensives include intravenous infusions of nicardipine or esmolol, or even sodium nitroprusside in extreme emergencies.[76] Maternal stabilization should be prioritized before proceeding for a planned cesarean.

Airway

Normal physiologic changes in pregnancy include laryngeal mucosal engorgement and edema. Airway edema may be particularly marked in parturients with preeclampsia, creating greater potential for difficult endotracheal intubation.[78-81] The American Society of Anesthesiologists Task Force on Obstetric Anesthesia and the Society for Obstetric Anesthesiology and Perinatology recommend to "consider early insertion of a neuraxial catheter for obstetric (e.g., twin gestation or preeclampsia) or anesthetic indications (e.g., anticipated difficult airway or obesity) to reduce the need for general anesthesia if an emergent procedure becomes necessary. In these cases, the insertion of a neuraxial catheter may precede the onset of labor or a patient's request for labor analgesia."[82] Furthermore, it is recommended that "labor and delivery units should have personnel and equipment readily available to manage airway emergencies consistent with the American Society of Anesthesiologists (ASA) Practice Guidelines for Management of the Difficult Airway."[83] Endotracheal tubes of varying size, especially smaller sizes, and supraglottic airways should be readily available.

Labor Analgesia for Vaginal Delivery

In the absence of contraindications, neuraxial analgesia is recommended as part of the management of preeclamptic patients in labor, as its effect of being the most complete mode of labor analgesia assists in blood pressure management. Additional benefits of neuraxial analgesia include the ability to utilize an epidural catheter for anesthesia to avoid potential complications of general anesthesia if the need for an emergency cesarean arises.

Coagulation status must be assessed prior to placement of neuraxial analgesia or anesthesia in the setting of preeclampsia. This includes assessment for thrombocytopenia and platelet count trend. It was found in a 2017 systematic review[84] that the risk of epidural hematoma was less than 0.2% for parturients with platelets counts from 70,000/mm³ to 100,000/mm³ in the absence of other coagulation abnormalities, but risk was poorly defined for platelet counts below 70,000/mm^3. The decision to proceed with neuraxial blockade in the setting of platelet counts below 70,000/mm^3 must be weighed against the risk of proceeding with general anesthesia. Additional coagulation studies, such as prothrombin time, partial thromboplastin time, and fibrinogen levels, may be helpful to assess coagulation status when platelet counts are below 100,000/mm^3, particularly for women with HELLP or concern for disseminated intravascular coagulation (DIC).[85]

Cesarean Delivery, Neuraxial Anesthesia, and General Anesthesia

Cesarean delivery in preeclamptic parturients should proceed with neuraxial anesthesia, if possible. Aspiration prophylaxis should be administered prior to cesarean delivery, to include nonparticulate antacid, as well as consideration of histamine-2-receptor antagonist and metoclopramide.[54] Vasopressors and crystalloids for volume expansion should be readily available to support maternal blood pressure and uteroplacental perfusion after neuraxial anesthesia, but the incidence of spinal hypotension is less in preeclampsia compared to healthy parturients.[86,87] When spinal anesthesia was compared to epidural anesthesia for preeclamptic patients undergoing cesarean delivery, there was found to be a higher incidence of hypotension after spinal anesthesia, but hypotension was quickly treated with small doses of vasopressors in all groups without adverse outcomes.[88]

Although crystalloid should be used for volume expansion after neuraxial anesthesia, fluid restriction is recommended. It has been found that the endothelial glycocalyx is disrupted during fluid loading in preparation for neuraxial anesthesia in healthy parturients. There is concern that disrupted pulmonary endothelial glycocalyx could put preeclamptic parturients at further risk for pulmonary edema with vigorous crystalloid preloading or coloading.[89,90]

General anesthesia is reserved for emergent cesarean without an epidural in place, hemodynamic instability, altered mental status (eclampsia, increased intracranial pressure), pulmonary edema, or any contraindication to neuraxial anesthesia. If general anesthesia is required, then induction of anesthesia and endotracheal intubation should be approached with caution. Potential complications of general anesthesia associated with preeclampsia include difficult or failed endotracheal intubation, as well as exacerbated hypertensive response and stroke during intubation or emergence from general anesthesia.[91] Special considerations for general anesthesia in the parturient with preeclampsia are summarized in Figure 7.4. The airway should be reassessed for potential worsening of airway edema and recognition of potential difficult intubation. Fasting guidelines should be followed unless the urgency of the cesarean does not allow. All parturients should be given aspiration prophylaxis. Magnesium for seizure prophylaxis should continue to infuse in the operating room.[69,92] Invasive hemodynamic monitoring can be considered, particularly in the setting of severe hypertension.

After adequate preoxygenation, induction should proceed by rapid sequence, and agents should be chosen based on individual clinical condition and hemodynamic status. An exaggerated hypertensive response following laryngoscopy could lead to stroke and even death. Drugs such as remifentanil, esmolol, and nicardipine have been utilized on induction of general anesthesia in preeclampsia to maintain hemodynamic stability during rapid sequence induction and endotracheal intubation.[93] It is important to maintain hemodynamic stability throughout the anesthetic, including upon emergence. Antihypertensive drugs such as labetalol and hydralazine may be titrated prior to emergence to prevent severe hypertension.

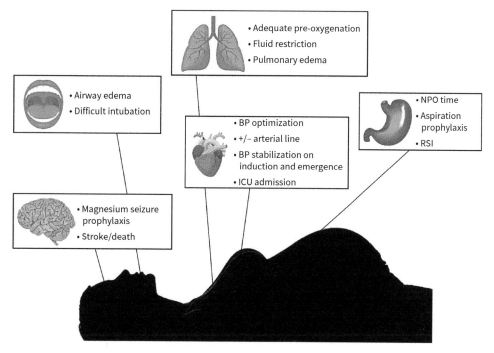

Figure 7.4 General anesthesia and preeclampsia: general anesthesia in the preeclamptic patient requires careful consideration of potential multisystemic manifestations of the disease to avoid serious adverse outcomes.

Volatile anesthetics used for anesthesia maintenance may contribute to uterine atony and postpartum hemorrhage. It has been suggested, however, that decreasing the volatile anesthetic concentration to 0.5 MAC of sevoflurane or 0.5–1 MAC of desflurane combined with oxytocin after delivery of the fetus will not increase the risk of uterine atony.[94] Additionally, nitrous oxide may be added to deepen the anesthetic.[95] If second-line uterotonics are used to help with uterine tone after delivery, methylergonovine should be avoided or used with caution due to the potential for exacerbated hypertension.[96] Magnesium potentiates the action of nondepolarizing neuromuscular blocking drugs.[97] Clinical deterioration or severe end-organ manifestations may require management in a critical care unit.

Intrauterine Fetal Demise

Introduction

Fetal demise, or stillbirth, is defined as fetal death at 20 weeks of gestation or later. The rate of fetal demise in the United States has remained relatively unchanged since 2006, and is illustrated in Figure 7.5. According to the latest National Vital Statistics Report on Fetal and Perinatal Mortality in the United States in 2013, the fetal mortality rate was 5.96 fetal deaths per 1,000 live births and fetal deaths.[98] Fetal mortality rates were highest in non-Hispanic

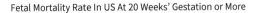

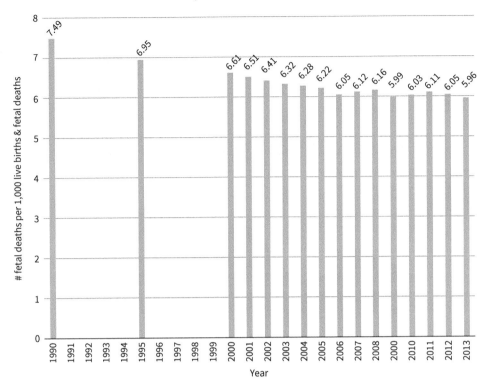

Figure 7.5   Fetal mortality rate in the United States at 20 weeks' gestation and more.
MacDorman MF, Gregory EC. Fetal and perinatal mortality: United States, 2013. *Natl Vital Stat Rep.* 2015;64(8):4, Table A.

black women, teenagers, women age 35 and older, unmarried women, and women with multiple pregnancies.[98] Risk factors for fetal demise include the following: advanced maternal age[99,100]; comorbidities such as hypertension,[71] diabetes,[101,102] or history of thromboembolism or thrombophilia[103,104]; obesity[105]; fetal growth restriction[106,107]; multiple gestation[108]; and previous pregnancy complications such as history of fetal demise, preterm delivery, fetal growth restriction, or preeclampsia.[109,110]

Causes of Fetal Demise

The cause of a fetal death is often difficult to identify, and is multifactorial in at least 25% of cases.[111] Figure 7.6 illustrates the most common causes of fetal demise. Between 14.3% and 47.4% of fetal deaths are unexplained.[112] Fetal demise may be associated with chromosomal or congenital abnormalities, infection, placental insufficiency, or cord events.[110] Genetic abnormalities have been associated with 6–12% of fetal deaths at 20 weeks' gestation or more.[113] Infection has been associated with 10–25% of fetal deaths in developed countries, and is more strongly associated with demise prior to 28 weeks' gestation.[114] Umbilical cord accidents were associated with 10% of stillbirths in a prospective, population-based,

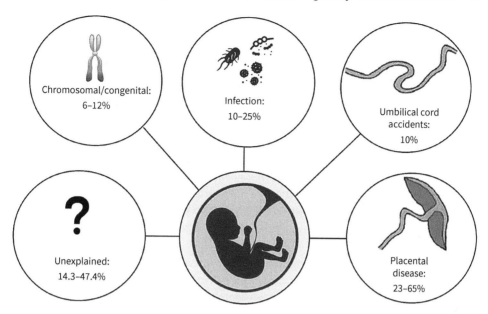

Figure 7.6 Cause of fetal demise: many times, fetal demise is multifactorial or unexplained. Specific causes of fetal demise include chromosomal or congenital abnormalities, infection, umbilical cord accidents, or placental disease.

case-control study by the Stillbirth Collaborative Research Network and are considered to be an important cause of fetal demise deserving further investigation.[115,116]

Placental disease has been associated with 23–65% of stillbirths.[115,117,118] Placental causes of fetal demise include abruption, infarction, hypoplasia, immaturity, and inflammatory.[118] Chronic fetal hypoxia may lead to heart failure by interrupting fetal heart development, as has been shown in mouse models, ultimately resulting in fetal death.[119] Placental abnormalities and other maternal factors such as smoking, illicit drug use, and anemia may cause prolonged fetal hypoxia.[119,120]

Obstetric Management

It is recommended that an investigation of potential causes of fetal demise be pursued, as it may provide closure for the family, reduce the risk for recurrence of fetal demise, and potentially direct management of subsequent pregnancies to minimize recurrence risk.[121] Delivery of the fetus is typically not urgent, and often both expectant management and induction of labor are offered to the parturient. Dilation and evacuation may be considered for early fetal demise. Early studies of fetal demise found that most women delivered within two weeks of fetal death, and 94% had delivered by five weeks. Spontaneous labor was experienced by 84% of the study group.[122]

Expectant management in the setting of fetal death carries risks of coagulopathy and infection. In early studies, hypofibrinogenemia was detected in 33% of parturients who had not delivered by 5 weeks and was associated with Rh incompatibility in Rh-negative mothers.[122] However, later studies indicated that hypofibrinogenemia and hemorrhage developed in Rh-positive mothers at 4 weeks from demise and even earlier.[123] Surveillance for coagu-lopathy and infection during expectant management should be considered, including weekly laboratory evaluation of coagulation status, although the usefulness has not been validated.

Anesthetic Management

In general, anesthetic management of the parturient with fetal demise is unchanged from standard care. It is important, however, to consider the potential for coagulopathy, particu-larly if the latency period between fetal demise and labor and delivery has been prolonged, or if associated with any other conditions that may further contribute to coagulopathy, such as placental abruption or preeclampsia. Initial evaluation for coagulopathy should focus on a subjective history of abnormal bleeding and objective findings, such as visible ecchymoses, or hematoma formation or bleeding from mucous membranes or venipuncture sites. Laboratory analysis may be considered, including platelet count, fibrinogen level, prothrombin time, and activated partial thromboplastin time. Serial measurements may prove more beneficial than any single measurement.[124] A decision regarding placement of neuraxial analgesia or anes-thesia requires clinical judgment and consideration of the potential risks and benefits.

Fetal demise is a risk factor for DIC, which should be promptly diagnosed and swiftly managed with supportive measures, blood product administration, and evacuation of the uterus to resolve the likely underlying cause of DIC.[124]

References

1. Buchanan TA, Xiang AH. Gestational diabetes mellitus. *J Clin Invest*. 2005;115 (3):485–491.
2. DeSisto CL, Kim SY, Sharma AJ. Prevalence estimates of gestational diabetes mellitus in the United States, Pregnancy Risk Assessment Monitoring System (PRAMS), 2007–2010. *Prev Chronic Dis*. 2014;11:E104.
3. Bouthoorn SH, Silva LM, Murray SE, et al. Low-educated women have an increased risk of ges-tational diabetes mellitus: the Generation R Study. *Acta Diabetol*. 2015;52(3):445–452.
4. Caughey AB, Cheng YW, Stotland NE, Washington AE, Escobar GJ. Maternal and pa-ternal race/ethnicity are both associated with gestational diabetes. *Am J Obstet Gynecol*. 2010;202(6):616.e1–5.
5. Berkowitz GS, Lapinski RH, Wein R, Lee D. Race/ethnicity and other risk factors for gesta-tional diabetes. *Am J Epidemiol*. 1992;135(9):965–973.
6. Crombach G, Siebolds M, and Mies R. Insulin use in pregnancy. Clinical pharmacokinetic considerations. *Clin Pharmacokinet*. 1993;24(2):89–100.
7. Barbour LA, McCurdy CE, Hernandez TL, Kirwan JP, Catalano PM, Friedman JE. Cellular mechanisms for insulin resistance in normal pregnancy and gestational diabetes. *Diabetes Care*. 2007;30 Suppl 2:S112–S119.
8. Lain KY, Catalano PM. Metabolic changes in pregnancy. *Clin Obstet Gynecol*. 2007;50(4): 938–948.
9. Moyer VA, U.S. Preventive Services Task Force. Screening for gestational diabetes mel-litus: U.S. Preventive Services Task Force recommendation statement. *Ann Intern Med*. 2014;160(6):414–420.

10. American Diabetes Association. 2. Classification and diagnosis of diabetes: standards of medical care in diabetes—2018. *Diabetes Care.* 2018;41(Suppl 1):S13–S27.

11. Carpenter MW, Coustan DR. Criteria for screening tests for gestational diabetes. *Am J Obstet Gynecol.* 1982;144(7):768–773.

12. National Diabetes Data Group. Classification and diagnosis of diabetes mellitus and other categories of glucose intolerance. *Diabetes.* 1979;28(12):1039–1057.

13. Metzger BE, Gabbe SG, Persson B, et al. International Association of Diabetes and Pregnancy Study Groups recommendations on the diagnosis and classification of hyperglycemia in pregnancy. International Association of Diabetes and Pregnancy Study Groups Consensus Panel. *Diabetes Care.* 2010;3;3(3):676–682.

14. Vandorsten JP, Dodson WC, Espeland MA, et al. NIH consensus development conference: diagnosing gestational diabetes mellitus. *NIH Consens State Sci Statements.* 2013;29(1):1–31.

15. Meltzer S, Snyder J, Penrod J, Nudi M, Morin L. Gestational diabetes mellitus screening and diagnosis: a prospective randomized controlled trial comparing costs of one-step and two-step methods. *BJOG.* 2010;117(4):407–415.

16. Farrar D, Duley L, Dowswell T, Lawlor DA. Different strategies for diagnosing gestational diabetes to improve maternal and infant health. *Cochrane Database Syst Rev.* 2017;8:CD007122.

17. Committee on Practice Bulletins—Obstetrics. ACOG Practice Bulletin No. 190: Gestational diabetes mellitus. *Obstet Gynecol.* 2018;131(2):e49–e64.

18. Han S, Middleton P, Shepherd E, Van Ryswyk E, Crowther CA. Different types of dietary advice for women with gestational diabetes mellitus. *Cochrane Database Syst Rev.* 2017;2:CD009275.

19. Moses RG, Barker M, Winter M, Petocz P, Brand-Miller JC. Can a low-glycemic index diet reduce the need for insulin in gestational diabetes mellitus? A randomized trial. *Diabetes Care.* 2009;32(6):996–1000.

20. Louie JC, Markovic TP, Perera N, et al. A randomized controlled trial investigating the effects of a low-glycemic index diet on pregnancy outcomes in gestational diabetes mellitus. *Diabetes Care.* 2011;34(11):2341–2346.

21. Barakat R, Pelaez M, Lopez C, Lucia A, Ruiz JR. Exercise during pregnancy and gestational diabetes-related adverse effects: a randomized controlled trial. *Br J Sports Med.* 2013;47(10):630–636.

22. Crowther CA, Hiller JE, Moss JR, McPhee AJ, Jeffries WS, Robinson JS. Effect of treatment of gestational diabetes mellitus on pregnancy outcomes. Australian Carbohydrate Intolerance Study in Pregnant Women (ACHOIS) Trial Group. *N Engl J Med.* 2005;352(24):2477–2486.

23. Landon MB, Spong CY, Thom E, et al. A multicenter, randomized trial of treatment for mild gestational diabetes. Eunice Kennedy Shriver National Institute of Child Health and Human Development Maternal-Fetal Medicine Units Network. *N Engl J Med.* 2009;361(14):1339–1348.

24. Hartling L, Dryden DM, Guthrie A, Muise M, Vandermeer B, Donovan L. Benefits and harms of treating gestational diabetes mellitus: a systematic review and meta-analysis for the U.S. Preventive Services Task Force and the National Institutes of Health Office of Medical Applications of Research. *Ann Intern Med.* 2013;159(2):123–129.

25. American Diabetes Association. 13. Management of diabetes in pregnancy: standards of medical care in diabetes—2018. *Diabetes Care.* 2018;41(Suppl 1):S137–S143.

26. Poolsup N, Suksomboon N, Amin M. Efficacy and safety of oral antidiabetic drugs in comparison to insulin in treating gestational diabetes mellitus: a meta-analysis. *PLoS One.* 2014;9(10): e109985.

27. National Institute for Health and Clinical Excellence. Diabetes in pregnancy: management of diabetes and its complications from preconception to the postnatal period. 2015. https://www.nice.org.uk/guidance/ng3.

28. Castillo WC, Boggess K, Sturmer T, Brookhart MA, Benjamin DK Jr, Funk MJ. Trends in glyburide compared with insulin use for gestational diabetes treatment in the United States, 2000–2011. *Obstet Gynecol.* 2014;123(6):1177–1184.

29. Farrar D, Simmonds M, Bryant M, et al. Treatments for gestational diabetes: a systematic review and meta-analysis. *BMJ Open.* 2017;7(6):e015557.

30. Butalia S, Gutierrez L, Lodha A, Aitken E, Zakariasen A, Donovan L. Short- and long-term outcomes of metformin compared with insulin alone in pregnancy: a systematic review and meta-analysis. *Diabet Med.* 2017;34(1):27–36.

31. Song R, Chen L, Chen Y, et al. Comparison of glyburide and insulin in the management of gestational diabetes: a meta-analysis. *PLoS One.* 2017;12(8):e0182488.

32. Metzger BE. Long-term outcomes in mothers diagnosed with gestational diabetes mellitus and their offspring. *Clin Obstet Gynecol.* 2007;50(4):972–979.

33. Bottalico JN. Recurrent gestational diabetes: risk factors, diagnosis, management and implications. *Semin Perinatol.* 2007;31(3):176–184.

34. Kim C, Newton KM, Knopp RH. Gestational diabetes and the incidence of type 2 diabetes: a systematic review. *Diabetes Care.* 2002;25(10):1862–1868.

35. Russell MA, Phipps MG, Olson CL, Welch HG, Carpenter MW. Rates of postpartum glucose testing after gestational diabetes mellitus. *Obstet Gynecol.* 2006;108(6):1456–1462.

36. Chodick G, Elchalal U, Sella T, et al. The risk of overt diabetes mellitus among women with gestational diabetes: a population-based study. *Diabet Med.* 2010;27(7):779–785.

37. England LG, Dietz PM, Njoroge T, et al. Preventing type 2 diabetes: public health implications for women with a history of gestational diabetes mellitus. *Am J Obstet Gynecol.* 2009;200(4):365.e1–8.

38. Sibai BM, and Viteri OA. Diabetic ketoacidosis in pregnancy. *Obstet Gynecol.* 2014;123(1):167–178.

39. Ehrenberg HM, Durnwald CP, Catalano P, Mercer BM. The influence of obesity and diabetes on the risk of cesarean delivery. *Am J Obstet Gynecol.* 2004;191(3):969–974.

40. Yogev Y, Xenakis EM, Langer O. The association between preeclampsia and the severity of gestational diabetes: the impact of glycemic control. *Am J Obstet Gynecol.* 2004;191(5):1655–1660.

41. Montoro MN, Kjos SL, Chandler M, Peters RK, Xiang AH, Buchanan TA. Insulin resistance and preeclampsia in gestational diabetes mellitus. *Diabetes Care.* 2005;28(8):1995–2000.

42. Coleman TL, Randall H, Graves W, and Lindsay M. Vaginal birth after cesarean among women with gestational diabetes. *Am J Obstet Gynecol.* 2001;184(6):1104–1107.

43. Sacks DA. Etiology, detection, and management of fetal macrosomia in pregnancies complicated by diabetes mellitus. *Clin Obstet Gynecol.* 2007;50(4):980–989.

44. Schaefer-Graf UM, Heuer R, Kilavuz O, Pandura A, Henrich W, Vetter K. Maternal obesity not maternal glucose values correlates best with high rates of fetal macrosomia in pregnancies complicated by gestational diabetes. *J Perinat Med.* 2002;30(4):313–321.

45. Johnstone FD, Nasrat AA, and Prescott RJ. The effect of established and gestational diabetes on pregnancy outcome. *Br J Obstet Gynaecol.* 1990;97(11):1009–1015.

46. Rosenstein MG, Cheng YW, Snowden JM, Nicholson JM, Doss AE, Caughey AB. The risk of stillbirth and infant death stratified by gestational age in women with gestational diabetes. *Am J Obstet Gynecol.* 2012;206(4):309.e1–7.

47. Persson B, Hanson U, Marcus C. Gestational diabetes mellitus and paradoxical fetal macrosomia—a case report. *Early Hum Dev.* 1995;41(3):203–213.

48. Thevarajah A, Simmons D. Risk factors and outcomes for neonatal hypoglycaemia and neonatal hyperbilirubinaemia in pregnancies complicated by gestational diabetes mellitus: a single centre retrospective 3-year review. *Diabet Med.* 2019;36(9):1109–1117.

49. Antepartum fetal surveillance. Practice Bulletin No. 145. American College of Obstetricians and Gynecologists. *Obstet Gynecol.* 2014;124(1):182–192.

50. ACOG Committee Opinion No. 764: Medically indicated late-preterm and early-term deliveries. *Obstet Gynecol.* 2019;133(2):e151–e155.

51. Spong CY, Mercer BM, D'alton M, Kilpatrick S, Blackwell S, Saade G. Timing of indicated late-preterm and early-term birth. *Obstet Gynecol.* 2011;118(2 Pt 1):323–333.

52. Practice Bulletin No. 173: Fetal macrosomia. American College of Obstetricians and Gynecologists' Committee on Practice Bulletins—Obstetrics. *Obstet Gynecol.* 2016;128(5):e195–209.

53. Shnider SM, Abboud T, Artal R, Henriksen E, Stefani SJ, Levinson G. Maternal endogenous catecholamines decrease during labor after lumbar epidural anesthesia. *Anesthesiology.* 1980;;53(3):S299.

54. Datta S. Anesthetic and obstetric management of high-risk pregnancy. 3rd ed. New York: Springer; 2004:343.

55. Naylor CD, Sermer M, Chen E, Sykora K. Cesarean delivery in relation to birth weight and gestational glucose tolerance: pathophysiology or practice style? Toronto Trihospital Gestational Diabetes Investigators. *JAMA.* 1996;275(15):1165–1170.

56. Malinow AM, Ostheimer GW. Anesthesia for the high-risk parturient. *Obstet Gynecol.* 1987;69(6):951–964.

57. Vohra A, Kumar S, Charlton AJ, Olukoga AO, Boulton AJ, McLeod D. Effect of diabetes mellitus on the cardiovascular responses to induction of anesthesia and tracheal intubation. *Br J Anaesth.* 1993;71(2):258–261.

58. Say L, Chou D, Gemmill A, et al: Global causes of maternal death: a WHO systematic analysis. *Lancet Glob Health.* 2014;2(6):e323–e333.

59. Creanga AA, Syverson C, Seed K, Callaghan WM. Pregnancy-related mortality in the United States, 2011–2013. *Obstet Gynecol.* 2017;130(2):366–373.

60. Redman CWG, Jacobson S-L, Russell R. Hypertension in pregnancy. In: Powrie R GM, Camann W, eds. De Swiet's Medical Disorders in Obstetric Practice. 5th ed. Chichester, West Sussex: Blackwell Publishing; 2010:153–181.

61. American College of Obstetricians and Gynecologists. Hypertension in Pregnancy: report of the American College of Obstetricians and Gynecologists' Task Force on Hypertension in Pregnancy. *Obstet Gynecol.* 2013;122(5):1122–1131.

62. Hauth JC, Ewell MG, Levine RJ, et al. Pregnancy outcomes in healthy nulliparas who developed hypertension. Calcium for Preeclampsia Prevention Study Group. *Obstet Gynecol.* 2000;;95(1):24–28.

63. Barton JR, O'Brien JM, Bergauer NK, Jacques DL, Sibai BM. Mild gestational hypertension remote from term: progression and outcome. *Am J Obstet Gynecol.* 2001;184(5):979–983.

64. Walker RL, Hemmelgarn B, and Quan H. Incidence of gestational hypertension in the Calgary Health Region from 1995 to 2004. *Can J Cardiol.* 2009;25(8):e284–e287.

65. Wallis AB, Saftlas AF, Hsia J, and Atrash HK. Secular trends in the rates of preeclampsia, eclampsia, and gestational hypertension, United States, 1987–2004. *Am J Hypertens.* 2008;21(5):521–526.

66. Saudan P, Brown MA, Buddle ML, Jones M. Does gestational hypertension become pre-eclampsia? *Br J Obstet Gynaecol.* 1998;105(11):1177–1184.

67. Sibai BM, Stella CL. Diagnosis and management of atypical preeclampsia-eclampsia. *Am J Obstet Gynecol.* 2009;200(5):481.e1–7.

68. Magee LA, von Dadelszen P, Bohyun CM, et al. Serious perinatal complications of non-proteinuric hypertension: an international, multicenter, retrospective cohort study. *J Obstet Gynaecol Can.* 2003;25(5):372–382.

69. ACOG Practice Bulletin No. 202: Gestational Hypertension and Preeclampsia. *Obstet Gynecol.* 2019;133(1):e1–25.

70. Tranquilli AL, Dekker G, Magee L, et al. The classification, diagnosis and management of the hypertensive disorders of pregnancy: A revised statement from the ISSHP. *Pregnancy Hypertens.* 2014;4(2):97–104.

71. Mol BWJ, Roberts CT, Thangaratinam S, Magee LA, de Groot CJM, Hofmeyr GJ. Pre-eclampsia. *Lancet.* 2016;387(10022):999–1011.

72. Brown MA. Pre-eclampsia: proteinuria in pre-eclampsia—does it matter any more? *Nat Rev Nephrol.* 2012:8(10):563–565.

73. Barton JR, Sibai BM. Diagnosis and management of hemolysis, elevated liver enzymes, and low platelets syndrome. *Clin Perinatol.* 2004;31(4):807–833, vii.

74. Zeeman GG. Neurologic complications of pre-eclampsia. *Semin Perinatol.* 2009;33(3): 166–172.

75. Altman D, Carroli G, Duley L, et al. Do women with pre-eclampsia, and their babies, benefit from magnesium sulphate? The Magpie Trial: a randomised placebo-controlled trial. *Lancet.* 2002;359(9321):1877–1890.

76. ACOG Committee Opinion No. 767: Emergent therapy for acute-onset, severe hypertension during pregnancy and the postpartum period. *Obstet Gynecol.* 2019;133(2):e174–e180.

77. Dhariwal NK, Lynde GC. Update in the management of patients with preeclampsia. *Anesthesiology Clin.* 2017;35(1):95–106.

78. Munnur U, de Boisblanc B, and Suresh MS. Airway problems in pregnancy. *Crit Care Med.* 2005;33(10 Suppl):S259–S268.

79. Brock-Utne JG, Downing JW, and Seedat F. Laryngeal oedema associated with pre-eclamptic toxaemia. *Anaesthesia.* 1977;32(6):556–558.

80. Seager SJ, and Macdonald R. Laryngeal oedema and pre-eclampsia. *Anaesthesia.* 1980;;35(4):360–362.

81. Brimacombe J. Acute pharyngolaryngeal oedema and pre-eclamptic toxaemia. *Anaesth Intensive Care.* 1992;20(1):97–98.

82. Practice guidelines for obstetric anesthesia: an updated report by the American Society of Anesthesiologists Task Force on Obstetric Anesthesia and the Society for Obstetric Anesthesia and Perinatology. *Anesthesiology.* 2016;124(2):270–300.

83. Apfelbaum JL, Hagberg CA, Caplan RA, et al. Practice guidelines for management of the difficult airway: an updated report by the American Society of Anesthesiologists Task Force on Management of the Difficult Airway. *Anesthesiology.* 2013;118(2):251–270.

84. Lee LO, Bateman BT, Kheterpal S, et al. Risk of epidural hematoma after neuraxial techniques in thrombocytopenic parturients: A report from the Multicenter Perioperative Outcomes Group. *Anesthesiology.* 2017;126(6):1053–1063.

85. Leduc L, Wheeler JM, Kirshon B, Mitchell P, Cotton DB. Coagulation profile in severe preeclampsia. *Obstet Gynecol.* 1992;79(1):14–18.

86. Aya AG, Mangin R, Vialles N, et al. Patients with severe preeclampsia experience less hypotension during spinal anesthesia for elective cesarean delivery than healthy parturients: a prospective cohort comparison. *Anesth Analg.* 2003;97(3):867–872.

87. Henke VG, Bateman BT, Leffert LR. Spinal anesthesia in severe preeclampsia. *Anesth Analg.* 2013;117(3):686–693.

88. Visalyaputra S, Rodanant O, Somboonviboon W, Tantivitayatan K, Thienthong S, Saengchote W. Spinal versus epidural anesthesia for cesarean delivery in severe preeclampsia: a prospective randomized, multicenter study. *Anesth Analg.* 2005;101(3):862–868.

89. Powell M, Mathru M, Brandon A, Patel R, Frolich MA. Assessment of endothelial glycocalyx disruption in term parturients receiving a fluid bolus before spinal anesthesia: a prospective observational study. *Int J Obstet Anesth.* 2014;23(4):330–334.

90. Hofmeyr R, Matjila M, Dyer R. Preeclampsia in 2017: Obstetric and anaesthesia management. *Best Pract Clin Anaesthesiol.* 2017;31(1):125–138.

91. Abir G, Mhyre J. Maternal mortality and the role of the obstetric anesthesiologist. *Best Pract Res Clin Anaesthesiol.* 2017;31(1):91–105.

92. Taber EB, Tan L, Chao CR, Beall MH, Ross MG. Pharmacokinetics of ionized versus total magnesium in subjects with preterm labor and preeclampsia. *Am J Obstet Gynecol.* 2002;186(5):1017–1021.

93. Pant M, Fong R, Scavone B. Prevention of peri-induction hypertension in preeclamptic patients: a focused review. *Anesth Analg.* 2014;119(6):1350–1356.

94. Yildiz K, Dogru K, Dalgic H, et al. Inhibitory effects of desflurane and sevoflurane on oxytocin-induced contractions of isolated pregnant human myometrium. *Acta Anaesthesiol Scand.* 2005;49(9):1355–1359.

95. Robins K, Lyons G. Intraoperative awareness during general anesthesia for cesarean delivery. *Anesth Analg.* 2009:109(3):886–890.

96. Vercauteren M, Palit S, Soetens F, Jacquemyn Y, Alahuhta S. Anaesthesiological considerations on tocolytic and uterotonic therapy in obstetrics. *Acta Anaesthesiol Scand.* 2009;53(6):701–709.

97. Kussman B, Shorten G, Uppington J, Comunale ME. Administration of magnesium sulphate before rocuronium: effects on speed of onset and duration of neuromuscular block. *Br J Anaesth.* 1997;79(1):122–124.

98. MacDorman MF, Gregory EC. Fetal and perinatal mortality: United States, 2013. *Natl Vital Stat Rep.* 2015;64(8):1–24.

99. Fretts RC, Schmittdiel J, McLean FH, Usher RH, Goldman MB. Increased maternal age and the risk of fetal death. *N Engl J Med.* 1995;333(15):953–957.

100. Reddy UM, Ko CW, Willinger M. Maternal age and the risk of stillbirth throughout pregnancy in the United States. *Am J Obstet Gynecol.* 2006;195(3):764–770.

101. Wientrob N, Karp M, Hod M. Short- and long-range complications in offspring of diabetic mothers. *J Diabetes Complications.* 1996;10(5):294–301.

102. Thung SF, Landon MB. Fetal surveillance and timing of delivery in pregnancy complicated by diabetes mellitus. *Clin Obstet Gynecol.* 2013;56(4):837–843.

103. Brenner B. Inherited thrombophilia and fetal loss. *Curr Opin Hematol.* 2000;;7(5):290–295.

104. Wu O, Robertson L, Twaddle S, et al. Screening for thrombophilia in high-risk situations: systematic review and cost-effectiveness analysis. The Thrombosis: Risk and Economic Assessment of Thrombophilia Screening (TREATS) study. *Health Technol Assess.* 2006;10(11):1–110.

105. Aune D, Saugstad OD, Henriksen T, Tonstad S. Maternal body mass index and the risk of fetal death, stillbirth, and infant death: a systematic review and meta-analysis. *JAMA.* 2014;311(15):1536–1546.

106. Lee C, Marlow N, Arabin B, et al. Perinatal morbidity and mortality in early-onset fetal growth restriction: cohort outcomes of the trial of randomized umbilical and fetal flow in Europe (TRUFFLE). *Ultrasound Obstet Gynecol.* 2013;42(4):400–408.

107. Temming LA, Dicke JM, Stout MJ, et al. Early second-trimester fetal growth restriction and adverse perinatal outcomes. *Obstet Gynecol.* 2017;130(4):865–869.

108. Devoe LD. Antenatal fetal assessment: multifetal gestation—an overview. *Semin Perinatol.* 2008;32(4):281–287.

109. Smith GC, Shah I, White IR, Pell JP, Dobbie R. Previous preeclampsia, preterm delivery, and delivery of a small for gestational age infant and the risk of unexplained stillbirth in the second pregnancy: a retrospective cohort study, Scotland, 1992-2001. *Am J Epidemiol.* 2007;165(2):194–202.

110. ACOG Practice Bulletin No. 102: management of stillbirth. *Obstet Gynecol.* 2009;113(3): 748–761.

111. Pacora P, Romero R, Jaiman S, et al. Mechanisms of death in structurally normal stillbirths. *J Perinat Med.* 2019;47(2):222–240.

112. Vergani P, Cozzolino S, Pozzi E, et al. Identifying the causes of stillbirth: a comparison of four classification systems. *Am J Obstet Gynecol.* 2008;199(3):319.e1–4.

113. Wapner RJ, Lewis D. Genetics and metabolic causes of stillbirth. *Semin Perinatol.* 2002;26(1):70–74.

114. Goldenberg RL, Thompson C. The infectious origins of stillbirth. *Am J Obstet Gynecol.* 2003;189(3):861–873.

115. Stillbirth Collaborative Research Network Writing Group. Causes of death among stillbirths. *JAMA.* 2011;306(22):2459–2468.

116. Collins JH. Umbilical cord accidents and legal implications. *Semin Fetal Neonatal Med.* 2014;19(5):285–289.

117. Varli IH, Petersson K, Bottinga R, et al. The Stockholm classification of stillbirth. *Acta Obstet Gynecol Scand.* 2008;87(11):1202–1212.

118. Korteweg FJ, Erwich JJHM, Holm JP, et al. Diverse placental pathologies as the main causes of fetal death. *Obstet Gynecol.* 2009;114(4):809–817.

119. Ream M, Ray AM, Chandra R, Chikaraishi DM. Early fetal hypoxia leads to growth restriction and myocardial thinning. *Am J Physiol Regul Integr Comp Physiol.* 2008;295(2):R583–R595.

120. Oyelese Y, Ananth CV. Placental abruption. *Obstet Gynecol.* 2006;108(4):1005–1016.

121. Silver, RM. Fetal death. *Obstet Gynecol.* 2007;109(1):153–167.

122. Goldstein DP, Johnson JP, Reid DE. Management of intrauterine fetal death. *Obstet Gynecol.* 1963;21:523–529.

123. Phillips LL, Skodelis V, King TA. Hypofibrinogenemia and intrauterine fetal death. *Am J Obstet Gynecol.* 1964;89:903–914.

124. Thachil J, Toh CH. Disseminated intravascular coagulation in obstetric disorders and its acute haematological management. *Blood Rev.* 2009;23(4):167–176.

Gestational diabetes mellitus is diagnosed if at least two plasma readings are elevated.

8

Intrapartum Monitoring and Fetal Assessment

Courtney Rhoades and Kristen Vanderhoef

Introduction

Intrapartum fetal monitoring allows real-time fetal evaluation during labor and delivery. This chapter will address the most common types of fetal monitoring, external and internal, as well as the interpretation and categorization of fetal heart rate (FHR) tracings. Fetal resuscitation will also be discussed, as well as how delivery planning is affected by monitoring and interpretation. The chapter will conclude with a discussion of common medications utilized during labor and delivery and their fetal effects.

Electronic Fetal Monitoring

The developing fetal parasympathetic and sympathetic forces modulate the FHR, which matures throughout gestation. The FHR pattern can reflect fetal well-being with heart rate accelerations or fetal compromise with decreased variability and abrupt decreases in the FHR, especially in the setting of stress or contractions.[1] The resulting heart rate patterns have been used in obstetrics for the past 70 years to look for signs of metabolic acidosis or lack thereof in the fetus. The use of electronic fetal monitoring (EFM) has reduced the risk of neonatal seizures but has not changed the national rate of cerebral palsy. Despite the evidence that EFM has increased the cesarean section (C/S) rate in the United States, EFM is still the most common obstetric procedure.[2] EFM pattern recognition in conjunction with clinical assessment conveys insight into the fetal metabolic status prior to and while in labor.

Electronic fetal monitoring in the intrapartum period is commonly started externally on the patient's belly with the patient in lateral recumbent, semi-Fowler's, or upright position (see Figure 8.1). The monitor consists of a monitoring unit and an ultrasound transducer that picks up the fetal heart movement or blood flow when placed over the fetal heart and another tocodynamometer (toco) that sits on the fundus of the uterus and tracks the myometrial tension to record the contraction frequency. While not required for the procedure, the maternal heart rate is often monitored with a pulse oximeter or heart-rate monitor to ensure that the tracing recorded is indeed the fetus and not a maternal heart-rate tracing. All three of these metrics are recorded either on paper or electronically or both.[1]

The rate of the tracing recording can affect the look of the pattern, so it is important to know the speed of transcription when traveling to other countries. In the United States, the speed is solely 3 centimeters per minute (cm/min). If there is difficulty with tracing the fetus

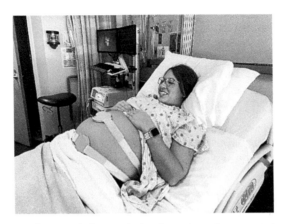

Figure 8.1 An example of external electronic fetal monitor placement during the intrapartum period.

due to fetal movement, heart rate drop off, maternal obesity, or fetal arrhythmia, internal fetal monitoring can be initiated. Internal monitoring requires the patient's amniotic sac be ruptured and a fetal scalp electrode applied. Contraindications to internal monitoring include an inability to rupture the patient due to a closed cervix, high fetal station, or transmission of infectious maternal conditions such as HIV, Hepatitis B and C, and active Herpes virus. The fetal scalp electrode is applied to the fetal scalp, avoiding fontanels, scalp sutures, and the face, and pierces the skin and transmits the R waves of the fetal ventricle depolarization. Internal monitoring of the FHR is more accurate but has contraindications that need to be taken in to account prior to placement.[3]

Internal monitoring of the contractions is also more accurate but more intrusive. The intrauterine pressure catheter (IUPC) lies between the fetus and the uterine wall inside the uterus after amniotic rupture. This fluid-filled catheter can precisely measure contraction timing, length, and strength, while the external monitor is limited to timing only. The IUPC also can be used to put more fluid back into the uterus and around the fetus as an amnioinfusion. The IUPC requires ruptured membranes and knowing the placental position in order to avoid placing it in or through the placenta. It carries the risk of uterine perforation, fetal injury, and infection. Studies on the regular use of IUPCs have not been shown to improve clinical outcome; however, it is helpful with patients that are being augmented or induced and falling off the labor curve or when the timing of fetal decelerations are in question and there is a potential for amnioinfusion to resuscitate the fetus.[3]

Ultrasound on labor and delivery is a useful adjunct to EFM. Most patients presenting to the labor floor have undergone at least one ultrasound during pregnancy. That ultrasound confirms fetal number, gestation, fetal anomalies, fetal growth, placental location, and amniotic fluid levels. The exam done between 18 and 22 weeks, rules out many issues that can compromise fetal well-being and the ability to have a vaginal delivery. Abnormalities found are followed up with ultrasounds and possibly antenatal fetal testing to confirm fetal well-being. Follow-up testing aids with delivery planning.[4]

When the patient presents to the labor unit, another ultrasound is often performed for presentation of the fetus, FHR, fluid level, and placental location. If this is the first ultrasound of the pregnancy, assessment of estimated gestational age, size, and gross fetal anomalies is performed as well. If the fetus is not vertex and needs delivery, the provider will need to decide whether to try to change the position of the fetus through a procedure called external cephalic version, plan for a cesarean delivery. Low amniotic fluid levels can be a sign of rupture of membranes, placental maturation or insufficiency. If the placenta is low lying near the cervical os, more bleeding may be expected in labor and it may preclude vaginal delivery, as would a placenta completely covering the cervical os, as in the case of placenta previa. All of these findings may change the management of the patient.[4]

Once the patient is admitted, the fetal heart should be monitored either intermittently or continuously. The decision on intermittent monitoring is based on hospital policy and the provider. Each hospital will have its own policy, but usually the fetus must have a reassuring fetal heart tracing, normal prenatal care, and no active medical issues. The recommendation from the American College of Obstetricians and Gynecologists (ACOG) and the Association of Women's Health, Obstetric and Neonatal Nurses (AWHONN) is for fetal assessment every 30 min in active labor and every 15 min in the second stage. With intermittent auscultation and fetal assessment, the recommendation from ACOG is every 15 min in active labor and every 5 min when pushing. Regardless, hospitals require some frequency of continuous fetal monitoring once interventions such as labor augmentation and regional anesthesia are initiated.[1]

Fetal Heart Monitoring and Interpretation

Evaluation of fetal heart tracings is fraught with differences in interpretation, making care of the patient a challenge. In 2008, a large partnership between ACOG, Society of Maternal-Fetal Medicine, and the Eunice Kennedy Shriver National Institute of Child Health and Human Development (NICHD) convened to attempt to standardize nomenclature and fetal tracing categories and to set goals for research. These standards have been adopted across the country and are used to interpret the fetal heart tracings during antepartum surveillance and in the intrapartum period.[5]

Fetal heart tracings show the FHR, and sometimes the maternal heart rate on the upper part of the tracing. The lower part of the tracing shows uterine contractions. The tracings are evaluated in 30-minute (min) increments to establish a baseline rate rounded to the nearest 5 beats per min during a 10-min segment. This can be difficult during marked fetal heart variability or baseline changes. The baseline must be a minimum of 2 min in any 10-min segment or defer to the prior 10-min segment. The normal heart rate range for a term fetus is 110 to 160 beats per min with anything above 160, for more than 2 min, classified as tachycardia. Bradycardia is a heart rate less than 110, for more than 2 min.

Variability refers to the small changes in amplitude and frequency near the baseline FHR. If the tracing looks like a straight, flat line, there is absent variability. If the variability is minimal, there are 5 beats or less of the small changes in the heartbeat. Moderate variability is considered normal for a term fetus and is 6–25 beats per min. Marked variability exists with an amplitude of 25 beats per min. Moderate variability is reassuring, but absent or minimal variability can be a sign of acidosis. Minimal variability can be normal during a sleep cycle or in response to medication.

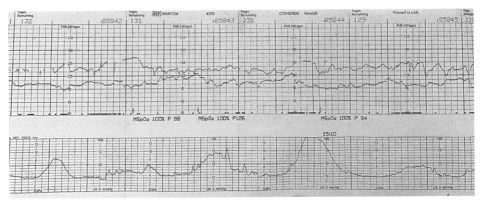

Figure 8.2 Fetal heart tracing showing a normal, category 1 tracing with acceleration and contractions without decelerations.

The tracing is also evaluated for accelerations and decelerations. These are changes that happen over a longer time than variability and are abrupt increases, in the case of accelerations, or decreases in the heart rate, in the case of decelerations.

Accelerations are visually apparent abrupt increases, 15 beats per min or more from baseline, lasting longer than 15 seconds and less than 2 min. If it lasts more than 2 min but less than 10 min, it is a prolonged acceleration and if it lasts more than 10 min it is a baseline change. Accelerations often occur with fetal movement and overall are reassuring that fetal acid-base status is normal (refer to Figure 8.2).

Decelerations are further categorized by the timing during a contraction. The majority of decelerations on fetal monitoring are variable decelerations. The abrupt FHR change is not consistent in onset in relationship to the contraction onset: it lasts at least 15 seconds and the decrease is at least 15 beats per min. Variable decelerations often have a "V" type pattern and are related to transient cord compression (see Figure 8.3). Unless they are recurrent and deep, they are only signs of transient interruption of the fetal oxygenation pathway and do not appear in conjunction with fetal acidemia. Recurrent variable decelerations can cause fetal hypoxia and lead to acidemia over time.

Early decelerations are usually due to vagal nerve stimulation with compression of the head. The timing mirrors in onset and completion of the contraction and the nadir tends to

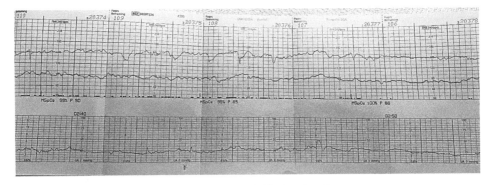

Figure 8.3 Fetal heart tracing demonstrating variable decelerations.

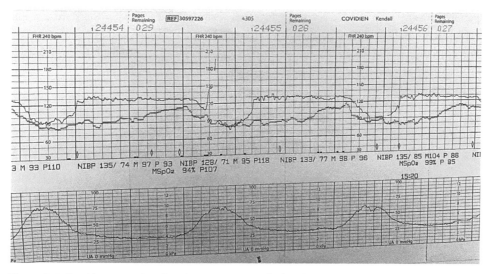

Figure 8.4 Fetal heart tracing showing recurrent early decelerations.

happen at the same time as the peak of the contraction (see Figure 8.4). Late decelerations are at least 15 beats per min of FHR decrease lasting 15 seconds or greater, but less than 2 min and the nadir is after the peak of the contraction. The onset is after the initiation of the contraction and the end of the deceleration is also after the contraction has finished (see Figure 8.5). Late decelerations signal placental insufficiency and a decrease in oxygenation pathway to the fetus.

If a deceleration lasts longer than 2 min but less than 10 min, it is considered a prolonged deceleration. If it lasts 10 min or longer, it is considered a baseline change. If the decelerations occur with more than half the contractions, then they are considered recurrent. Sinusoidal

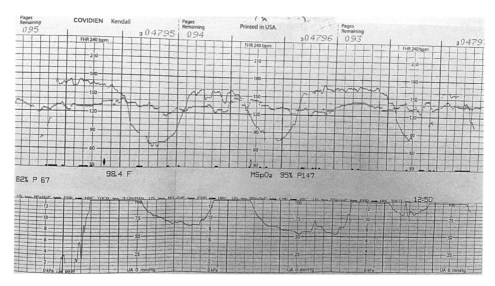

Figure 8.5 These are examples of late decelerations and occurred as the patient was being wheeled to the operating room for an urgent cesarean delivery.

patterns are also seen and are due to medications or severe fetal acidemia. These are sine-like waves in an undulating pattern, lasting longer than 20 min with a cycle frequency of 3–5 beats per min. Using these definitions, the fetal heart tracings are broken into three categories to communicate between teams and standardize care.[5]

NICHD Fetal Categories

Category 1

Baseline: 110–160 beats per min (normal)
Variability: 6–25 beats per min (moderate)
Accelerations: present or absent
Late or variable decelerations: absent
Early decelerations: present or absent

Category 2

This includes all tracings that cannot be defined as Category 1 or 3.

Baseline: may have bradycardia or tachycardia, if normal variability
Variability: may have minimal or marked; if absent may not have decelerations
Accelerations: none to stimulation (vibroacoustic or scalp stimulation)
Decelerations: periodic or episodic—recurrent variables with minimal or moderate variability; prolonged decelerations; recurrent late decelerations with moderate variability; variables with shoulders or slow return to baseline

Category 3

Baseline: any including bradycardia
Variability: absent with decelerations or bradycardia
Decelerations: recurrent late decelerations; recurrent variable decelerations; sinusoidal pattern.[6]

When Category 2 or 3 tracings occur, intervention is needed. The patient and fetus should be evaluated to determine reasons for the concerning tracing. Resuscitation measures need to be taken to address the presumed cause and reevaluation of the fetal tracing should occur. Resuscitation measures address the common causes of Category 2 and 3 tracings. Depending on the clinical picture, the resuscitative measures can occur in any order. If the patient's blood pressure is low, measures to increase the blood pressure should be attempted. Intravenous fluids can be given and, if hypotension is due to regional anesthesia, medications can be given to increase blood pressure to baseline. Maternal repositioning from supine to left or right side lateral recumbent or even on hands and knees may help with changing fetal position and placental perfusion (see Figures 8.6 and 8.7).

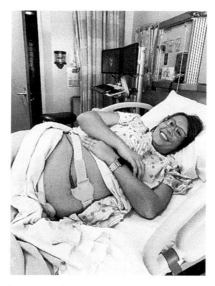

Figure 8.6 Left lateral positioning of a laboring parturient.

There is little evidence that oxygen is helpful unless maternal oxygenation is abnormal; therefore, oxygen saturation should be evaluated. Attention should also be turned to uterine activity. Uterine tachysystole (more than 5 contractions in a 10-min period averaged over 30 min) can cause fetal tracing changes due to uterine tone affecting placental perfusion. If this is the case, uterine tocolytics should be given and any uterotonics, such as oxytocin, stopped. If there is difficulty in assessing the timing of contractions in relationship to the fetal heart reaction, and there are no contraindications, internal monitors can be placed. Amnioinfusion can be started to place more fluid between the fetus and uterus, decreasing variable decelerations with increasing the cushion of fluid inside the uterus.

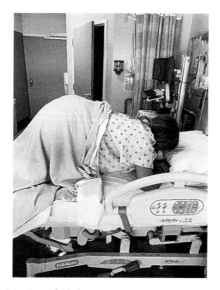

Figure 8.7 Knee-chest positioning of a laboring parturient.

Gestational age and reserve of the fetus have effects on fetal monitoring. Earlier gestation means the nervous system will be less developed. Accelerations in a fetus that is less than 32 weeks only has to meet the criterion of 10 beats per min above the baseline for 10 seconds. In a preterm fetus the baseline is often at the upper limits of normal, and variability lessens the earlier the fetus. Variable decelerations that are mild and quick are often present and unrelated to contractions and fetal acid base status during the premature time period. Changes in the premature fetal status can happen more quickly and be more dramatic because there is less fetal reserve compared to a term pregnancy. Fetal tachycardia in a premature fetus may lead to acidemia, low Apgar scores, and adverse outcomes in addition to things seen in a term fetus, such as infection and maternal fever.

The fetal heart tracing should be re-evaluated after appropriate interventions. If the tracing does not improve, a delivery plan needs to be discussed. This plan needs to take into account the risks and benefits to the patient and fetus, and the possibility that the condition may improve or quickly and dramatically worsen. The differences in labor units and the availability of teams needed for a safe delivery need to be taken in to account. Communication with the nursing, obstetric, anesthesia, and pediatric teams is critical to the best outcome for the patient.[5]

Fetal Impact of Common Obstetric and Anesthetic Medications

Many medications are given on labor and delivery to augment labor and alleviate pain. Maternal comorbidities also require pharmacologic therapy leading up to and during the intrapartum period. Though the primary focus is maternal condition, the fetus must always be considered. Choosing the medication that treats the mother with the fewest fetal side effects is of utmost importance. Here, we will discuss the most common medications utilized during the intrapartum period and their fetal effects.

Gestational Hypertension-Preeclampsia-Eclampsia Pharmacologic Treatment

Gestational hypertension is defined as a systolic blood pressure (SBP) > 140 mm Hg or a diastolic blood pressure (DBP) > 90 mm Hg after 20 weeks' gestation. Preeclampsia is gestational hypertension with other signs of organ system involvement, such as proteinuria. Eclampsia is preeclampsia with seizures. Goals of pharmacologic therapy include controlling hypertension, preventing seizures, maintaining placental blood flow, and preventing fetal toxicity.[7] Titration of medications is of utmost importance because rapid decrease in mean arterial blood pressure (MAP) can decrease utero-placental perfusion and stress the fetus. The goal[8] of MAP reduction in preeclampsia is 15–25%, with an SBP goal of 120–160 mm Hg and a DBP goal 80–105 mm Hg. First-line agents include labetalol, hydralazine, and nifedipine. Labetalol is a combined alpha and beta adrenergic antagonist, with much greater beta activity. Hydralazine is a potent direct vasodilator. Nifedipine is a calcium channel blocker. When titrated appropriately, fetal effects are negligible.

Another important aspect of managing patients with preeclampsia is seizure prophylaxis utilizing magnesium sulfate. Magnesium's mechanism of action in eclamptic seizure prevention is not completely understood. Typical protocols involve a 4–6 gram loading dose over 20 min, followed by 1–2 grams per hour given via IV infusion. Maternal levels must be watched closely because high serum concentrations can lead to respiratory depression and even cardiac arrest.[7]

Induction of Labor

Cervical ripening is the first phase of labor induction, if this has not occurred naturally. Ripening can be accomplished either mechanically utilizing a Foley bulb, or pharmacologically with synthetic prostaglandins such as misoprostol, or a combination of both.[9] Misoprostol can be administered vaginally or orally, with similar results.[9] The most common complication of misoprostol use for cervical ripening is uterine hyperstimulation.[7] If hyperstimulation is not reversed, signs of impaired uteroplacental perfusion will appear, such as decreased FHR variability, fetal bradycardia, and FHR decelerations. Hyperstimulation, if left unchecked, could progress to placental abruption or even uterine rupture.[10] Lower doses and longer administration intervals decrease the risk of hyperstimulation. Terbutaline, a beta-agonist, effectively decreases the frequency of uterine contractions in most cases when uterine hyperstimulation occurs.[7] Foley bulb placement carries a reduced risk of uterine hyperstimulation when compared with misoprostol.[9] The combination of misoprostol plus a Foley bulb also decreases the risk of uterine hyperstimulation when compared to misoprostol alone.[9]

The second stage of labor induction is initiation of contractions and is accomplished using oxytocin, an endogenous peptide hormone. Oxytocin is administered intravenously as a continuous infusion. Both low- and high-dose regimens are used and titrated as necessary, using cervical dilation to assess efficacy. A dilation rate of 1 cm/hour is considered adequate progression of active labor.[7] Like misoprostol, a common side effect of oxytocin is uterine hyperstimulation. The first line of treatment involves decreasing or stopping the oxytocin infusion. If FHR changes accompany uterine hyperstimulation, the infusion is stopped, the patient is repositioned, oxygen is administered, and terbulatine is given.[10]

Labor Analgesia and Fetal Effects

Parenteral opioids are the most commonly used systemic medications for labor analgesia. They are inexpensive and do not require additional personnel or equipment. They do readily cross the placenta and cause many maternal and fetal side effects. Opioids provide a dissociation from pain, but not complete pain control. Opioids tend to decrease the variability of FHR tracings, though this generally does not signal fetal distress. Postdelivery neonatal respiratory depression is a function of which opioid was administered and when.[8]

Nitrous oxide is the most common inhalational agent used for labor analgesia. It is used extensively outside of the United States (US) and is gaining in popularity within the US currently. It is self-administered as a 50% nitrous/50% oxygen mixture. It provides incomplete labor analgesia, but it is an alternative when epidural analgesia is not available or contraindicated. It has no FHR effects and is quickly eliminated through respirations in the newborn.[11]

Neuraxial analgesia is the most effective method of treating labor pain. Epidural placement is the most common form of labor analgesia, but combined spinal epidural (CSE) analgesia as well as spinal analgesia can also be utilized. When labor pain is controlled with epidural analgesia, maternal plasma catecholamine levels decrease, which can improve utero-placental perfusion. Maternal hyperventilation is often reduced with epidural analgesia, improving oxygen delivery to the fetus. Epidural analgesia-induced hypotension has an incidence of 14%. If left untreated, utero-placental perfusion can become impaired.[8] Blood pressure (BP) should be monitored every 2–3 minutes after initiation of epidural analgesia until BP is deemed stable. Patient position plays a large role, with supine position being worst and lateral being best. First-line treatments include crystalloid fluid administration, full lateral position, and vasopressor administration. Ephedrine was the historic vasopressor of choice; however, recent studies suggest that phenylephrine is as safe and can also be utilized to treat hypotension in laboring patients with epidural analgesia in place. Ephedrine readily crosses the placenta and can increase FHR and variability.[8] Most epidurals are maintained with an infusion consisting of a dilute local anesthetic in combination with a low-dose opioid. Neither of these medications, given via the epidural route, seem to cause FHR changes in the absence of maternal hypotension or uterine hypertonus.[12] Indirectly, epidural analgesia decreases maternal plasma catecholamines. Epinephrine causes uterine relaxation. If epinephrine levels are reduced, uterine tachysystole can result, impairing utero-placental blood flow and leading to FHR decelerations. Prompt treatment is necessary with tocolytic medications such as terbutaline or nitroglycerin.

Summary

Intrapartum fetal monitoring techniques allow for real-time fetal evaluation. External monitoring is most common and generally adequate, but more invasive monitoring is available when necessary. The biggest challenge pertaining to intrapartum fetal monitoring is differences of interpretation. Many societies have worked to standardize interpretation and categorization and continue to do so, hopefully improving outcomes moving forward. Fetal monitoring enables delivery plan changes in real time to ensure the best outcome for mom and baby. Fetal monitoring allows health care teams to treat maternal conditions while monitoring fetal effects. Based on fetal tolerance, medications can be adjusted or changed.

References

1. American College of Obstetricians and Gynecologists. Intrapartum fetal heart rate monitoring: nomenclature, interpretation, and general management principles. 2009;114:192–202.
2. Wolfberg AJ, The future of fetal monitoring. *Reviews in Obstetrics & Gynecology.* 2012;5(3/4):e132–e136.
3. Diogo Ayres-de-Campos CY, FIGO consensus guidelines on intrapartum fetal monitoring: cardiotocography. International Journal of Gynecology and Obstetrics. 2015:13–24.

4. American College of Obstetrics and Gynecology. Practice bulletin no. 175: ultrasound in pregnancy. *Obstetrics and Gynecology.* 2016;128:e241–e256.

5. Miller LA, Mosby's pocket guide to fetal monitoring: a multidisciplinary approach. 8th ed. St. Louis, MO: Elsevier; 2017.

6. Macones GA, et al. The 2008 National Institute of Child Health and Human Development workshop report on electronic fetal monitoring: update on definitions, interpretation, and research guidelines. *Obstetrics and Gynecology.* 2008;112:661–666.

7. Briggs GG, Wan SR, Drug therapy during labor and delivery, part 2. *American Journal of Health-System Pharmacy.* 2006;63(12): 1131–1139.

8. Chestnut DH, Polley LS, Tsen LC, Wong CA. Chestnut's obstetric anesthesia principles and practice. 6th ed. Philadelphia, PA: Mosby Elsevier; 2019:453–454, 475, 498, 520, 853–855.

9. Chen W, et al. Meta-Analysis of Foley catheter plus misoprostol versus misoprostol alone for cervical ripening. Review article. *International Journal of Gynecology and Obstetrics.* 2015;129:193–198.

10. Pacheco LD, et al. Management of uterine hyperstimulation with concomitant use of oxytocin and terbutaline. *American Journal of Perinatology.* 2006;23(6):377–380.

11. Vallejo MC, Zakowski MI, Pro-con debate: nitrous oxide for labor analgesia. Review article. *Hindawi BioMed Research International.* 2019;4618798. https://doi.org/10.1155/2019/4618798.

12. Capogna G, Effect of epidural analgesia on the fetal heart rate. Review. *European Journal of Obstetrics & Gynecology and Reproductive Biology.* 2001;98:160–164.

9

Obstetric Management of Labor and Vaginal Delivery

Marianne David, Geoffrey Ho, Daniel Fisher, Laura Roland, Everett Chu, and Michelle S. Burnette

Introduction

Labor and delivery are complex processes characterized by painful uterine contractions and cervical dilation that ultimately result in the expulsion of the fetus. The trigger for labor is not fully understood but a diverse hormonal interplay, including a rise in prostaglandin production and an increase in the number of oxytocin receptors, are believed to be involved.[1] The estimated date of delivery (EDD) is the expected onset of labor based on the number of gestational weeks and is divided into four categories: preterm (< 37 weeks), early-term (37 weeks 0 days to 38 weeks 6 days), term (39 weeks 0 days to 40 weeks 6 days), late term (41 weeks 0 days to 41 weeks 6 days), and postterm (> 42 weeks).

In the United States, preterm births occurred between 9–14% of pregnancies, while postterm births occurred between 5–8%.[2]

Components of Labor and Delivery

Maternal Components

Days to weeks prior to the onset of labor, the cervix undergoes remodeling of connective tissue, or *ripening*. The condition of the cervix can be predictive of the proximity and the likely success of labor.

The uterus is a smooth muscle organ which can be divided into the active upper and the passive lower segments. During labor, the muscle fibers within the myometrium of the upper segment shorten sequentially with every contraction, pushing the contents of the uterus against the lower segment. This coordinated segmental contraction causes the uterus to distend and forces the cervix to efface and eventually dilate. Periods of relaxation between contractions are important to allow for uteroplacental blood flow.

The dimensions of the maternal bony pelvis may pose mechanical obstruction to the fetus and, in theory, early identification of mothers with less favorable pelvic types could predict potential difficulty with vaginal delivery. However, in clinical practice, radiographic investigations have insufficient evidence for improved outcomes and are instead associated with increased cesarean section rates.[3]

Fetal Components

At the onset of labor, the relation of the fetus to birth canal—including fetal *lie*, *presentation*, and *position*—are crucial to the eventual success of delivery.

Fetal lie describes the long axis of the fetus in relation to the mother, and can either be longitudinal, transverse, or oblique. Of these, the longitudinal lie is the most common, and is essential for the fetus to be delivered vaginally. An oblique lie, where the axes of the mother and fetus cross at 45 degrees, is otherwise known as an unstable lie, and resolves to either a longitudinal or transverse lie during labor.

Fetal presentation describes the part of the fetus closest to the birth canal. Accordingly, longitudinal lies can be either cephalic (head) or breech (rear) presentations, and transverse lies are shoulder presentations. Cephalic presentations can be further subdivided, depending on the degree of neck flexion of the fetus, into vertex (full flexion), brow (neutral) or face (full extension).

Fetal position describes the bony landmark of the presenting part of the fetus in relation to the maternal pelvis. This is determined on vaginal examination by palpating the sagittal suture and fontanelles of the fetus. Bony landmarks differ according to the presentation: the occiput for vertex, the mentum for face, and the sacrum for breech. Current evidence suggests that vaginal delivery of a singleton breech fetus may be reasonable under hospital-specific protocol guidelines for eligibility and labor management. However, detailed informed consent should be documented, including risks that perinatal or neonatal mortality or short-term serious neonatal morbidity may be higher than in cesarean delivery.[4]

Stages of Labor

Labor has four stages: the first stage, or the clinical onset of labor until full cervical dilation; the second stage, or full cervical dilation and fetal descent until delivery; the third stage, or the delivery of the placenta and membranes; and the fourth stage, defined as the immediate postpartum period of recovery when the parturient is most at risk of hemorrhage.

Signs that herald the beginning of labor include extrusion of a mucus plug, rupture of the amniotic sac, and onset of contractions. Fetal fibronectin (fFN) test is used to rule out preterm labor. A positive test suggests the likelihood of labor within the next 7–14 days and need for closer monitoring. A negative test, on the other hand, is associated with a < 1% chance of delivery within the next 14 days.[5]

First Stage: Cervical Effacement and Dilatation

Historically, the first stage of labor is divided into two phases—*latent* and *active*. This definition is based on landmark studies performed by Emanuel Friedman in the 1950s who analyzed the rate of cervical dilation and fetal descent in thousands of nulliparous and multiparous women. The Friedman curve is a graphical representation of expected cervical dilation against time.[6]

The latent phase signals the onset of labor and occurs with maternal perception of uterine contractions occurring at regular intervals. At this phase, the rate of cervical dilation is slow, but significant changes occur in the cervical connective tissue components. The active phase, on the other hand, is characterized by a significant increase in the rate of change of cervical dilation and ends at full cervical dilation and retraction.

Abnormalities during the first stage of labor were previously defined using the 95th percentile on the Friedman curve as threshold.[6] A *prolonged latent phase* is one that lasts > 20 hours in nulliparous women and > 14 hours in multiparous women. In a *protracted active phase*, progress occurs more slowly than normal and the cervix dilates at a rate of < 1.2 cm/hr in nulliparous women and < 1.5 cm/hr in multiparous women. In *active phase arrest*, there is complete cessation of progress. This is defined as an absence of cervical change > 2 hours despite adequate uterine contractions in a cervix that is at least 4 cm dilated.

However, there have been many changes in obstetrics since the Friedman labor curve was introduced more than 50 years ago. Today, induction of labor is more widespread, as well as the augmentation of labor with oxytocin and the use of epidurals for labor analgesia.[7] This prompted the reassessment of the labor curve and its applicability in modern obstetric practice. More recently, driven by the increased rate of cesarean delivery despite no measurable improvement in maternal and fetal outcomes, the traditional definition of labor has been revised in favor of a more contemporary one. Data from the Consortium of Safe Labor, a multicenter retrospective study of 62,415 deliveries, found that labor progresses more slowly than previously described. Cervical dilation to 4–6 cm occurs far slower than the Friedman curve suggests and the maximal change in cervical dilation does not occur until after 6 cm of cervical dilation.[8] Moreover, both nulliparous and multiparous women dilate to 6 cm at the same rate but multiparous women undergo a more rapid cervical dilation once this threshold is reached.[8] Accordingly, protraction and arrest disorders have been redefined by the American College of Obstetricians and Gynecologists (ACOG) in that neither should be diagnosed before 6 cm of dilation because allowing labor to continue for a longer period may reduce the rate of cesarean deliveries.[9]

Admission in the latent phase of labor is associated with more arrests of labor, cesarean births in the active phase, increased oxytocin, and the use of antibiotics for intrapartum fever.[10–12] Women in the latent phase of labor, who have an otherwise uncomplicated course, may have their admission for labor and delivery delayed.[13]

Second Stage: Fetal Delivery

The second stage of labor encompasses full cervical dilatation to delivery of the fetus. The length of this stage is highly variable but the median duration is approximately 50 minutes and 20 minutes for nulliparous and multiparous parturients, respectively.[14] A second stage that lasts greater than 3–4 hours is associated with adverse maternal outcomes, such as puerperal infection, third-degree and fourth-degree perineal lacerations, and postpartum hemorrhage (PPH).[15] Moreover, for each hour in the second stage of labor, the chance for spontaneous vaginal delivery decreases. After 3 hours or more, only about a quarter of nulliparous women and a third of multiparous women give birth spontaneously and up to 30–50% of those may require operative delivery.[16] If the fetus is low enough in the birth canal, an operative vaginal delivery, or delivery assisted by forceps or vacuum, may be attempted. For patients with epidural anesthesia, the presence of an epidural catheter may enable the anesthesia provider to administer fast-onset, dense analgesia to aid in instrumental delivery and perhaps reduce the need for cesarean section.

Episiotomy, a surgical incision used to extend the vaginal opening, is rarely used in modern obstetrics in the absence of fetal distress or shoulder dystocia as it carries the risk of severe perineal trauma, perineal pain, and dyspareunia.[17] Shoulder dystocia, an obstetric emergency of the second stage, occurs when the fetal anterior shoulder becomes impacted behind the maternal pubic symphysis after delivery of the of the fetal head. The presence of neuraxial analgesia can facilitate interventions such as extending an episiotomy, adding suprapubic pressure, delivering the posterior fetal arm, or cephalic replacement of the fetal head for possible emergent cesarean delivery.[18–20] Causes of arrest of descent include cephalopelvic disproportion, labor dysfunction, malposition, and macrosomia. Operative vaginal or cesarean delivery should be considered.

Four human pelvic types have been described. The most common is the gynecoid pelvis, thought to be most ideal for vaginal childbirth. A gynecoid pelvis shape may permit rotation of the baby into an occiput anterior position, which allows for fetal neck flexion and facilitates passage of the smaller suboccipitobregmatic head diameter through the birth canal.[21] Occiput posterior fetal presentation, possibly related to an android pelvis shape, may result in a more difficult vaginal delivery secondary to the larger head diameter (occipitofrontal or occipitomental).

Third Stage: Placental Separation and Delivery

The third stage begins with delivery of the fetus and ends with the expulsion of the placenta. The uterus contracts rapidly after the fetus is delivered, causing a decrease in surface area for placental implantation. As the size of the placenta remains unchanged, this causes it to detach from the surface of the uterus. Delivery of the placenta is also aided by increased maternal intra-abdominal pressure or by fundal pressure with gentle traction on the umbilical cord.

A placenta that fails to separate immediately postpartum prevents the uterus from contracting adequately and can result in hemorrhage. Retained placenta could be due to trapped or *incarcerated placenta,* when the placenta is separated from the uterine wall but remains in the uterine cavity because the cervix has closed; *placenta adherens,* when the placenta is adhered to the uterine wall; or *placenta accreta,* when the placenta has grown through the wall of the myometrium. When the placenta does not separate freely from the uterus within 30 minutes of delivery, or when an immediate PPH ensues, manual extraction of the placenta may be indicated. The obstetric provider will place his or her hand within the uterine cavity and physically separate the placenta from the wall of the uterus. If this is unsuccessful, especially in the setting of uterine bleeding, dilation and curettage (D&C) may be necessary, with a hysterectomy reserved for rare cases. Neuraxial analgesia can be extended to anesthesia and can be used to facilitate uterine relaxation and patient tolerance of placental extraction. When significant blood loss has occurred, general anesthesia should be considered to avoid the hypotension caused by the vasodilation and sympathectomy of a neuraxial block and facilitate resuscitation. Once the placenta has been delivered, uterotonics should be administered to encourage uterine contraction. Oxytocin is the first-line agent and is most commonly administered by a continuous infusion. The efficacy of oxytocin may be decreased in patients who have been exposed to it during labor. Other options for uterine atony include the ergot analog methylergonovine, and the prostoglandins carboprost and misoprostol.

Fourth Stage of Labor: Uterine Contraction and Tamponade

The fourth stage of labor is generally regarded as the first hour after delivery, when significant PPH can occur. During this stage, parturients are monitored closely to assure the uterus remains contracted and lacerations, if present, are repaired and surgical hemostasis achieved.

Primary PPH is blood loss occurring during the first 24 hours after delivery that is greater than 1000 mL regardless of mode of delivery, or blood loss that is accompanied by symptomatic hypovolemia. PPH accounts for 11% of maternal deaths in the United States.[22] Risk factors for hemorrhage include hypertensive diseases of pregnancy, polyhydramnios, intrauterine infection, multiple gestation, retained placenta, and antepartum hemorrhage.[23] Secondary PPH is that which occurs beyond 24 hours after birth.

Quantitative Blood Loss

Visual estimates are thought to underestimate blood loss by up to 50%.[24] In determining quantitative blood loss (QBL), blood-soaked drapes, lap pads, and tapes are weighed to give a measured determination of blood loss. Calibrated under-buttock drapes help collect and quantify blood loss in vaginal deliveries. Determining QBL allows for a more accurate assessment compared to estimated blood loss (EBL) and may help in the prompt identification of PPH.

Shock Index

In addition to blood loss, the shock index (SI) is a tool that can be used to quickly identify patients in need of resuscitation. SI is defined as heart rate divided by systolic blood pressure. The normal range is 0.5 to 0.7 in healthy adults. Shock index < 0.9 is correlated with a parturient who is likely not in need of ICU admission. Conversely, shock index > 1.7 points to a patient in extremis who needs urgent intervention.[25]

Postpartum Pain

Pain is an inevitable feature of childbirth and continues to be one of the most commonly reported concerns by women in the immediate postpartum period. Prevention and treatment are especially important in patients who underwent cesarean section or who sustained severe perineal lacerations during vaginal delivery. Acute postpartum pain can affect the mother's ability to care for herself and her infant and increase the risk of opioid abuse, postpartum depression, and the development of chronic pain.[26] The assessment of recovery from postpartum pain is recommended as part of the patient's postpartum evaluation.[27]

Management

ACOG recommends using multimodal analgesics along with nonpharmacologic therapies in managing postpartum pain.[26] This should include nonopioid alternatives such as acetaminophen and nonsteroidal anti-inflammatory drugs (NSAIDs). Opioids should be reserved for breakthrough pain when other options are inadequate. Multimodal analgesia results in the additive or synergistic effects of different modes of medications while minimizing the side effects of individual drugs. There is also superior pain relief when oral analgesics are given at scheduled intervals rather than on demand. The combination of NSAIDs and acetaminophen has been shown to be synergistic for pain relief. When the use of opioids becomes necessary, the goal is to achieve the best pain relief possible while minimizing side effects. Oral opioid administration is still the preferred route when tolerated.

An important consideration in choosing pharmacologic agents is to minimize the drug transfer to breast milk. Lactation is not fully established during the first several days postpartum, and little drug is excreted through milk at this time. However, neonatal metabolism and elimination are also poorly developed, and maternal opioid analgesia can easily accumulate in the neonate.[28] While NSAIDs are generally avoided during pregnancy, they are considered safe for nursing mothers. Ibuprofen specifically has limited transfer into breast milk.[29]

The most common sources of pain after a vaginal delivery are uterine contractions, breast engorgement, and perineal lacerations.[26] In the first few days after childbirth, myometrial contractions occur as the uterus continues to involute, resulting in afterpains. Oxytocin release, stimulated by nursing, can increase the strength of the contractions.[30] These contractions will decrease in intensity and frequency as the uterus returns to prepregnancy size. Afterpains can be treated with heading pads and NSAIDs. Breast engorgement pain is most commonly associated with onset of lactation and can be treated nonpharmacologically with ice packs.

Neuraxial analgesia with infusions using lower drug concentrations may be protective against instrumented vaginal deliveries.[31,32] Severe perineal laceration should be repaired under neuraxial or general anesthesia to allow for maximum sphincter relaxation. After repair, nonopioid medications should be used to reduce the risk of constipation and avoid suture breakdown.

Neuraxial opioids remain the most effective at managing postcesarean section pain.[26] In patients who cannot receive neuraxial analgesia, other regional techniques, such as transversus abdominus plane (TAP) blocks or quadratus lumborum (QL) blocks, as well as local anesthetic wound infiltration, are alternatives. Because TAP blocks only relieve somatic but not visceral pain after cesarean delivery, they are not superior to intrathecal morphine.[31] QL blocks, on the other hand, deposit local anesthetics closer to the paravertebral space and offer some visceral coverage.

Postpartum Depression

Postpartum depression (PPD) is defined as clinical depression occurring any time within the first year after delivery. Pain is a risk factor for developing postpartum depression. Women who developed advance perineal lacerations or severe pain after cesarean delivery are more likely to experience postpartum depression, whereas those who received adequate labor pain relief are at a lower risk.[33,34] Risk factors found to contribute to PPD included body mass index (BMI), chronic pain, and history of anxiety or depression, as well as expectation-to-reality mismatch (see Box 9.1). Whether or not a woman delivered as she intended affected

---

Box 9.1 Breech Presentation

Psychiatric risk factors
- History of anxiety or depression
- History of other psychiatric disorders

Obstetric complications
- History of miscarriage
- Known fetal anomalies
- Injury during delivery, perineal lacerations

Maternal comorbidities
- Increased BMI
- History of chronic pain
- Antepartum anemia

Social factors
- History of domestic violence or abuse
- History of substance abuse

---

her risk of developing PPD.[33] By helping the patient anticipate and prepare for labor pains and avoid unmatched expectations, the anesthesiologist can play a role in decreasing the incidence of PPD.

Special Considerations

Vaginal Birth After Cesarean (VBAC) and Trial of Labor After Cesarean (TOLAC)

The early 20th-century adage of "once a cesarean, always a cesarean" is not a 21st-century guideline. Cesarean rates have steadily increased in the last several decades, and trial of labor after cesarean (TOLAC) is encouraged by ACOG.[35] Many large studies have demonstrated that for women who attempt TOLAC, 60–80% will go on to have a successful vaginal birth after cesarean (VBAC).[36–40] However, of the women who are considered good candidates, only 30% choose TOLAC.[41]

Individual circumstances must be considered when helping women understand their possible success when undergoing TOLAC. Women who are more likely to achieve a VBAC are those who are of a normal weight (BMI 18.5–24.9), do not have a need for induction of labor, and did not have a previous cesarean indication of dystocia.[36,37] The greatest predictor of successful VBAC is a history of a previous vaginal delivery, resulting in a VBAC success rate of 85–90%.[36,39,42]

Beyond providing the experience of vaginal birth to women and the well-studied benefits to the neonate, VBAC is associated with several health advantages to the parturient. Women who achieve VBAC have shorter recovery periods and lower risk of PPH, infection, thromboembolic events, and they avoid major abdominal surgery when compared to both TOLAC requiring repeat cesarean and elective repeat cesarean.[40,43]

TOLAC carries a 0.5–0.9% uterine rupture rate with one previous low-transverse hysterotomy.[44] Data is limited and inconsistent on the increased morbidity of women undergoing TOLAC after multiple low-transverse hysterotomy cesareans. However, there is a significant associated risk of uterine rupture in women who have a history of uterine rupture, transmural myomectomy, or previous cesarean with a classical or T-incision hysterotomy.[35,36]

Obstetrical Considerations

Women who have a calculated 60–70% chance of successful VBAC have equal or less morbidity than elective repeat cesarean if they undergo TOLAC.[35] Multiple gestations have not been found to be a contraindication to TOLAC, and outcomes of singleton pregnancies to twin pregnancies who undergo TOLAC are similar.[35,45] Induction and augmentation of labor are associated with an increased risk of uterine rupture when compared with spontaneous labor. Moreover, patients who have an induced or augmented labor are less likely to have a successful VBAC.

Anesthetic Management

The anesthesia provider must consider the possibility of abnormal placentation or uterine rupture when caring for the parturient attempting a TOLAC. The American Society of Anesthesiologists (ASA) recommends offering placement of an early neuraxial catheter in these patients.[46] Having neuraxial anesthesia may avoid the need for general anesthesia in the case of uterine rupture or conversion to repeat cesarean.[46] Moreover, neuraxial anesthesia does not mask the pain symptoms of lower uterine rupture because the most sensitive diagnostic sign is fetal heart rate tracing (FHR) showing severe variable decelerations.[35] Previous cesarean scars predispose a patient to abnormal placentation and an increased risk of peripartum hemorrhage. Radiographic imaging and antenatal ultrasound may identify an accreta spectrum. In these cases, a planned cesarean delivery may be indicated and the anesthesiologist must be prepared for resuscitation in the event of a massive hemorrhage.

Multiple Gestation

Prior to the early 1980s, twin births were relatively stable at approximately 2% of all births. Twin rates began climbing in the United States and, by 2009, 1 in 30 babies born in the United States was a twin, effectively raising the twin rate 76% in that time period.[47] This increase has been observed to be due to women who have delayed childbearing until after the age of 30 spontaneously having twins, as well as greater utilization of reproductive technology.[47] A study in the Netherlands found that women with multiple pregnancies had four times the risk of severe acute maternal morbidity than women with a singleton pregnancy.[48]

Obstetrical Considerations

Fetal complications are more commonly encountered in multiple-gestation pregnancies, with higher rates of preterm delivery, twin-to-twin transfusion, umbilical cord prolapse, polyhydramnios, malpresentation, and congenital abnormalities when compared to singleton pregnancies.

Parturients of multiple gestations have magnified physiologic changes when compared to their singleton counterparts. Not only are the cardiovascular demands more pronounced, but also even in uncomplicated twin pregnancies, systemic vascular resistance was found to be lower than in singleton pregnancies. Near term, the larger gravid uterus decreases total lung capacity and functional residual capacity to a greater extent than singleton pregnancies. The larger uterus also applies greater aortocaval compression, predisposing multiple gestation parturients to more severe supine hypotension syndrome.

Beyond the physiologic changes of multiple-gestation pregnancies, mechanical stress from increased stretching of the uterus puts the parturient at a much greater risk of uterine atony and PPH compared to their singleton counterparts. The incidence of PPH is 9.1% in multiple gestations compared to 4.7% in singletons.[49]

Anesthetic Management

Early epidural analgesia is recommended for laboring patients with multiple gestation. An epidural can provide pelvic relaxation and pain relief in the event of instrument assisted delivery and internal podalic version. Moreover, if immediate cesarean is indicated, surgical anesthesia can be rapidly obtained with 3% 2-chloroprocaine.

After delivery, the patient is at an increased risk of PPH from uterine distention. Intravenous oxytocin should be administered to prevent and treat uterine atony. Methergine, carboprost, and misoprostol can be added if adequate uterine contraction is not achieved, but it is unclear which uterotonic in addition to oxytocin is most efficacious.[50] Continued uterine atony despite uterotonic administration and fundal/uterine massage may require surgical intervention.

External Cephalic Version (ECV)

During normal active labor, the fetal head is the presenting feature. Breech presentation occurs when the fetal buttocks and/or lower extremities overlie the pelvic outlet in a longitudinal lie. Breech presentation can be frank breech (knees are extended and hips are flexed), complete breech (knees and hips are flexed), or incomplete breech (one or both lower extremities are extended at the hips).

Twenty five percent of fetuses are in a breech position at 28 weeks of gestation.[51] However, many will convert spontaneously to a vertex position by 34 weeks. Of the 3–4% that remain in a breech position into labor, there are significant increased risks, including intrapartum fetal death/asphyxiation, birth trauma, umbilical cord prolapse, arrested descent, spinal cord injuries, and preterm delivery.[52]

Obstetrical Considerations

In order for the parturient to attempt a vertex vaginal birth and therefore obviate the risks associated with a breech delivery or a cesarean section, ACOG recommends that all women who are near term with breech presentations should be offered an external cephalic version (ECV) attempt if there are no contraindications.[52] ECV has an average success rate of 58% and is likely to be most successful if done after 36–37 weeks gestation.[52] If the procedure is successful at this gestational age, the fetus is less likely to revert back to breech position. Moreover, if complications ensue and an emergency cesarean section is warranted, delivery does not present a premature infant. ECV is most likely to be successful in patients presenting in frank breech or transverse lie, the patient is of a normal BMI and parous, amniotic fluid is normal, presenting fetal part is not in the pelvis, and the fetal back is not posteriorly positioned.[53]

Several interventions have been shown to increase ECV success rates including the use of tocolytic therapy, specifically beta stimulants, especially when combined with neuraxial analgesia.[54] Moreover, the use of neuraxial analgesia for ECV has increased rates of vertex presentation at labor.[55]

Anesthetic Management

Neuraxial analgesia can be offered to patients undergoing ECV. If the patient elects to have a neuraxial block, placing an epidural or a combined spinal epidural (CSE) is prudent because having a catheter allows for a rapid conversion of analgesia to anesthesia and may prevent general endotracheal anesthesia in the event of an emergency cesarean delivery. A low-dose spinal of 2.5mg of heavy bupivacaine has been shown to increase the success rate of ECV and results in a more timely discharge. However, higher dose spinals have relatively lower pain scores with the procedure.[56]

References

1. Casey ML, MacDonald PC. Biomolecular processes of the initiation of parturition: decidual activation. *Clin Obstet Gynecol.* 1988;31(3):533–552.
2. Martin JA, Hamilton BE, Osterman MJK. Births in the United States, 2018. NCHS Data Brief, no 346. Hyattsville, MD: National Center for Health Statistics. 2019.
3. Pattison R, Cuthbert A, Vanneval A. Pelvimetry for fetal cephalic presentations at or near term for deciding on mode of delivery. *Cochrane Database Syst Rev.* 2017;3:CD000161. doi:10.1002/14651858.CD000161.pub2.
4. ACOG Committee Opinion No 745. Mode of term singleton breech delivery. *Obstet Gynecol.* 2018;132(2):e60–e63. doi:10.1097/AOG.0000000000002755.
5. Ruma M, Bittner C, Soh C. Current perspectives on the use of fetal fibronectin testing in preterm labor diagnosis and management. *Am J Manag Care.* 2017;23(19 Suppl):S356–S362.
6. Friedman EA. Patterns of labor as indicators of risk. *Clin Obstet Gynecol.* 1973;16(1):172–183.
7. Zhang J, Troendle J, Yancey M. Reassessing the labor curve in nulliparous women. *Am J Obstet Gynecol.* 2002;187(4):824–828.
8. Zhang J, Landy HJ, Branch DW, et al. Contemporary patterns of spontaneous labor with normal neonatal outcomes. *Obstet Gynecol.* 2010;116(6):1281–1287.
9. American College of Obstetricians and Gynecologists (College); Society for Maternal-Fetal Medicine, Caughey AB, Cahill AG, Guise JM, Rouse DJ. Safe prevention of the primary cesarean delivery. *Am J Obstet Gynecol.* 2014;210(3):179–193.
10. Bailit JL, Dierker L, Blanchard MH, Mercer BM. Outcomes of women presenting in active versus latent phase of spontaneous labor. *Obstet Gynecol.* 2005;105(1):77–79.

11. Neal JL, Lamp JM, Buck JS, Lowe NK, Gillespie SL, Ryan SL. Outcomes of nulliparous women with spontaneous labor onset admitted to hospitals in preactive versus active labor. *J Midwifery Womens Health.* 2014;59(1):28–34.

12. Wood AM, Frey HA, Tuuli MG, et al. Optimal admission cervical dilation in spontaneously laboring women. *Am J Perinatol.* 2016;33(2):188–194.

13. ACOG Committee Opinion No. 766: Approaches to Limit Intervention During Labor and Birth. *Obstet Gynecol.* 2019;133(2):e164–e173.

14. Kilpatrick SJ, Laros RK Jr. Characteristics of normal labor. *Obstet Gynecol.* 1989;74(1):85–87.

15. Rouse DJ, Weiner SJ, Bloom SL, et al. Second-stage labor duration in nulliparous women: relationship to maternal and perinatal outcomes. *Am J Obstet Gynecol.* 2009;201(4):357.

16. Cheng YW, Hopkins LM, Laros RK Jr, Caughey AB. Duration of the second stage of labor in multiparous women: maternal and neonatal outcomes. *Am J Obstet Gynecol.* 2007;196(6):585. e1–6.

17. American College of Obstetricians and Gynecologists. Practice Bulletin No. 198: Prevention and management of obstetric lacerations at vaginal delivery. *Obstet Gynecol.* 2018;132(3): e87–e102.

18. O'Leary JA, Leonetti HB. Shoulder dystocia: prevention and treatment. *Am J Obstet Gynecol.* 1990;162(1):5–9.

19. American College of Obstetricians and Gynecologists. Practice Bulletin No. 178: Shoulder dystocia. *Obstet Gynecol.* 2017;129:e12333.

20. Sandberg EC. The Zavanelli maneuver: 12 years of recorded experience. *Obstet Gynecol.* 1999;93(2):312–317.

21. Barth Jr WH. Persistent occiput posterior. *Obstet Gynecol.* 2015;125(3):695–709.

22. Quantitative blood loss in obstetric hemorrhage. ACOG Committee Opinion No. 794. American College of Obstetricians and Gynecologists. *Obstet Gynecol.* 2019;134:e150–6.

23. Bateman BT, Berman MF, Riley LE, Leffert LR. The epidemiology of postpartum hemorrhage in a large, nationwide sample of deliveries. *Anesth Analg.* 2010;110(5):1368–1373.

24. Patel A, Goudar SS, Geller SE, et al. Drape estimation vs. visual assessment for estimating postpartum hemorrhage. *Int J Gynaecol Obstet.* 2006;93(3):220–224.

25. Nathan HL, El Ayadi A, Hezelgrave NL, et al. Shock index: an effective predictor of outcome in postpartum haemmorrhage? *BJOG.* 2015;122(2):268–275.

26. ACOG Committee Opinion No 742: Postpartum pain management. *Obstet Gynecol.* 2018;132(1):e35–e43.

27. McKinney J, Keyser L, Clinton S, Pagliano C. ACOG Committee Opinion No 736: Optimizing postpartum care. *Obstet Gynecol.* 2018;132(3):784–785.

28. Hale TW. Maternal medications during breastfeeding. *Clin Obstet Gynecol.* 2004;47(3): 696–711.

29. Spencer JP, Gonzalez III LS, Barnhart DJ. Medications in the breast feeding mother. *Am Fam Physician.* 2001;64(1):119–126.

30. Deussen AR, Ashwood P, Martis R. Analgesia for relief of pain due to uterine cramping/involution after birth. *Cochrane Database Syst Rev.* 2011;(5):CD004908. doi:10.1002/14651858. CD004908.pub2.

31. Lim G, Facco FL, Nathan N, et al. A review of the impact of obstetric anesthesia on maternal and neonatal outcomes. *Anesthesiology.* 2018;129(1):192–215.

32. Peralta F, Bavaro JB. Severe perineal lacerations after vaginal delivery: are they an anesthesiologist's problem? *Curr Opin Anaesthesiol.* 2018;31(3):258–261.

33. Orbach-Zinger S, Landau R, Harousch AB, et al. The relationship between women's intention to request a labor epidural analgesia, actually delivering with labor epidural analgesia, and postpartum depression at 6 weeks: a prospective observational study. *Anesth Analg.* 2018;126(5):1590–1597.

34. Lim G, Farrell LM, Facco FL, Gold MS, Wasan AD. Labor analgesia as a predictor for reduced postpartum depression scores: A retrospective observational study. *Anesth Analg.* 2018;126(5):1598–1605.

35. ACOG Practice Bulletin No. 205 Summary: Vaginal birth after cesarean delivery. *Obstet Gynecol.* 2019;133(2):393–395.

36. Landon M, Grobman W. What we have learned about trial of labor after cesarean delivery from the maternal-fetal medicine units cesarean registry. *Semin Perinatol.* 2016;40(5):281–286.

37. Silver RM, Landon MB, Rouse DJ, et al. Maternal morbidity associated with multiple repeat cesarean deliveries. *Obstet Gynecol.* 2006;107(6):1226–1232.

38. Cunningham FG, Bangdiwala S, Brown SS, Dean TM, Frederiksen M, Rowland Hogue CJ, King T, Spencer Lukacz E, McCullough LB, Nicholson W, Petit N, Probstfield JL, Viguera AC, Wong CA, Zimmet SC. National Institutes of Health Consensus Development Conference Statement: Vaginal Birth After Cesarean: New Insights. March 8–10, 2010. *Obstetrics & Gynecology.* 2010;115(6):1279–1295.

39. Royal College of Obstetricians and Gynaecologists. Birth after previous caesarean birth. Green-top Guideline No 45, 2015. https://www.rcog.org.uk/globalassets/documents/guidelines/gtg_45.pdf. Accessed Sep 12, 2019.

40. Flamm, BL, Goings, JR, Liu, Y, Wolde-Tsadik, G. Elective repeat cesarean delivery versus trial of labor: a prospective multicenter study. *Obstet Gynecol.* 1994;83(6):927–932.

41. Metz TD, Stoddard GJ, Henry E, Jackson M, Holmgren C, Esplin S. How do good candidates for trial of labor after cesarean (TOLAC) who undergo elective repeat cesarean differ from those who choose TOLAC? *Am J Obstet Gynecol.* 2013;208(6):458.e1–6.

42. Mercer BM, Gilbert S, Landon MB, et al. Labor outcomes with increasing number of prior vaginal births after cesarean delivery. *Obstet Gynecol.* 2008;111(2 Pt 1):285–291.

43. Guise JM, Denman MA, Emeis C, et al. Vaginal birth after cesarean: new insights on maternal and neonatal outcomes. *Obstet Gynecol.* 2010;115(6):1267–1278.

44. Landon MB, Hauth JC, Leveno KJ, et al. Maternal and perinatal outcomes associated with a trial of labor after prior cesarean delivery. *N Engl J Med.* 2004;351(25):2581–2589.

45. Ford, AD, Bateman, BT, Simpson, LL. Vaginal birth after cesarean delivery in twin gestations: a large, nationwide sample of deliveries. *Am J Obstet Gynecol.* 2006;195(4):1138–1142.

46. Practice guidelines for obstetric anesthesia: an updated report by the American Society of Anesthesiologists Task Force on Obstetric Anesthesia and the Society for Obstetric Anesthesia and Perinatology. *Anesthesiology.* 2016;124(2):270–300.

47. Martin JA, Hamilton BE, Osterman MJK. Three decades of twin births in the United States, 1980–2009. *NCHS Data Brief.* 2012;(80):1–8.

48. Witteveen T, Van Den Akker T, Zwart JJ, Bloemenkamp KW, Van Roosmalen, J. Severe acute maternal morbidity in multiple pregnancies: a nationwide cohort study. *Am J Obstet Gynecol.* 2016;214(5):641.e1–641.e10.

49. Conde-Agudelo A, Belizán JM, Lindmark G. Maternal morbidity and mortality associated with multiple gestations. *Obstet Gynecol.* 2000;95(6 Pt 1):899–904.

50. Practice Bulletin No. 183 Summary: Postpartum hemorrhage. *Obstet Gynecol.* 2017;130(4):923–925.

51. Hickok DE, Gordon DC, Milberg JA, Williams MA, Daling JR. The frequency of breech presentation by gestational age at birth: a large population-based study. *Am J Obstet Gynecol.* 1992;166(3):851–852.

52. Practice Bulletin No. 161 Summary: External cephalic version. *Obstet Gynecol.* 2016;127(2): 412–413.

53. Kok M, Cnossen J, Gravendeel L, van der Post J, Opmeer B, Mol BW. Clinical factors to predict the outcome of external cephalic version: a metaanalysis. *Am J Obstet Gynecol.* 2008;199(6):630.e1–7; discussion e1–5.

54. Cluver C, Gyte GM, Sinclair M, Dowswell T, Hofmeyr GJ. Interventions for helping to turn term breech babies to head first presentation when using external cephalic version. *Cochrane Database Syst Rev.* 2015;(2):CD000184. doi:10.1002/14651858.CD000184.pub4.

55. Goetzinger KR, Harper LM, Tuuli MG, Macones GA, Colditz GA. Effect of regional anesthesia on the success rate of external cephalic version: a systematic review and meta-analysis. *Obstet Gynecol.* 2011;118(5):1137–1144.

56. Chalifoux LA, Bauchat JR, Higgins N, et al. Effect of intrathecal bupivacaine dose on the success of external cephalic version for breech presentation: a prospective, randomized, blinded clinical trial. *Anesthesiology.* 2017;127(4):625–632.

10

Pharmacology and Non-anesthetic Drugs During Pregnancy and Lactation

Adam L. Wendling

Introduction

Medication use during pregnancy and lactation is very common, yet understanding the potential impacts of such use on pregnancy, lactation, and fetal or neonatal development is far from complete. Very nearly every medication used during pregnancy and lactation has not been specifically tested in this population. This creates a paradox: many pregnant/lactating women use medications that have not been tested in their cohort, potentially leading to adverse events that may not be detected until thousands of patients have been exposed to the offending medications years later. In contrast, the lack of understanding and knowledge regarding these medications often results in fear of harm, which leads to the unnecessary avoidance of potentially beneficial medications during pregnancy and lactation. In this chapter, we will discuss the scope of the problem, pharmacologic factors potentially influencing drug transfer, and specific medications of concern in pregnancy and lactation.

Background

The Hippocratic Oath pledges physicians "to abstain from doing harm;" the Latin maxim *primum non nocere* means "first, do no harm." Physicians have used medications to try to cure disease, alleviate pain, and relieve suffering for literally thousands of years. In so doing, we have potentially exposed countless generations to risks that are not well understood. The history of two medications, diethylstilbestrol (DES) and thalidomide, has served as a glaring warning to society and resulted in a sea change in our approach to medication development and subsequent use.[1]

The use of DES was meant to reduce pregnancy complications such as preterm deliveries and pregnancy losses.[2] Later, it was recognized that exposed women suffered a 30% increase in breast cancer rates. Concomitantly, the female offspring of women who used DES during their pregnancies were found to have significant increases in rare genitourinary cancers. Female offspring exposed in utero to DES also suffered genitourinary tract malformations, increased infertility rates (nearly double that of unexposed women), and, among those exposed women who became pregnant, their pregnancies had a significantly higher rate of complications such as premature birth, miscarriage, and preeclampsia. The American Cancer Society estimates between 5 and 10 million people have been exposed to DES. In essence, DES exposure in utero has led to the suffering of more than two generations of people. Thalidomide was used between the years 1959 and 1962 to treat pregnancy-related morning sickness; later thalidomide-exposed offspring were found to have a significant increase in limb malformations and peripheral neuritis.

The story of these two drugs awakened society to both the immediate and delayed risks of medication exposure during pregnancy. In response, the US Food and Drug Administration in the 1970s introduced a policy of exclusion of women capable of becoming pregnant from phase I and II clinical trials, which had the result of excluding virtually all women from drug development. Since then, medication developed and tested on men was assumed to have the same outcomes on women. However, we know this to not be true: there are numerous pharmacokinetic and pharmacodynamic differences between men and women due to differences in body size and composition and hormone levels. For example, women have increased activity in cytochrome P3A4, which results in a decreased effect of a number of antidepressants, anxiolytics, opioids, and antiepileptic drugs. As a result, women potentially suffer from untreated or undertreated disease, which contributes to, at the very least, a disparity in health outcomes and, more than likely, adverse health outcomes.

The recognition of these differences has resulted in the gradual inclusion of women in medication trials. However, there remains a stark gap in knowledge of treatment outcomes for women, especially pregnant and breastfeeding women. Women represented less than 20% of subjects in industry-sponsored trials from the 1990s, and although this disparity in representation has decreased, between 2010 and 2012, only 45% of participants were women.[3] Still, of these industry-sponsored trials between 2010 and 2012, 95% explicitly excluded pregnant women. The teratogenicity of medications approved by the FDA from 2000 to 2010 was "undetermined" for 97.7%; there was "no data regarding safety in pregnancy" in 73.3% and "very limited data" for 19.2% (Figure 10.1).[4] The mean time between a drug being classified as "undetermined" to a more precise risk category

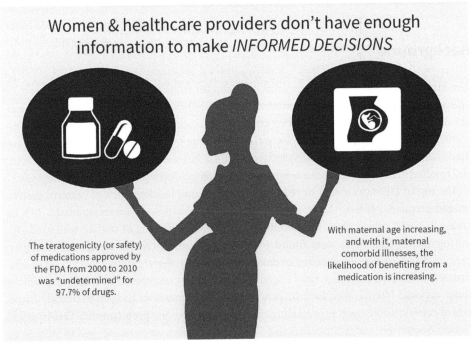

Figure 10.1 An aging maternal population with increasing comorbid illnesses is more likely to need a medication to manage a comorbid illness, but women and healthcare providers do not have enough knowledge of the effects of pregnancy on medication pharmacokinetics, or what is teratogenic and what is safe.

was 27 years. This lack of inclusion of pregnant women results in abundant "contraindications" and "special warnings" on medication labeling (potentially limiting the availability of safe and effective treatments), and treatments that are thought to be safe are years later found to in fact cause harm.

Scope of the Problem

Around the world, maternal age and comorbid conditions are increasing, thereby increasing the likelihood of women potentially benefiting from medication use during pregnancy and lactation. Today, it is commonly estimated that at least three out of five pregnant women use four to five medications during pregnancy (Figure 10.2). According to Stock and Norman, "In high-income countries, four out of five women are prescribed one or more medications during pregnancy and even more pregnant women self-medicate with both prescription and over-the-counter medications."[5] The safety of currently available medications is almost exclusively determined by surveillance studies after drug approval (pregnancy exposure registries), leading to a significant delay in the recognition of both safe and unsafe medications for use during pregnancy. Further, surveillance studies are invariably nonrandomized or lack any comparison group, thereby making it difficult to determine the impact of the condition meant to be treated versus the medication. These studies are frequently small, limiting their ability to detect anything but the largest treatment effects.

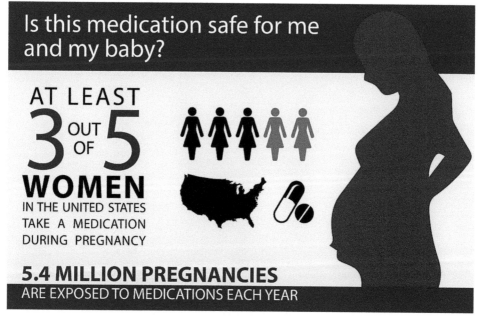

Figure 10.2 At least 3 out of 5 pregnant women use 4 to 5 medications during pregnancy despite the fact that the safety of currently available medications is almost exclusively determined by surveillance studies after drug approval, leading to a significant delay in the recognition of both safe and unsafe medications for use during pregnancy.

Rate of Pregnancy Loss and Major Birth Defects

Approximately 10 to 15% of all pregnancies result in miscarriage, while just under 1% result in stillbirth. The rate of miscarriage increases with maternal age, as does the rate of comorbid illnesses and medication use during pregnancy; this further complicates the detection of complications due to medication use versus age or comorbid illness. The Centers for Disease Control states that approximately 1 in 33 pregnancies is complicated by one or more birth defects.[6] Detecting adverse pregnancy outcomes that result from medication exposure during pregnancy is complicated by these frequently concomitant conditions.

Indications for Maternal Medication Use During Pregnancy and Lactation

As previously mentioned, maternal age and comorbid illnesses are increasing. Medication use during pregnancy may be necessary for the benefit of the mother, and thereby potentially benefit the fetus, since untreated maternal conditions frequently lead to adverse pregnancy outcomes. Conversely, because there are safe alternatives to breastfeeding, medication use during lactation may not have the same risk-to-benefit ratio (Figure 10.3).

Pharmacology of Drug Transfer During Pregnancy

Pregnancy Physiologic Changes and Impact on Pharmacokinetics and Pharmacodynamics

Numerous physiologic changes of pregnancy (Table 10.1) have the potential to impact drug pharmacokinetics.

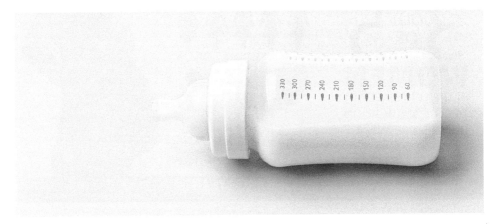

Figure 10.3 Frequently, there is no alternative to medication use during pregnancy for the benefit of the mother and thereby the benefit of the baby until delivery. After delivery, there are safe alternatives to breastfeeding when medication use is necessary for the mother.

Table 10.1 Physiologic Changes of Pregnancy and Their Results

Physiologic Change	Result
Decreased gastric emptying/gut motility	Increased time and potentially decreased peak levels
Decreased gastric pH	Decreased absorption
Increased vascularity of respiratory mucosa	Increased absorption of inhalational drugs
Increased minute ventilation leads to increased arterial pH	Decreased protein binding
Increased total body water	Increased volume of distribution of water-soluble drugs
Increased renal blood flow	Increased renal clearance of drugs
Decreased serum albumin leads to decreased protein binding	Increased free fraction of drugs
Increased cytochrome P450	Increased metabolism of drugs

There are also factors involved in antepartum medication exposure (Figure 10.4) and those involved in neonatal medication exposure during breastfeeding (Figure 10.5).

Gestational Age/Stage of Development

The timing of the exposure to medication during pregnancy or lactation has a degree of influence on the outcome. Generally speaking, exposure to truly teratogenic medications during the first trimester manifests as miscarriage; exposure during the second trimester (during organogenesis) may result in major malformations; and exposure during the third trimester may result in preterm labor and delivery, stillbirth, or other pregnancy

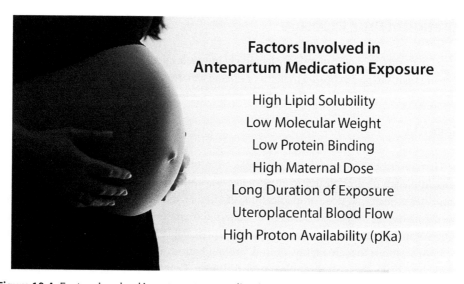

Figure 10.4 Factors involved in antepartum medication exposure.

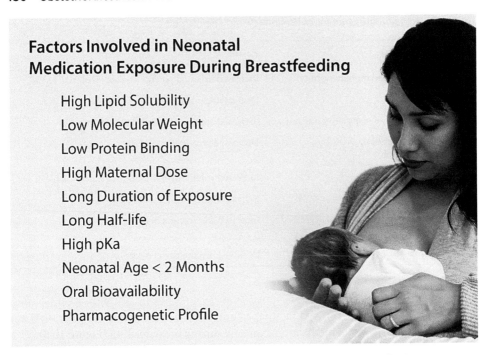

Factors Involved in Neonatal Medication Exposure During Breastfeeding

High Lipid Solubility

Low Molecular Weight

Low Protein Binding

High Maternal Dose

Long Duration of Exposure

Long Half-life

High pKa

Neonatal Age < 2 Months

Oral Bioavailability

Pharmacogenetic Profile

Figure 10.5 Factors involved in neonatal medication exposure during breastfeeding.

complications (see "Specific Medications"). Exposure during lactation is similar, with younger, smaller neonates potentially at greater risk due to factors such as smaller size, an immature liver, and reduced protein binding. Adverse events due to medication exposure through lactation primarily occur in neonates less than 2 months of age and are uncommon after the age of 6 months.[7]

Duration of Drug Exposure

A brief exposure to medication is far less likely to result in detectable manifestations in the offspring than a longer exposure in utero or during lactation.

Placenta

The characteristics of the placenta, uteroplacental blood flow, maternal plasma, and fetal status influence fetal exposure to maternally administered medications.[8] The higher the administered maternal dose of medication, the higher the chance for fetal/neonatal exposure. Similarly, the longer the duration of maternal treatment, the higher fetal/neonatal exposure. Maternal medications cross the placenta primarily through passive diffusion (Figure 10.6). Medications that are highly ionized, protein bound, and of high molecular weight are less likely to reach the fetus through passive diffusion. Conversely, medications that are lipid soluble are more likely to reach the fetus. Some medications are transported by facilitated

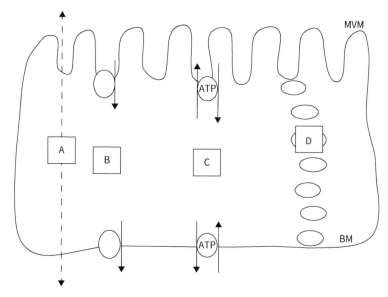

Figure 10.6 Diagram showing mechanisms of placental drug transfer: (A) simple diffusion; (B) facilitated diffusion using a carrier; (C) active transport using ATP; (D) pinocytosis. BM = basal membrane of the syncytiotrophoblast, MVM = microvillous membrane of the syncytiotrophoblast.

Adapted from a diagram in Desforges and Sibley with permission from the International Journal of Developmental Biology. Copyright obtained from BJA Education.

diffusion. These medications tend to be related to endogenous compounds such as glucocorticoids and cephalosporins. For only a few medications are there known active transports through the placenta; most rely on passive diffusion. Active transport across the placenta involves energy expenditure to move medications into the fetal circulation. Drugs with known active transport include dopamine, norepinephrine, and digoxin. Uteroplacental blood flow directly correlates to drug exposure to the fetus. Elimination of medications after they have reached the fetus occurs primarily through redistribution back to the maternal circulation and clearance from maternal blood. Frequently, drugs that rely on passive diffusion will become ionized in the obligatory lower pH environment of the fetus, delaying their redistribution out of the fetus to the mother.

Medication Use and Lactation

Many of the same factors involved in antenatal medication exposure are similar to maternal medication use during lactation, with some additional factors. In general, maternal medication use during lactation results in far lower neonatal exposure than occurs during the antepartum period. Pharmacologic characteristics that increase drug transfer into breast milk include high lipid solubility, low protein binding, lack of ionization, low molecular weight, and long half-life. Increasing the maternal dose and duration of exposure increases the drug accumulation into breast milk. Certain medications may alter or reduce breast milk production (such as antihistamines, anticholinergics, estrogen-containing

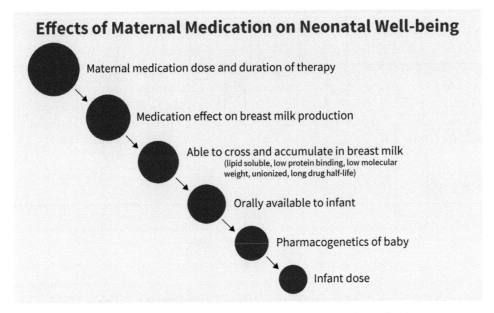

Effects of Maternal Medication on Neonatal Well-being

Maternal medication dose and duration of therapy

Medication effect on breast milk production

Able to cross and accumulate in breast milk
(lipid soluble, low protein binding, low molecular
weight, unionized, long drug half-life)

Orally available to infant

Pharmacogenetics of baby

Infant dose

Figure 10.7   Diagram illustrating the effect of medication on breastmilk production.

substances, and uncommonly dopaminergic medications). Factors that are unique concerns regarding neonatal drug exposure from breastmilk include the oral bioavailability of the excreted drug, the age and condition of the neonate, and drug pharmacogenetics (Figure 10.7). Not only must a drug accumulate in breastmilk—it also must be orally bioavailable to the neonate. The risks of adverse reactions are greater among premature neonates or neonates with significant chronic medical illnesses. Neonates with specific genetic profiles such as cytochrome P450 2D6 ultra-rapid metabolizers may have dramatically different reactions to medications than the mother (see the reference to codeine in "Specific Medications").

Specific Medications

Warfarin

Maternal warfarin use may be indicated due to conditions such as thromboprophylaxis in the setting of mechanical heart valves (especially mechanical mitral valves), where alternate anticoagulants have been found to be inferior. Warfarin has similar anticoagulant effects in the fetus. Warfarin exposure during the first trimester frequently results in either miscarriage or inhibition of fetal bone growth, and later exposure may lead to serious, frequently fatal, fetal and maternal hemorrhagic complications (fetal hemorrhage in utero or intracranial hemorrhage during birth; life-threatening maternal postpartum hemorrhage). Warfarin has very low levels of excretion into breastmilk and no measurable anticoagulant effect among breastfed neonates whose mothers consumed up to 12 mg per day.[9]

Insulin

Due to insulin's high molecular weight, there is no known direct fetal exposure to maternally administered insulin. Conversely, maternal insulin administration may reduce maternal blood glucose levels. Blood glucose rapidly crosses the placenta and un- or undertreated maternal hyperglycemia has obvious immediate and delayed adverse impacts on the pregnancy and the fetus.

Heparin

Pregnancy-related physiologic changes have a significant impact on the pharmacokinetics of heparin that include pregnancy-related thrombophilia and decreases in circulating antithrombin to an increased volume of distribution and increased clearance. These pregnancy-related changes result in increased dosing requirements for a therapeutic effect. Similar to insulin, both unfractionated and low-molecular-weight heparin have sufficiently high molecular weight and polarization that neither cross the placenta nor accumulate in breastmilk.

Steroids

Corticosteroids pass through the placenta through facilitated diffusion. Older data suggested a possible link between maternal corticosteroid use and cleft lip, as well as adverse pregnancy outcomes such as gestational diabetes. However, the association between corticosteroid use and cleft lip is limited at best, and the indication for maternal corticosteroid use must be considered. For example, corticosteroids are frequently administered for maternal autoimmune disorders, and untreated disease may have serious maternal health impacts. During breastfeeding, no neonatal adverse effects from maternal corticosteroid administration have been detected.

Opioids

Chemically, opioids possess many of the characteristics that lead to in-utero exposure and accumulation in breastmilk. Limited evidence hints at chronic in-utero exposure to opioids during the first trimester being associated with an increase in the incidence of neural tube defects; however, the absolute increased risk is small and inconsistently detected.[10] In women maintained on buprenorphine or methadone for opioid use disorder, no increase in malformations has been detected. Conversely, women with untreated substance abuse disorder frequently suffer adverse pregnancy outcomes, including intrauterine growth restriction, preterm labor and delivery, abruption, and fetal death. It is recommended that pregnant women with opioid use disorder undergo opioid agonist therapy rather than medically supervised withdrawal because of the risk of relapse and adverse outcomes with substance abuse. Due to increased hepatic clearance, methadone requirements to prevent withdrawal symptoms typically increase during pregnancy. Regarding lactation, although

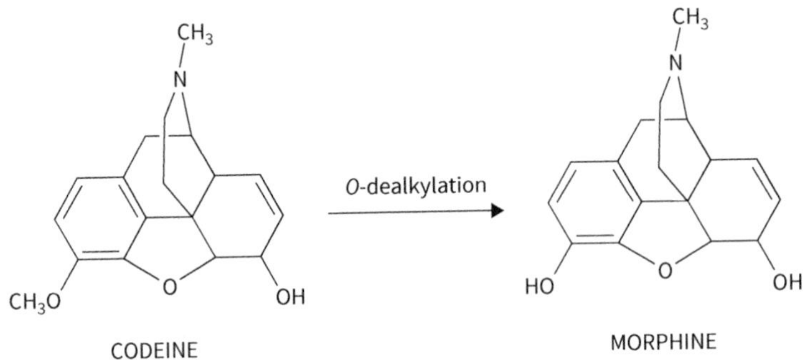

Figure 10.8 Five percent of the population are null metabolizers and will not make any morphine from codeine. Another 5% of the population are ultrarapid metabolizers and will take all of the codeine and make it into morphine. The worst possible combination is that the mother is a null metabolizer and ingests a large amount of codeine without analgesic effect and the breastfeeding baby is an ultrarapid metabolizer, taking all of that codeine in breastmilk and turning it all into morphine. O-dealkylation is by CYP450 2D6.

many opioids are excreted into breastmilk, once present in breastmilk, not all opioids are orally bioavailable to the neonate. Generally speaking, women stable on chronic opioid agonist therapy should be encouraged to breastfeed due to the benefits, including reduced neonatal abstinence syndrome.[9] The Agency for Healthcare Research and Quality guideline for analgesia in the breastfeeding mother states, in reference to opioid analgesics in opioid-naïve mothers, that "In general, opioids of any type should be used with caution and for the shortest reasonable course in a breastfeeding mother."[11] One in five breastfeeding neonates of mothers prescribed oxycodone experienced sedation. Limit the dose of hydrocodone and oxycodone analgesics to less than 30 mg/day for less than 4 days whenever possible. Meperidine has active metabolites that accumulate in breastmilk. Codeine and tramadol require metabolism by cytochrome p450 to the active drug; approximately 5% of the population are ultra-rapid metabolizers, converting all of the prodrug to the active form and may experience excessive sedation and respiratory depression after routine dosages. Consequently, codeine and tramadol are not recommended for breastfeeding mothers (Figure 10.8).

Benzodiazepines

Early studies of diazepam exposure suggested an increased incidence of cleft palate among exposed neonates. Other studies revealed that prenatal exposure to benzodiazepines increased the incidence of cleft palate from 6 out of 1000 to 7 out of 1000 births. Other studies were unable to detect any impact of in utero benzodiazepine exposure on congenital malformations. However, in-utero exposure does increase the risk of "neonatal floppy baby syndrome" and neonatal withdrawal. Neonatal withdrawal may occur for up to 3 months after birth. Breastfeeding while on benzodiazepines may typically be continued unless the neonate develops symptoms of depression.

Nonsteroidal Anti-inflammatory Drugs

Exposure to nonsteroidal anti-inflammatory drugs (NSAIDs) early in pregnancy may increase the risk of miscarriage and malformations. The use of NSAIDs after 30 weeks of gestation may result in the temporary closure of the ductus arteriosus of unclear significance and oligohydramnios. Indomethacin is still used as tocolytic therapy where the benefit of prolonging the pregnancy is deemed to outweigh the risk. Ibuprofen is excreted into breastmilk in very low levels, far below the dose that is deemed safe in neonates.

Antidepressants

The physiologic changes of pregnancy contribute to a decreased serum concentration of common selective serotonin reuptake inhibitors (SSRIs), selective norepinephrine reuptake inhibitors (SNRIs), and tricyclic antidepressants (TCAs). The SSRI paroxetine has a possible association with cardiac malformations, craniosynostosis, omphalocele, and anencephaly.[12] The SSRI sertraline has a possible association with cardiac malformations and omphalocele. These associations are weak and inconsistently found in surveillance studies. Neonates may experience a transient withdrawal syndrome from SSRIs manifested by jitteriness, mild respiratory distress, weak cry, and poor tone. TCAs may be associated with limb abnormalities and a transient withdrawal syndrome similar to SSRIs. Again, these associations are weak and inconsistent. SNRIs and atypical antidepressants have not been found to be associated with any adverse outcome. These medications are transferred into breastmilk at very low levels that are not likely to be clinically relevant.

Antiepileptics/Mood Stabilizers

Lithium seems to increase the risk of congenital heart disease, especially Ebstein's abnormality, in exposed neonates. Breastfeeding infants of mothers taking lithium have been found to have neonatal depression. Lithium treatment generally contraindicates breastfeeding due to neonatal depression. Valproate has been linked to neural tube defects, limb and facial abnormalities, cardiac defects, and long-term cognitive defects. Carbamazepine has been associated with facial abnormalities and fingernail hypoplasia. Lamotrigine has not been associated with congenital abnormalities.

Antihypertensive Agents

All hypertensive agents have been associated with neonates that are small for their gestational age, low birth weight, and preterm birth. Labetolol treatment has a tenuous link to attention deficit disorder in exposed offspring. A very limited body of evidence suggests an increased incidence of sleep disorders in offspring exposed in utero to methyldopa and clonidine.[13] These findings are derived from study designs that cannot differentiate the impact of hypertension from the impact of treatment of hypertension; just having hypertension may lead to these outcomes just as easily as the treatment of hypertension. Even the commonly held assumption that angiotensin-converting enzyme inhibitors and angiotensin receptor blockers result in miscarriages and fetal malformations is based on limited data. Un- or undertreated maternal hypertension poses significant risk to both mother and fetus, so risks of treatment must be balanced against risks of an untreated medical condition.

Summary/Recommendations

In the past, mothers and neonates have been harmed by medication use during pregnancy and lactation (e.g., DES, thalidomide, and codeine). However, mothers and neonates continue to potentially suffer from either withholding beneficial treatments or using medications with an incomplete knowledge of the risk(s). Whenever possible, the risk of potential fetal or neonatal harm should be weighed against the risk of harm due to untreated disease. The physiologic changes of pregnancy alter the pharmacokinetics of several medications. Generally speaking, the lowest effective dose of a single agent for the shortest duration feasible is likely the safest choice. While the likely neonatal exposure in breastmilk to maternal medications is less than that during pregnancy, the risk-to-benefit analysis is skewed by the fact that there are alternatives to breastfeeding while there is not an alternative to pregnancy until delivery.

References

1. Yakerson A. Women in clinical trials: a review of policy development and health equity in the Canadian context. *J Equity Health*. 2019;18:56.
2. American Cancer Society. DES exposure: questions and answers. Available at https://www.cancer.org/cancer/cancer-causes/medical-treatments/des-exposure.html. Accessed October 11, 2019.
3. Shields KE, Lyerly AD. Exclusion of pregnant women from industry sponsored clinical trials. *J Obstet Gynaecol*. 2013;122:1077–1081.
4. Adam MP, Plifka JE, Friedman JM. Evolving knowledge of the teratogenicity of medications in human pregnancy. *Am J Med Genet C Semin Med Genet*. 2011;157:175–182.
5. Stock SJ, Norman JE. Medicines in pregnancy. *F1000 Res*. 2019;8:211.
6. National Center on Birth Defects and Developmental Disabilities, Centers for Disease Control and Prevention. Data & statistics on birth defects. Available at https://www.cdc.gov/ncbddd/birthdefects/data.html. Accessed October 11, 2019.
7. Sachs HC, Committee on Drugs. The transfer of drugs and therapeutics into human breast milk: an update on selected topics. *Pediatrics*. 2013;132:e796–e809.
8. Griffiths SK, Campbell JP. Placental structure, function and drug transfer. *Contin Educ Anaesth Crit Care Pain*. 2015;15:84–89.
9. Drugs and Lactation Database (LactMed) [Internet]. Bethesda, MD: National Library of Medicine (US); 2006-2018. Available at: https://www.ncbi.nlm.nih.gov/books/NBK501137/. Accessed October 25, 2019.

10. Mascola MA, Borders AE, Terplan M. Committee Opinion No. 711. American College of Obstetricians and Gynecologists. *Obstet Gynecol.* 2017;130:e81–e94.

11. Agency for Healthcare Research and Quality National Guideline Clearinghouse. Analgesia and anesthesia for the breastfeeding mother, revised 2012. Available at https://www.guidelinecentral.com/summaries/analgesia-and-anesthesia-for-the-breastfeeding-mother-revised-2012/#section-society. Accessed October 25, 2019.

12. ACOG Committee on Practice Bulletins. Committee opinion number 711. Use of psychiatric medications during pregnancy and lactation. *Obstet Gynecol.* 2017;130:e81–e94.

13. Fitton CA, Steiner MFC, Aucott L, et al. In-utero exposure to antihypertensive medication and neonatal child health outcomes. *J Hypertens.* 2017;35:2123–2137.

11
Local Anesthetics

Michelle Eddins

Introduction

Within the realm of obstetric anesthesiology, local anesthetics are most commonly used in conjunction with neuraxial techniques (spinal, epidural, combined spinal epidural) to achieve labor analgesia as well as surgical anesthesia. They are also used for pudendal nerve blocks and for soft tissue infiltration (cervical/vaginal laceration repair, cesarean section incision, etc.). Local anesthetics work by transiently inhibiting sensory, motor, and autonomic nerve impulses, thereby allowing obstetric patients to deliver comfortably. With local anesthetics being the most widely used pharmacologic anesthetic agent in obstetric anesthesiology, it is imperative that the anesthesia provider be well versed in the clinical application of these agents.

Mechanism of Action

Local anesthetics work by binding to and inhibiting voltage-gated sodium channels on axonal nerve fibers.[1] Under normal conditions, the neural membrane has a negative resting potential of -90 mV.[2] This negative membrane potential is due to the outward transport of sodium ions (Na+) and the inward transport of potassium ions (K+), as well as the relatively permeability of the membrane to potassium and its relative impermeability to sodium.[2] With nerve excitation, membrane permeability to sodium ions increases, resulting in an influx of sodium and an increase in the resting membrane potential. If the threshold potential is reached, depolarization occurs.[2] Blockage of sodium channels by local anesthetics inhibits the sodium influx that is required for membrane depolarization and achievement of an action potential.[2]

Classification

There are two major types of local anesthetics—the aminoamides and the aminoesters.[1] These two groups differ based on their chemical structure and mode of metabolism.[1]

All local anesthetics consist of a desaturated carbon ring and a tertiary amine connected by an alkyl chain.[2] The aminoester group of local anesthetics consists of an ester linkage that connects the carbon ring to the alkyl chain and tertiary amine, whereas the aminoamide group consists of an amide linkage (Figure 11.1).

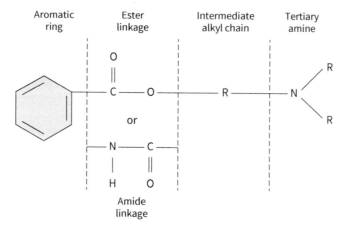

Figure 11.1 Local anesthetic molecular structure.

From: Bucklin BA, Santos AC. Local anesthetics and opioids. In: Chestnut DH, Wong CA, Tsen LC, Ngan Kee WD, Beilin Y, Mhyre JM, Bateman BT, eds. *Chestnut's obstetric anesthesia: principles and practice.* 6th ed. Philadelphia, PA: Elsevier; 2020:271.

The aminoesters are metabolized by plasma pseudocholinesterase, and, therefore, have a shorter duration of action compared to the aminoamide group, which undergoes hepatic metabolism.[3]

Both groups of local anesthetics have four main physiochemical properties that determine their pharmacokinetics—molecular weight, pKa, lipid solubility, and protein binding (Table 11.1).

Table 11.1 Physiochemical Properties of Local Anesthetics Commonly Used in Obstetric Anesthesia

	Molecular Weight (Base) (Da)	pK_a	Lipid Solubility	% Protein Bound
Esters:				
2-Chloroprocaine	271	8.9	0.14	–
Tetracaine	264	8.6	4.1	–
Amides:				
Lidocaine	234	7.9	2.9	64
Bupivacaine (and levobupivacaine)	288	8.2	28	96
Ropivacaine	274	8.0	3	90–5

Modified From Bucklin BA, Santos AC. Local Anesthetics and Opioids. In: Chestnut DH, Wong CA, Tsen LC, Ngan Kee WD, Beilin Y, Mhyre JM, Bateman BT, eds. *Chestnut's obstetric anesthesia: principles and practice.* 6th ed. Philadelphia, PA: Elsevier; 2020: 271.

Table 11.2 Local Anesthetics Commonly Used for Spinal Anesthesia

Drug	Dose (mg)			Duration (min)		
	Concentration (%)	T10	T4	Time to Onset (min)	Plain	Epinephrine (0.2 mg)
Lidocaine	5*	40–50	60–75	2–4	45–75	NR
Tetracaine	0.5	8–10	12–15	4–6	60–120	120–180
Bupivacaine	0.5–0.75	8–10	12–15	4–6	60–120	NR
Ropivacaine	0.5–0.75	10–14	15–20	-6	60–90	NR
Chloroprocaine	2–3	40–50	60	2–4	30–60	NR

*Must be diluted to 2.5% or less before administration.

NR = not recommended.

From Drasner K, Larson MD. Spinal and epidural anesthesia. In: Miller RD, Pardo, Jr. MC, eds. *Basics of anesthesia.* 6th ed. Philadelphia, PA: Elsevier; 2011: 266.

Local anesthetics typically used for spinal anesthesia include lidocaine, tetracaine, bupivacaine, ropivacaine, and chloroprocaine (Table 11.2). For epidural anesthesia, chloroprocaine, lidocaine, bupivacaine, and ropivacaine are most commonly used (Table 11.3).

Aminoamides

Lidocaine

Lidocaine has an intermediate onset and duration of action. It is routinely used for epidural analgesia and anesthesia.[4] Lidocaine is rarely used for subarachnoid anesthesia, due to the high incidence of transient neurologic symptoms (TNS).[5] TNS is the result of direct neurotoxicity of the lumbosacral nerves and is characterized by severe lower back pain and dysesthesia that radiates to the buttock and lower extremities.

Table 11.3 Local Anesthetics Commonly Used for Epidural Anesthesia

Drug	Duration (min)			
	Concentration (%)	Time to Onset (min)	Plain	Epinephrine (1:200,000)
Chloroprocaine	2–3	5–10	45–60	60–90
Lidocaine	1–2	10–15	60–120	90–180
Bupivacaine	0.25–0.5	15–20	120–200	150–240
Ropivacaine	0.25–1.0	10–20	120–180	150–200

From Drasner K, Larson MD. Spinal and epidural anesthesia. In: Miller RD, Pardo, Jr. MC, eds. *Basics of anesthesia.* 6th ed. Philadelphia, PA: Elsevier; 2011: 277.

Bupivacaine

Bupivacaine is the most widely used local anesthetic for labor epidural analgesia due to its prolonged duration of action and its ability to provide sensory blockade that outlasts the intensity and duration of its motor blockade.[5] It is also the agent that is most commonly used for spinal anesthesia due to its lack of association with TNS.[5]

Ropivacaine

Ropivacaine is the S enantiomer of bupivacaine.[6] It is less cardiotoxic and has a more preferential sensorimotor differential blockade (more motor sparing) compared to bupivacaine.[5] It has intrinsic vasoconstrictive properties, which likely contributes to its reduced cardiotoxicity.[5] The potency of ropivacaine is 61% that of bupivacaine for labor analgesia.[1]

Aminoesters

2-Chloroprocaine

2-Chloroprocaine is most commonly used when rapid surgical epidural anesthesia must be obtained, such as an urgent cesarean section.[5] It is formulated in high concentrations of 2% and 3% due to its relatively low potency. Despite its high pKa, it has a fast onset of action due to this high concentration.[4] Its rapid metabolism by plasma pseudocholinesterase makes the risk of systemic toxicity low despite its high concentration.[4] Many clinicians reserve the use of chloroprocaine exclusively for urgent cases due to the fact that it impairs the analgesic effects of epidural bupivacaine and opioids administered concurrently or subsequently thereafter. Currently, 2-chloroprocaine is only FDA approved for epidural administration.[5] This is due to neurotoxic injury that has occurred with subarachnoid administration.[5] It is believed that the preservative, sodium bisulfite, is responsible for this neurotoxicity.[5] Preservative-free formulations of 2-chloroprocaine are available, but its use for spinal anesthesia remains off-label in the United States.[5]

Tetracaine

Tetracaine is commonly used for spinal anesthesia.[5] It has a long duration of action, especially with the addition of a vasoconstrictor. Although it is an ester, it has a relatively slow rate of metabolism (about one tenth that of chloroprocaine). It is rarely used for epidural anesthesia due to its profound motor blockade and slow onset of action.[6]

Adjuvants

Epinephrine

Epinephrine is a vasoconstrictor that is commonly added to local anesthetics. By inducing local vasoconstriction, epinephrine reduces systemic absorption of the local anesthetic, thereby, prolonging its duration of action.[6] Slowing systemic absorption also reduces the risk of toxicity. Epinephrine is most commonly added to lidocaine.[6] The duration of epidural anesthesia with lidocaine is doubled with the addition of an epinephrine concentration of 5 mcg/ml (1:200,000).[5] Due to the long duration of action of both bupivacaine and ropivacaine, epinephrine is not routinely added to these local anesthetics.[6]

Via its central α_2 adrenergic agonist affects, epinephrine also increases the intensity of epidural analgesia.[1] These receptors are located in superficial laminae of the spinal cord as well as several brainstem nuclei.[1]

Epinephrine also serves as an intravascular marker, allowing for early detection of inadvertent administration of local anesthetic intravenously. Inadvertent intravenous administration of lidocaine with epinephrine will result in hypertension and tachycardia. Epinephrine's α_1 adrenergic agonistic effects produce vasoconstriction and hypertension, whereas its β_2 adrenergic agonistic effects result in tachycardia.[1]

> **Important!** Prior to the initiation of epidural analgesia or anesthesia, a test dose of 3 ml of 1.5% lidocaine with 1:200,000 epinephrine should be administered to check for inadvertent intravascular injection. An increase in heart rate or blood pressure by 20% or more defines a positive test dose. In addition to the hemodynamic changes that result from the epinephrine, patients may also complain of dizziness, tinnitus, circumoral numbness, or metallic taste due to the systemic effects of the local anesthetic itself. In the event of a positive test dose, the intravascular catheter should be removed immediately.

Sodium Bicarbonate

Sodium Bicarbonate can be added to local anesthetics to raise the pH, which brings the pH closer to the pKa. The closer the pH is to the pKa, the higher the proportion of the drug exists in the unionized form.[2] Only the unionized form of the local anesthetic can penetrate the nerve sheath and cell membrane, thus blocking nerve conduction (Figure 11.2). Therefore, the addition of sodium bicarbonate to local anesthetics increases the amount of the unionized form of the local anesthetic, which hastens the onset of action of nerve blockade.[6] The addition of sodium bicarbonate tends to have the greatest effect on local anesthetics containing epinephrine, because of the more acidic formulation by which they are manufactured.[1] For plain lidocaine, bupivacaine, and 2-chloroprocaine, alkalization with sodium bicarbonate hastens the onset of action by approximately 10 minutes.[1] For ropivacaine, however, the addition of sodium bicarbonate has no effect on onset of action.[1]

> **Warning!** Alkalization of local anesthetics with the addition of sodium bicarbonate can result in precipitation of the local anesthetic. Bupivacaine in particular has a narrow margin of safety between successful alkalization and precipitation. Always inspect the local anesthetic for precipitation prior to administration.

Sodium bicarbonate is not produced premixed with local anesthetics by manufacturers and therefore, must be mixed by the clinician. When performing alkalization of local anesthetics, 8.4% sodium bicarbonate (1mEq/mL) should be used.[1] The mixture should then be administered soon after it is prepared.

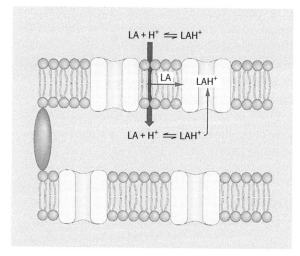

Figure 11.2 Diffusion of unionized form of local anesthetic across nerve sheath.
From: Drasner, K. Local Anesthetics. In: Miller RD, Pardo, Jr. MC, eds. *Basics of anesthesia*. 6th ed. Philadelphia, PA: Elsevier; 2011:131.

The amount of sodium bicarbonate needed to effectively raise the pH varies by local anesthetic (Table 11.4).

Local Anesthetic Systemic Toxicity

Systemic absorption of high levels of local anesthetic can result in local anesthetic systemic toxicity (LAST).[1] In general, pregnancy results in increased sensitivity to local anesthetics.[1] Therefore, staying under the maximum dose of a particular anesthetic is critical in preventing toxicity.[1] Toxicity usually occurs in the context of inadvertent intravenous administration of local anesthetics intended for neuraxial use. Therefore, a test dose should always be performed prior to the initiation of epidural analgesia or anesthesia. LAST can also occur when large doses of local anesthetic are rapidly administered through the epidural catheter or when standard doses of aminoamide local anesthetics are administered to patients with impaired liver function due to slowed hepatic clearance.

Table 11.4 Amount (mL) of Sodium Bicarbonate Needed to Effectively Raise the pH of Various Local Anesthetics

Local Anesthetic	Sodium Bicarbonate (mL)
Lidocaine	10.0
Bupivacaine	0.1
1-Chloroprocaine	0.3

From Bucklin BA, Santos AC. Local anesthetics and opioids. In: Chestnut DH, Wong CA, Tsen LC, Ngan Kee WD, Beilin Y, Mhyre JM, Bateman BT, eds. Chestnut's obstetric anesthesia: principles and practice. 6th ed. Philadelphia, PA: Elsevier; 2020: 299.

Toxicity occurs most commonly with aminoamide local anesthetics due to their long duration of action compared to aminoesters.[1] Aminoester local anesthetics are rapidly metabolized in the blood stream by RBC esterases, therefore blood concentration levels do not become high enough to cause LAST.[7] Ranking of commonly used local anesthetics in obstetric practice from most toxic to least toxic are as follows: bupivacaine, ropivacaine, lidocaine, and 2-chloroprocaine.[1] Bupivacaine's potent neurotoxicity is due to its high lipid solubility, which facilitates rapid transport across the blood-brain barrier. The profound cardiotoxicity of bupivacaine, however, is due to its strong affinity for myocardial sodium channels.

Signs and Symptoms

Local anesthetics exert toxic systemic effects via blockade of voltage-gated sodium channels.[4] The two systems that are affected by LAST are the central nervous system (CNS) and cardiovascular system.[4] CNS sequelae usually present first due to the high sensitivity of the CNS to local anesthetics.[1] The severity of CNS symptoms is proportional to the local anesthetic concentration in the bloodstream. This relationship has been well-defined for lidocaine (Figure 11.3). If toxicity is not recognized and treated, cardiovascular collapse quickly ensues.

Initial CNS symptoms include tinnitus, circumoral numbness, facial twitching, metallic taste in the mouth, and vertigo.[3] As local anesthetic plasma concentrations rise, CNS excitation occurs in the form of tonic-clonic seizures.[3] This initial excitatory phase is due to

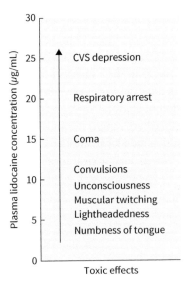

Figure 11.3 Signs and symptoms of local anesthetic systemic toxicity with increasing plasma concentrations of lidocaine.

From: Bucklin BA, Santos AC. Local Anesthetics and Opioids. In: Chestnut DH, Wong CA, Tsen LC, Ngan Kee WD, Beilin Y, Mhyre JM, Bateman BT, eds. Chestnut's *Obstetric anesthesia: principles and practice*. 6th ed. Philadelphia, PA: Elsevier; 2020:275.

blockade of specific cortical inhibitory receptors by the local anesthetic.[1] Further increase in local anesthetic concentration results in CNS depression due to blockade of both inhibitory and excitatory pathways.[1] This CNS depression typically presents as loss of consciousness.

As LAST progresses, cardiovascular collapse quickly follows neurologic toxicity.[7] Profound hypotension develops due to both arteriolar vascular smooth muscle relaxation as well as direct myocardial depression.[7] Blockade of sodium ion channels on cardiac myocytes results in impaired conduction and automaticity. Early electrocardiogram findings typically include a prolonged PR interval and widening of the QRS complex.[7] Delayed conduction can lead to severe sinus bradycardia and even asystole. Ventricular arrhythmias most commonly occur with bupivacaine toxicity.[1]

Treatment

The treatment for LAST is 20% lipid emulsion.[1] Intravenous lipid emulsion essentially functions as a "lipid sink" by actively binding to lipophilic local anesthetics, thereby reducing the overall plasma concentration.[1] An initial bolus dose of 1.5 ml/kg (approximately 100 ml for average 70 kg adult) should be immediately administered at the first signs of LAST.[1] An infusion of 0.25 ml/kg/min should then be initiated.[1] Up to two additional boluses may be administered in the setting of persistent cardiovascular collapse.[7]

> **Warning!** Although propofol is a lipid containing agent, it should **NOT** be used as a substitute for 20% lipid emulsion. The actual lipid concentration of propofol is so low that enormous amounts of propofol would have to be administered to successfully treat LAST. In addition, propofol will exacerbate the cardiovascular collapse present in the setting of local anesthetic toxicity.

In addition to the administration of 20% lipid emulsion, the patient's airway, breathing, and circulation must be supported. Administer 100% oxygen to the patient. If the patient has inadequate respiratory effort, proceed with bag mask ventilation or tracheal intubation. Seizure activity should be terminated as quickly as possible with the administration of a benzodiazepine.[1] Advanced cardiac life support should be instituted in the setting of hemodynamic instability. There are, however, a few modifications that should occur in the setting of LAST. The epinephrine dose should be reduced to < 1 mcg/kg.[7] Vasopressin, beta blockers, calcium channel blockers, and local anesthetics must be avoided.[7]

LAST typically requires prolonged resuscitation, and cardiopulmonary bypass may be necessary.[1] Therefore, it is important to alert the nearest facility with cardiopulmonary bypass capabilities as soon as resuscitative efforts begin. If return of spontaneous circulation has not been achieved within 5 minutes of cardiac arrest, then a perimortem cesarean section should be performed at the bedside.[1] Delivery of the fetus increases the effectiveness of maternal resuscitative efforts by relieving aortocaval compression and improves outcomes for both mother and baby.[1]

The American Society of Regional Anesthesia and Pain Medicine has created a checklist for the management of LAST (Box 11.1). All cases of LAST should be reported to the national database at www.lipidrescue.org.

Box 11.1 Management of Local Anesthetic Systemic Toxicity

- Stop injecting local anesthetic.
- Call for help.
- Position patient with left uterine displacement.
- Prepare for emergency delivery. Consider delivery of the infant if the mother is not resuscitated within several minutes.
- Administer 20% lipid emulsion administration at the first sign of LAST.
  - Bolus: 1.5ml/kg over 2–3 min (approximately 100ml)
  - Infusion: 200–250 ml over 15–20 min
  - Repeat bolus dose once or twice for persistent cardiovascular collapse
  - Recommended maximum dose: 12 ml/kg
- Control seizure (benzodiazepine is preferred). Beware that hypoxemia and acidosis develop rapidly during a seizure.
- Alert the nearest facility capable of cardiopulmonary bypass.
- Monitor maternal vital signs and fetal heart rate.
- Support maternal blood pressure with fluids and pressures.
- Initiate advanced cardiac life support.
  - **AVOID** vasopressin, calcium entry-blocking agents, beta-adrenergic receptor antagonist, and local anesthetics.
  - **REDUCE** individual epinephrine doses to less than 1 mcg/kg.

Modified from Bucklin BA, Santos AC. Local anesthetics and opioids. In: Chestnut DH, Wong CA, Tsen LC, Ngan Kee WD, Beilin Y, Mhyre JM, Bateman BT, eds. *Chestnut's obstetric anesthesia: principles and practice.* 6th ed. Philadelphia, PA: Elsevier; 2020: 277.

Allergic Reactions

Allergic reactions to local anesthetics are rare to occur. Less than 1% of adverse reactions to local anesthetics are anaphylactic in nature.[6] The aminoester local anesthetics trigger allergic reactions more commonly than the aminoamides due to the fact that aminoesters produce the metabolite para-aminobenzoic acid.[6] Cross sensitivity does not occur between the two classes of local anesthetics. Therefore, patients who are allergic to aminoester local anesthetics can still receive aminoamide local anesthetics. However, allergic reactions to aminoamide local anesthetics can still occur if the preservative methylparaben is used.[6] This is because methylparaben is structurally similar to para-aminobenzoic acid. Should anaphylaxis to a local anesthetic occur, administer epinephrine and support the patient's airway, breathing, and circulation.

References

1. Bucklin BA, Santos AC. Local anesthetics and opioids. In: Chestnut DH, Wong CA, Tsen LC, et al., eds. Chestnut's obstetric anesthesia: principles and practice. 6th ed. Philadelphia, PA: Elsevier; 2020:271–311.

2. Butterworth JF, Mackey DC, Wasnick JD. Local anesthetics. In: *Morgan and Mikhail's clinical anesthesiology.* 5th ed. United States: McGraw-Hill Education; 2013:263–276.

3. Cunningham FG, Leveno KJ, Bloom SL, et al. Obstetrical analgesia and anesthesia. In: *Williams obstetrics.* 25th ed. United States: McGraw-Hill Education; 2018:485–502.

4. Drasner K. Local anesthetics. In: Miller RD, Pardo MC Jr., eds. *Basics of anesthesia.* 6th ed. Philadelphia, PA: Elsevier; 2011:130–142.

5. Drasner K, Larson MD. Spinal and epidural anesthesia. In: Miller RD, Pardo MC Jr., eds. *Basics of anesthesia.* 6th ed. Philadelphia, PA: Elsevier; 2011:253–283.

6. Freeman BS. Local anesthetics. In: Freeman, BS, Berger JS, eds. *Anesthesiology core review.* United States: McGraw-Hill Education; 2014:161–165.

7. Salinas F, Local anesthetics. In: Barash PG, Cullen BF, Stoelting RK, et al., eds. *Clinical anesthesia fundamentals.* Philadelphia, PA: Wolters Kluwer; 2015:209–227.

12
Opioid Analgesia

Najmeh Izadpanah, Seung Lee, Kanchana Gattu, and Blake Watterworth

Introduction

The field of obstetric anesthesiology began in 1847 with the use of ether for labor analgesia by an obstetrician named James Young Simpson. There were concerns over the safety of ether during labor and its effects on the fetus. Subsequently "twilight sleep," which was a combination of morphine and scopolamine, was used for labor analgesia but lost its appeal due to concern for neonatal sedation. General anesthesia was used for cesarean sections in the mid-twentieth century but was associated with both maternal and fetal complications such as failed endotracheal intubations, maternal aspiration, and neonatal depression.[1] As a result, neuraxial anesthesia became a popular choice for labor analgesia and cesarean sections. Neuraxial analgesia can be administered via different mechanisms such as spinal, epidural, or combined-spinal-epidural. There are advantages and disadvantages to each method and the approach chosen to deliver neuraxial analgesia is patient specific.

Although neuraxial analgesia is the most commonly employed method for labor analgesia given lower systemic effects on the mother and the fetus, non-neuraxial analgesia can also be used during labor when neuraxial analgesia is contraindicated, undesired, unsuccessful, or unavailable. Non-neuraxial analgesia can be offered through nonpharmacological and pharmacological methods. Examples of analgesic options used in labor are summarized in Table 12.1. The choice of analgesia during labor is patient dependent and determined by combined decision-making between the patient, obstetric anesthesiologist, and the obstetrician. There are many instances where neuraxial analgesia may not be possible. Box 12.1 lists the absolute and relative contraindications to neuraxial analgesia. If this method cannot be utilized, a mainstay of labor analgesia includes the use of opioid medications.

Systemic Opioids

Systemic opioids are the most widely used non-neuraxial labor analgesia worldwide.[2] Systemic opioids during labor offer several advantages including lower cost, ease of administration, lack of specialized equipment, placement or administration, higher breast-feeding success rates, improved motility, and decreased instances of instrumentation during vaginal delivery (Box 12.2). Furthermore, some women choose to avoid neuraxial analgesia during labor due to fear of development of back pain and the perceived increased risk of cesarean delivery.[3]

Several disadvantages exist to the use of systemic opioids for labor pain. One major disadvantage is the inability to provide adequate analgesia during labor. Other potential disadvantages include side effects such as nausea, vomiting, pruritus, and sedation. Systemic opioids can cross the placenta by passive diffusion, causing neonatal side effects such as decreased fetal heart rate variability, decreased fetal movement, respiratory depression, and sedation (Box 12.3). Due to the risks of opioid use, smaller drug doses with minimal active

Table 12.1 Analgesic Options During Labor

Neuraxial	Non-neuraxial	

• Epidural
• Spinal
• Combined Spinal-Epidural
	Nonpharmacological
	  • Music
	  • Breathing exercises
	  • Massage
	  • Acupuncture
	  • Hypnosis
	  • Hydrotherapy
	  • Transcutaneous Electrical Nerve
	   Stimulation (TENS)
		Pharmacological
		  • Opioids
		  • Acetaminophen
		  • Ketamine
		  • Benzodiazepine
		  • Inhalational agents

Box 12.1 Contraindications to Neuraxial Techniques

Absolute
- Patient refusal
- Anticoagulation
- Coagulopathy
- Bacteremia or epidural site infection

Relative
- Elevated intracranial pressure
- Maternal Cardiac Disease
- Local anesthetic allergy
- Skeletal anomalies

Box 12.2 Advantages of Opioids During Labor

1. Lower cost
2. Ease of administration
3. No need for specialized equipment or personnel
4. Higher breast-feeding success rates
5. Improved maternal motility

Box 12.3 Disadvantages of Opioids During Labor

- Inability to provide adequate analgesia
  - Poor patient satisfaction
- Maternal side effects
  - nausea, vomiting, pruritus, sedation
- Fetal side effects
  - low APGAR scores, respiratory depression

Table 12.2 Parenteral Opioids: Typical Dosages, Frequency of Administration, Onset of Action, and Duration of Action

Opioid	Dose	Frequency	Onset of Action	Duration of Action
Meperidine	25–50 mg IV 50–100 mg IM	Every 4 hours	10–15 minutes	2–3 hours
Morphine	0.05–0.1 mg/kg IV 0.1–0.2 mg/kg IM	Every 4 hours	2–3 minutes IV 20–40 minutes IM	3–6 hours
Fentanyl	50–100 mcg IV	Every 1–2 hours	2–4 minutes	30–60 minutes
Alfentanil	10 mcg/kg IV	Every 1–2 min via PCA	1 minute	1–2 minutes
Remifentanil	20–40 mcg IV	Every 2–3 min via PCA	1 minute	2–3 minutes
Tramadol	50–100 mg IV	Every 6 hours	60 minutes	4–6 hours
Codeine	30–60mg PO or IM	Every 4–6 hours	15–30 minutes	4–6 hours
Nalbuphine	10–20 mg IV or IM	Every 4–6 hours	2–3 minutes	3–6 hours
Butorphanol	1–2 mg IV or IM	Every 3–4 hours	30–60 minutes	3–4 hours

metabolites are preferred. When large doses of opioids or long-acting opioids are administered close to delivery, the neonatal side effects become more prevalent. To decrease the prevalence of these side effects, dosing schedules are used to limit the amount, frequency, and timing of medications administered. Common schedules are summarized in Table 12.2. Particular attention should be given to administration in relation to the timing of anticipated birth.[4] Side effects and toxicity, however, may create a situation that limits the analgesic potential of systemic opioids during labor. Boxes 12.4 and 12.5 summarize potential maternal and fetal side effects of opioids.

Systemic opioids can be administered through a variety of routes. Common methods include patient-controlled analgesia (PCA), intravenous (IV) via nurse-administered boluses, or intramuscular (IM) administration. Advantages to PCA include a more reliable analgesic effect and more stable plasma concentration of the drug due to smaller and more frequent self-administered dosing. IV administration has faster onset with ability to titrate to effect. An advantage of IM administration is easy administration, but it may increase pain and have a variable drug absorption.

Box 12.4 Maternal Side Effects Associated With Opioids

Nausea
Vomiting
Pruritus
Sedation
Drowsiness
Respiratory Depression

Box 12.5 Fetal Side Effects Associated With Opioids

Decreased fetal heart rate variability
Decreased fetal movement
Neonatal respiratory depression
Changes in neonatal neurobehavior
Low APGAR scores
Impairment of early breastfeeding

There are many different systemic opioids that can be used during labor. Each has variable pharmacologic properties that may be advantageous in a specific setting for an individual parturient. One must take into account differences in pharmacokinetics, pharmacodynamics, and resulting consequences to maternal and fetal well-being. Commonly used opioid agonists include meperidine, morphine, fentanyl, alfentanil, remifentanil, tramadol, and codeine. Mixed opioid agonist-antagonists like nalbuphine and butorphanol can also be used for pain management during labor.

Meperidine

Meperidine is a synthetic opioid which, unpopular in the United States, is the most commonly used systemic opioid for labor analgesia worldwide despite several drawbacks. Meperidine is metabolized in the liver to an active metabolite called normeperidine. Meperidine and normeperidine are lipid soluble and thus can cross the placenta and can cause fetal side effects such as reduced variability in fetal heart rate and neonatal respiratory depression. Other neonatal side effects include decreased APGAR scores, abnormal behavior, and difficulty initiating breastfeeding due to both decreased alertness and inhibition of sucking.[5] The maternal half-life of meperidine is 2–3 hours while the half-life of meperidine in newborns can be >12 hours. Maternal side effects include nausea, vomiting, sedation, and respiratory depression.

In a review by Smith et al., the effect of IM meperidine vs. placebo during labor was assessed. One study showed no clear difference in maternal satisfaction with pain control 30 minutes after administration. Out of the 25 women who received IM meperidine, only 3 reported to be "satisfied" or "very satisfied" with pain relief. Furthermore, out of the 25 women who received placebo, none reported to be "satisfied" or "very satisfied" 30 minutes after the administration of medication. Another study discussed includes 116 laboring participants, of which more women in the IM meperidine group reported "fair" or "good" pain relief within an hour of receiving the drug (RR 1.75, 95% CI 1.24 to 2.47, low-quality evidence).[4]

Morphine

Morphine is a mu opioid receptor agonist that is infrequently used for labor analgesia. It is metabolized in the liver to both an active metabolite, morphine-6-glucuronide, and an

Table 12.3 Relative Potency of Morphine vs. Fentanyl Comparing IV vs. Epidural vs. IT Administration

	Intravenous	Epidural	Intrathecal
Morphine	10 mg	1 mg	0.1 mg
Fentanyl	100 mcg	33 mcg	5 mcg

inactive metabolite, morphine-3-glucuronide, both of which are excreted by the kidneys. Due to its lipid solubility, morphine readily crosses the placenta. Side effects of morphine include nausea, vomiting, pruritus, sedation, and both maternal and neonatal respiratory depression.

Morphine is frequently administered epidurally and intrathecally for labor pain, which can produce less systemic side effects due to lower overall dose. Relative doses and potency comparisons of morphine are shown in Table 12.3. There still remains a risk of respiratory depression with the use of neuraxial morphine due to its duration of action. Depending on patient risk factors, route of administration, and dose of administration, there is variability in recommended assessment frequencies that are outlined in Table 12.4.[9]

Fentanyl

Fentanyl is a synthetic, potent, mu opioid-receptor agonist that is frequently utilized in neuraxial analgesia, but may also be administered systemically during labor. There are several advantages of using fentanyl during labor including high potency, about 50–100x more potent than morphine, fast onset of action, and short duration of action. Furthermore, fentanyl is metabolized by the liver to an inactive metabolite that is eliminated by the kidneys. Fentanyl does, however, have the ability to accumulate in the body after repeated doses due to prolonged clearance. Like other opioids, fentanyl can readily cross the placenta and cause neonatal respiratory depression.

Fentanyl, if used systemically, is usually administered in small IV doses of 50 to 100 mcg. At these doses, given at appropriate intervals, there was found to be no difference in APGAR scores, respiratory depression, or neonatal neurobehavior scores of neonates born to women who received IV fentanyl compared to those who did not receive IV fentanyl. Comparing women who received equivalent doses of IV fentanyl and IV meperidine, those that received IV fentanyl experienced fewer side effects such as nausea, vomiting, and sedation than those who received IV meperidine.[5]

Table 12.4 Recommended Monitoring Following Neuraxial Morphine Use

Risk Characteristics	Low-Dose and Healthy	High Dose or Risk Factors
Morphine Dose	IT > 0.05 and ≤ 0.15 mg Epidural >1 and ≤ 3 mg	IT > 0.15 mg Epidural > 3 mg
Respiratory Rate and Sedation Assessment	Q2 hours for 12 hours	Q1 hour for 12 hours then Q2 hours for 12–24 hours

Alfentanil

Alfentanil is a synthetic phenylpiperidine derivative that is less potent than fentanyl. It is highly protein-bound and thus less lipophilic than fentanyl. It does not cross the placenta as readily as fentanyl. It is also metabolized in the liver and excreted by the kidneys. In a study done by Morley-Foster et al. comparing the use of PCA fentanyl vs. PCA alfentanil, PCA fentanyl provided better pain relief than PCA alfentanil although the results were not statistically significant.[6]

Remifentanil

Remifentanil is an ultra-short-acting mu opioid receptor agonist that is rapidly hydrolyzed by tissue and plasma esterases into inactive metabolites. Remifentanil has become a suitable option for the cyclic pain of labor analgesia due to its fast onset of action of 1–2.5 minutes and a short context-sensitive half-life of 3 minutes. Typically, remifentanil is administered as a PCA when neuraxial analgesia is contraindicated or undesired by the patient.[5] Because of its short duration of action, remifentanil can be administered throughout labor and even close to anticipated birth without fear of neonatal respiratory depression, sedation, or neuro-behavioral changes.[5]

Due to the larger volume of distribution and higher clearance rate of remifentanil during pregnancy, the plasma concentration of one dose of remifentanil in a pregnant patient is about half that of nonpregnant patients. As mentioned previously, like other opioids, remifentanil can cross the placenta, but it is readily and rapidly broken down by fetal plasma and tissue esterases. Although there is limited data comparing remifentanil to neuraxial analgesia, it has been reported that there was no significant difference between APGAR scores, heart rate variability, need for neonatal resuscitation, or concerning cord gases when remifentanil was used during the second stage of labor.[5] It is worth mentioning that although remifentanil has become an attractive option for opioid labor analgesia due to its fast onset, short duration of action, and short context-sensitive half-life, laboring women receiving remifentanil need to be monitored closely as the doses required to achieve labor analgesia place the mother at risk for respiratory depression.[4]

There are several published administration regimens of remifentanil including PCA bolus with lockout, continuous infusion, and combined strategies. The PCA bolus dose that is typically given ranges between 0.1 and 1.0 mcg/kg, the lockout period is between 1 and 5 minutes, and continuous infusion rates are between 0.05 and 0.2 mcg/kg/ min. Consequently, the optimal drug administration dose and lockout settings have not yet been determined. Patients are educated to use their PCA button for a bolus administration with each contraction, and that no other individual, including healthcare providers or support persons, should push the PCA button.[5]

It has been noted that remifentanil is able to provide more pain relief than inhalational agents like nitrous oxide but is less effective at labor analgesia compared to neuraxial analgesia. Several small randomized controlled trials were able to show that in terms of satisfaction and perception of "pain relief," the use of a remifentanil PCA had similar results compared to neuraxial analgesia techniques despite a reduced analgesic efficacy. In those studies it was noted that maternal respiratory depression with decreased oxygen saturation was more common with remifentanil PCA compared with neuraxial analgesia.[5]

There are other studies comparing the use of IV PCA remifentanil to other systemic opioids and neuraxial analgesia techniques. In a double-blind, controlled trial, Evron et al. analyzed 88 patients who were randomly assigned to receive either IV PCA remifentanil or IV infusion of meperidine. Authors concluded that patients who received IV PCA remifentanil had more effective and reliable analgesia during labor, lower pain scores, higher satisfaction with pain relief, less oxygen desaturation, and less opioid analgesia failure requiring conversion to epidural analgesia.[7]

Codeine

Codeine is a naturally occurring opioid that is less potent than morphine yet there remains high potential for both maternal and neonatal opioid-related side effects such as sedation and respiratory depression. It may be administered orally or intramuscularly. Much of the evidence related to codeine's use during labor associates it with an increased risk of cesarean delivery, thus routine use of codeine during labor is not recommended over other drug choices.

Tramadol

Tramadol is a weak, synthetic opioid that not only is a mu receptor agonist but also inhibits the reuptake of norepinephrine and increases the release of serotonin. Tramadol can be administered orally, intravenously, or intramuscularly. Tramadol causes less cardiovascular and respiratory depression compared to equipotent doses of morphine. A review by Smith et al, includes a comparison of IM tramadol vs. no treatment. Among the 30 women who received IM tramadol, only five reported "satisfactory" analgesia.[4]

Nalbuphine

Nalbuphine is a partial opioid agonist-antagonist: it is an agonist at the kappa opioid receptor and an antagonist or partial agonist at the mu opioid receptor. Routes of administration can be subcutaneous, intramuscular, or intravenous. Its onset of action is 2–3 minutes with a duration of action of 3–6 hours. It is metabolized in the liver to inactive metabolites that are secreted in bile and excreted in feces. Compared to morphine, nalbuphine causes less respiratory depression. Four studies were included in a review by Smith et al that compared IM nalbuphine to IM meperidine. Outcomes showed that there was no difference in maternal satisfaction during labor and postnatal period, no difference in maternal pain scores, no difference in rates of cesarean delivery, and no difference in assisted vaginal births between nalbuphine and meperidine.[4] In terms of neonatal side effects, there was also no clear difference in need for neonatal naloxone administration, APGAR scores <7, or NICU admission when comparing nalbuphine to meperdine.[4]

Butorphanol

Butorphanol is a partial opioid agonist-antagonist with agonistic properties at the kappa opioid receptor and partial agonistic or antagonistic properties at the mu opioid receptor. It is five times more potent than morphine. It is metabolized in the liver to inactive metabolites and excreted in urine. Evidence indicates IV butorphanol provides more pain relief and lower pain scores compared to IV meperidine. Furthermore, nausea and vomiting was less with IV butorphanol compared to IV meperidine.[4] Compared to IV fentanyl, women were less likely to request additional analgesic doses if using butorphanol. Additionally, women in the IV fentanyl group were twice as likely to request an epidural compared to women in the IV butorphanol group. There is no evidence indicating significant differences regarding neonatal resuscitation, neonatal naloxone administration, and APGAR scores.[4]

The Opioid Tolerant Parturient

Opioid use and misuse in the United States has risen drastically in the last two decades and trends have been mirrored in the obstetric population. The diagnostic criteria for opioid use disorder (OUD) can be found in Box 12.6. Opioid use disorder diagnosed at delivery had increased four-fold from 1999 to 2014. Medication-assisted treatment has been the standard therapy for pregnant patients with OUD. It is thought a long-acting maintenance

---

Box 12.6 DSM-V Opioid Use Disorder

1. Taking larger amounts or taking drugs over a longer period than intended.
2. Persistent desire or unsuccessful efforts to cut down or control opioid use.
3. Spending a great deal of time obtaining or using the opioid or recovering from its effects.
4. Craving, or a strong desire or urge to use opioids
5. Problems fulfilling obligations at work, school, or home.
6. Continued opioid use despite having recurring social or interpersonal problems.
7. Giving up or reducing activities because of opioid use.
8. Using opioids in physically hazardous situations.
9. Continued opioid use despite ongoing physical or psychological problem likely to have been caused or worsened by opioids.
10. Tolerance (i.e., need for increased amounts or diminished effect with continued use of the same amount).
11. Experiencing withdrawal (opioid withdrawal syndrome) or taking opioids (or a closely related substance) to relieve or avoid withdrawal symptoms.

The Diagnostic and Statistical Manual of Mental Disorders (5th ed.) describes opioid use disorder as a problematic pattern of opioid use leading to problems or distress, with at least two of the following occurring within a 12-month period. One point for each item. 2–3 points: mild opioid use disorder. 3–4 points: moderate opioid use disorder. 5–6 points: severe opioid use disorder.

drug can prevent opioid use fluctuations and behaviors that risk harm to the mother and fetus. Fluctuations in opioid use and withdrawal, or risky drug-use behaviors, can lead to catecholamine surges, uterine contractions, changes in placental blood flow, and infection. The currently FDA-approved medications for OUD include methadone, buprenorphine, and naltrexone.

Methadone is a synthetic mu opioid receptor agonist and a potent, long-acting analgesic for use in chronic pain management and opioid dependence. Peak plasma levels occur at 2–4 hours with variable duration due to a biphasic elimination: analgesia associated with alpha-elimination of 8–12 hours and withdrawal suppression associated with beta-elimination of 30–60 hours. An increase in the corrected QT interval (Tc) of the electrocardiogram is a known side effect which can lead to arrhythmias such as torsade de pointes and should be monitored. Buprenorphine is a long-acting mixed agonist-antagonist opioid analgesic with high receptor affinity that is also used in OUD. There may be some advantages to buprenorphine use over methadone in neonatal outcomes related to lessened severity of neonatal withdrawal syndrome.

It is generally recommended to continue opioid maintenance medications throughout the peripartum period with attention to changing pharmacokinetics during pregnancy and individual pain requirements. Multimodal analgesia is recommended with an approach that maximizes neuraxial analgesia, but consideration should be given to these patients' elevated tolerance to opioid medications. They may require increased or more frequent dosing of short-acting opioid in the setting of cesarean delivery[8].

Summary

Opioid analgesics continue to be a mainstay in providing labor analgesia. They can be administered via multiple different routes and modalities. Neuraxial analgesia remains the most common and most effective methods of providing pain relief during labor, but there are instances where neuraxial analgesia is contraindicated, undesired, unavailable, or unsuccessful. In this chapter we described the benefits and risks of commonly used opioids for labor pain. The choice of labor analgesia should be a joint decision made by the anesthesiologist, obstetrician, and parturient and individualized to patient-specific risks, comorbidities, and goals.

References

1. Lim G, Facco FL, Nathan N, et al. A review of the impact of obstetric anesthesia on maternal and neonatal outcomes. *Anesthesiology*. 2018;129:192–215.
2. Bucklin BA, Hawkins JL, Anderson JR, Ullrich FA. Obstetric anesthesia workforce survey: twenty-year update. *Anesthesiology*. 2005;103(3):645–653.
3. Harkins J, Carvalho B, Evers A, Mehta S, Riley ET. Survey of the factors associated with a woman's choice to have an epidural for labor analgesia. *Anesthesiol Res Pract*. 2010;2010:356789. doi:10.1155/2010/356789. Epub 2010 Jun 29.
4. Smith LA, Burns E, Cuthbert A. Parenteral opioids for maternal pain relief in labour. *Cochrane Database of Systematic Reviews*. 2018;(6):CD007396.

5. Markley JC, Rollins MD. Non-neuraxial labor analgesia: options. *Clin Obstet Gynecol.* 2017;60(2):350–364.

6. Morley-Forster PK, Reid DW, Vandeberghe H. A comparison of patient-controlled analgesia fentanyl and alfentanil for labour analgesia. *Can J Anaesth.* 2000;47(2):113–119.

7. Evron S, Glezerman M, Sadan O, Boaz M, Ezri T. Remifentanil: a novel systemic analgesic for labor pain. *Anesth Analg.* 2005;100(1):233–238.

8. Landau R. Post-cesarean delivery pain. Management of the opioid-dependent patient before, during and after cesarean delivery. *Int J Obstet Anesth.* 2019;39:105–116.

9. Bauchat JR, Weiniger CF, Sultan P, et al. Society for Obstetric Anesthesia and Perinatology consensus statement. *Anesth Analg.* 2019;129(2):1.

13
Neuraxial Anesthesia

Paulina Cardenas

Neuraxial Anesthesia

Neuraxial anesthesia is the gold standard when providing pain relief for the parturient. The 1980s saw a dramatic increase in the use of neuraxial anesthesia. The increased use of neuraxial blocks and the decreased use of general anesthesia improved maternal safety.[1] The use of dilute solutions of local anesthetic for labor analgesia with the synergism of opioids allows for a sensory block that spares motor function during labor. When using a neuraxial catheter technique, the labor analgesia can be converted to provide surgical anesthesia in the event of a cesarean delivery. Furthermore, the Society of Obstetric Anesthesia and Perinatology (SOAP) recommends that neuraxial morphine should be the preferred method for postcesarean analgesia in healthy women.[2] It provides superior analgesia after cesarean when compared to intravenous opioids. Neuraxial anesthesia for cesarean delivery has the added advantage of allowing the mother to participate in childbirth and establish immediate skin-to-skin bonding and breastfeeding. It also allows for paternal participation and greater satisfaction with the birth experience. In addition, the provider can reassure patients that the use of neuraxial analgesia for labor does not increase the incidence of cesarean delivery.[3]

Anatomy

Neuraxial Anatomy

The spinal canal is surrounded by the bony structures of the vertebrae (Figure 13.1). It contains the structures targeted by neuraxial anesthesia. The innermost component is the spinal cord which emerges from the foramen magnum and ends at L1 in most adult patients as the conus medullaris. The spinal cord is covered by pia mater. The nerve roots for the lumbosacral dermatomes extend caudad from the conus medullaris and are referred to as the cauda equina (Figure 13.2). The spinal cord and nerve roots are surrounded by cerebral spinal fluid (CSF), and all of these structures are encased by the arachnoid mater and dura mater, which are closely adhered to one another. A potential space exists between the arachnoid mater and the dura mater, which is the subdural space. The pia mater, arachnoid mater, and dura mater make up the meninges. A fibrous band called the filum terminale emerges from the end of the spinal cord and attaches to the coccyx.

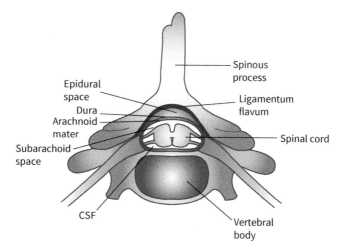

Figure 13.1 Vertebral and spinal anatomy.

Neuraxial Anatomic Changes in the Parturient

Pregnancy causes several anatomical changes to the neuraxis. There is engorgement of the epidural venous plexus due to venous congestion caused by the gravid uterus compressing on the inferior vena cava. This makes inadvertent puncture of a blood vessel more likely. The parturient also experiences a more pronounced lumbar lordosis during pregnancy and this can cause the intervertebral spaces to narrow compared to the nonpregnant patient. As the pelvis rotates forward the line between the iliac crests may cross at a higher vertebral body (L3–L4) than it would in a patient who is not pregnant (L4–L5). The thoracic kyphosis is flattened during pregnancy, resulting in more rostral spread of a hyperbaric solution after

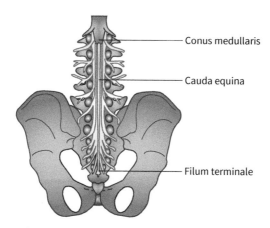

Figure 13.2 Lumbosacral spine.

administration of a spinal. Increased edema and obesity during pregnancy can also make placement of the neuraxial anesthesia more challenging.

Physiology

Neuraxial analgesia must provide pain relief during the first and second stages of labor. Pain during the first stage of labor is primarily visceral in nature and occurs due to uterine contractions and cervical dilation. Pain is transmitted through visceral afferent nerve fibers that enter the spinal cord from the T10–L1 nerve roots (Figure 13.3). Pain from the second stage of labor occurs from distension of the vaginal canal and perineum. The pain is somatic in nature and is carried by the pudendal nerve, which emerges from the S2–S4 nerve roots. Neuraxial anesthesia placed in the lower lumbar region provides initial relief for the first stage of labor and can be extended to provide relief for the second stage of labor as the fetus descends in the birth canal. The ideal lumbar space for labor analgesia is L2–3 or L3–4 since, in the event of an accidental dural puncture, this is below the level where the spinal cord ends. Effective blockade for both stages of labor should include T10–S4 dermatomes. Sensory block for a cesarean delivery should include the sacral dermatomes and extend cephalad to T4. Maternal discomfort may occur despite a T4 sensory block due to irritation of the undersurface of the diaphragm (C3–C5).

Techniques

The American College of Obstetricians and Gynecologists (ACOG) states that maternal request is a sufficient indication for pain relief during labor.[4] There are numerous neuraxial techniques that are used both during labor and for cesarean delivery (Figure 13.4). Early placement of the neuraxial (i.e., before the onset of labor or in early labor) may be beneficial for patients who have a higher risk of needing a cesarean delivery. This would include patients with multiple gestation, preeclampsia, or those who are undergoing a trial of labor after cesarean. When a neuraxial anesthetic is used during labor it can help avoid the need for a general anesthetic in the event of an emergent cesarean delivery.

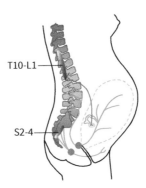

Figure 13.3 Pain pathways of labor.

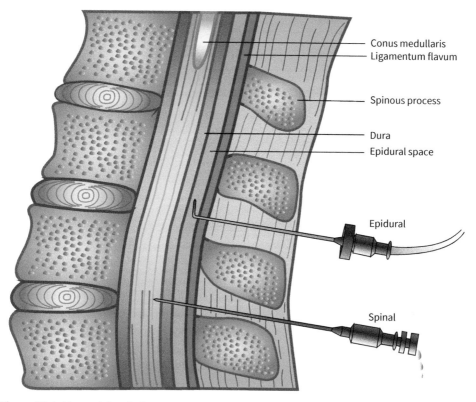

Figure 13.4 Neuraxial techniques.

Single-Shot Spinal Anesthesia

Spinal anesthesia provides a rapid onset neuroblockade. This technique is confirmed by the visualization of CSF in the hub of the spinal needle. This is the most commonly used technique for elective cesarean delivery. It is rarely used for labor analgesia since it does not provide continuous dosing. The use of pencil-point spinal needles reduces the incidence of postdural puncture headache (Figure 13.5). It is common to add both a lipophilic and a hydrophilic opioid when dosing the spinal for cesarean delivery. A spinal is typically performed below the level of L1 in order to avoid direct spinal cord trauma from the spinal needle.

Continuous Spinal Anesthesia

Continuous spinal anesthesia (CSA) involves puncturing the dura with the epidural needle and placing the epidural catheter in the intrathecal (subarachnoid) space. This may take place purposefully or after an inadvertent dural puncture where one notes a "wet tap." There would be no test dose in this situation because aspiration of CSF from the catheter would be evident and would confirm placement of the catheter in the intrathecal space. Spinal microcatheters used in the 1990s were withdrawn from the market due to concerns about cauda equine syndrome. Recently these have been reintroduced in US market but have not gained widespread use.

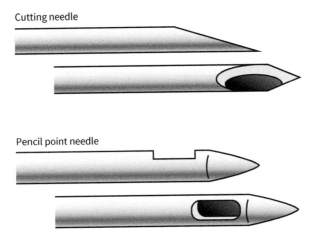

Figure 13.5 Pencil point vs. cutting spinal needle.

Intentional CSA is used sparingly since it would require a large bore puncture of the dura with an epidural needle. This would predispose the patient to a postdural puncture headache. It is used at times for the morbidly obese, those with known difficult airways, or patients who have significant cardiac comorbidities. The CSA allows for slow titration of medication and mitigates the abrupt onset of hemodynamic changes seen with a single-shot spinal. This may be beneficial in the patient where a slow onset of hemodynamic changes is essential.

Epidural Anesthesia

An epidural can be used during labor to provide analgesia. It can also be converted to provide surgical anesthesia for cesarean delivery should the patient require an operative delivery. It is not commonly used for elective cesarean deliveries since the block is less reliable than a single-shot spinal. A loss of resistance (LOR) technique is commonly used to find the epidural space (Figure 13.6). The LOR can be found with either saline or air in the syringe. The hanging drop technique is another technique to locate the epidural space. This is done with fluid in the hub of the needle; the fluid in the hub is aspirated into the epidural space as the needle is advanced past the ligamentum flavum. A dilute solution of local anesthetic is used to achieve analgesia. The epidural may be dosed in the following ways:

1. Intermittent bolus injection: this method requires periodic interventions by the provider. This can be done when the patient begins to feel discomfort between doses or at preset time intervals. No pump is required for this dosing regimen.
2. Continuous epidural infusion: an infusion pump is set at a continuous rate. CEI allows for a stable anesthetic level to be achieved.
3. Patient-controlled epidural analgesia: the infusion pump can be set at a continuous rate with bolus doses available upon patient request with lockout intervals. It can also be run without a background infusion. PCEA allows the patient more autonomy over her pain relief and requires less top-up interventions by the provider.

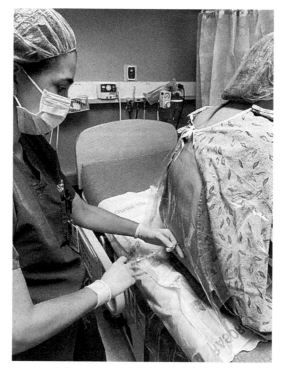

Figure 13.6 Loss of resistance technique.

4. Programmed intermittent epidural bolus: this protocol delivers a preset volume of medication as a bolus at preset intervals by the infusion pump. The volume and pressure of this intermittent bolus may allow for better distribution of the local anesthetic in the epidural space and less overall medication used.

Combined Spinal-Epidural

In a combined spinal-epidural (CSE), a needle-through-needle technique allows for a spinal to be performed through the epidural needle after the loss of resistance has been found. The epidural catheter is then threaded into the epidural space. This technique provides fast-onset relief in the event of a precipitous labor. When this technique is used for a cesarean delivery, it allows for extension of the duration of the analgesia in case the spinal begins to wear off. The disadvantage of this technique is that the epidural catheter is untested.

Low-dose Combined Spinal-Epidural

This technique involves a reduced dose for the spinal component of the CSE followed by epidurally injected local anesthetic to achieve a T4 level. This would result in a slower onset of hemodynamic changes.

Dural Puncture Epidural

Dural puncture epidural is a modification of the CSE technique where the dura is punctured with the spinal needle. There is confirmation of CSF flow, but no intrathecal medication is administered. The epidural catheter is then placed into the epidural space. The advantage of this technique is the confirmation of midline position and that the epidural needle is indeed in the epidural space. The dural puncture allows for translocation of epidural medications into the intrathecal space. This technique provides better sacral coverage, fewer physician top-ups, and lower incidence of unilateral block compared to traditional epidural techniques.[5]

Test Dose

Careful aspiration of the epidural catheter should occur after initial placement. Placement of the epidural catheter can be complicated by inadvertent dural puncture. It can also be complicated by inadvertent placement of the catheter in a blood vessel. The engorgement of the epidural venous plexus during pregnancy increases the likelihood of this occurring in parturients. An epidural test dose is commonly used. The test dose is used to assess that the epidural catheter has not inadvertently crossed the dura and thus occupied the intrathecal space. To test for intrathecal placement a common test dose includes 45 mg of lidocaine (3mL of 1.5% lidocaine) which would result in the patient experiencing symptoms of a spinal anesthetic. The epidural test dose also assesses for inadvertent placement of the catheter in a blood vessel. A dose of 15mcg of epinephrine (3mL of 1:200,000 solution) would result in a sharp increase of maternal heart rate, indicating intravascular placement.

Contraindications to Neuraxial

Absolute contraindications include patient refusal, anticoagulation, uncooperative patient, coagulopathy/thrombocytopenia, known allergy to anesthetic agents, hypovolemic shock/hemorrhage, untreated systemic infection, or infection at the site of needle insertion. SOAP has published a consensus statement regarding the management of parturients who are receiving thromboprophylaxis, which should be referenced anytime a parturient is anticoagulated.[6] The precise cutoff for placement of a neuraxial anesthetic in patients with thrombocytopenia is debated. When the platelet count is stable and between 80,000–100,000/mm^3, most practitioners are comfortable proceeding.[7]

Relative contraindications include preexisting neurologic disease, elevated ICP due to mass lesion, and skeletal abnormalities.

Equipment

Spinal needles with pencil-point tips are preferred over needles with a cutting bevel. Pencil-point needles have a reduced incidence of postdural puncture headache. Equipment necessary for airway management and/or general anesthesia should be readily available in the

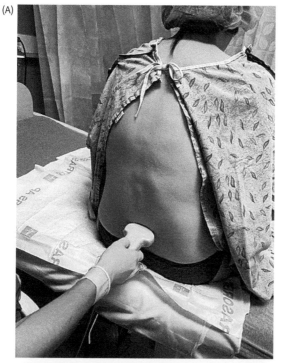

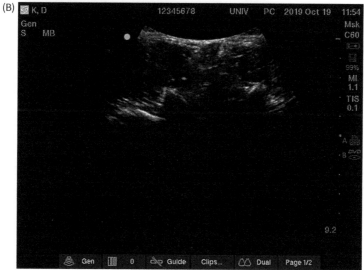

Figure 13.7 A. Transverse scan. B. "Flying bat."

event of a high spinal or unrecognized intrathecal catheter. Lipid emulsion in the event of local anesthesia systemic toxicity should always be available as well.

Ultrasonography for Neuraxial Anesthesia

Neuraxial ultrasonography has increasingly been adopted as a tool in regional anesthesia. Despite the bony anatomy of the spine it can help to identify the midline and the

(A)

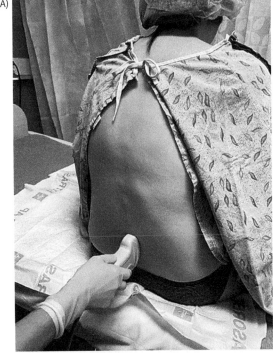

(B)

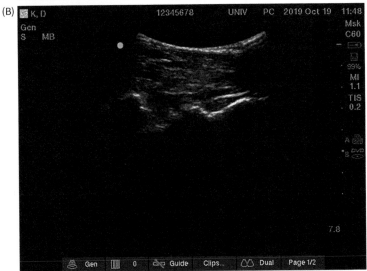

Figure 13.8 A. Longitudinal scan. B. "Saw-tooth" pattern.

intervertebral spaces. Real-time ultrasound guidance is challenging due to the extensive bony anatomy of the neuraxis. When ultrasonography is used, it is performed with imaging followed by the procedure. Preprocedural ultrasonography allows for the marking of the relevant spaces followed by sterile preparation of the skin and drape application.

There are two acoustic windows that are useful when visualizing the lumbar spine.[8] The curvilinear probe is used to obtain the transverse midline view and the longitudinal view.

The transverse view (Figure 13.7A) can help identify the depth of the ligamentum flavum/ dural complex. The transverse view will reveal a "flying bat" when the probe is in the middle of the intervertebral space (Figure 13.7B). The longitudinal approach (Figure 13.8A) can help identify the desired interspace more accurately than the anatomical estimates traditionally used. The longitudinal view will easily identify the sacrum and the lumbar interspaces as the probe is moved cephalad (Figure 13.8B); the image will resemble a "saw-tooth" pattern. Using a transverse and a longitudinal view of the lumbar spine may reduce the number of needle insertions and redirections.

Further Reading

Nathan N, Wong CA. Spinal, epidural, and caudal anesthesia: anatomy, physiology, and technique. In: Chestnut DH, Wong CA, Tsen L, et al., eds. *Chestnut's obstetric anesthesia: principles and practice.* 6th ed. Philadelphia: Elsevier; 2019:238–270.

References

1. Birnbach DJ, Bateman BT. Obstetric anesthesia: leading the way in patient safety. *Obstet Gynecol Clin North Am.* 2019;46(2):329–337.
2. Bauchat JR, Weiniger CF, Sultan P, et al. Society for Obstetric Anesthesia and Perinatology consensus statement: monitoring recommendations for prevention and detection of respiratory depression associated with administration of neuraxial morphine for cesarean delivery analgesia. *Anesth Analg.* 2019;129(2):458–474.
3. Practice guidelines for obstetric anesthesia: an updated report by the American Society of Anesthesiologists task force on obstetric anesthesia and the Society for Obstetric Anesthesia and Perinatology. *Anesthesiology.* 2016;124(2):270–300.
4. ACOG Practice Bulletin No. 209: Obstetric analgesia and anesthesia. *Obstet Gynecol.* 2019;133(3):595–597.
5. Chau A, Bibbo C, Huang C, et al. Dural puncture epidural technique improves labor analgesia quality with fewer side effects compared with epidural and combined spinal epidural techniques: a randomized clinical trial. *Anesth Analg.* 2017;124(2):560–569.
6. Leffert L, Butwick A, Carvalho B, et al. The Society for Obstetric Anesthesia and Perinatology consensus statement on the anesthetic management of pregnant and postpartum women receiving thromboprophylaxis or higher dose anticoagulants. *Anesth Analg.* 2018;126(3):928–944.
7. Bernstein J, Hua B, Kahana M, Shaparin N, Yu S, Davila-Velazquez J. Neuraxial anesthesia in parturients with low platelet counts. *Anesth Analg.* 2016;123(1):165–167.
8. Carvalho JC. Ultrasound-facilitated epidurals and spinals in obstetrics. *Anesthesiol Clin.* 2008; 26(1):145–158.

14

Alternative Regional Anesthetic Techniques

Michelle S. Burnette, Laura Roland, Everett Chu, and Marianne David

Introduction

While neuraxial techniques receive the bulk of the ink in the obstetric anesthetic literature, there are patients for whom neuraxial analgesia is undesirable, contraindicated, or not available. Classically in obstetric anesthesia there are three techniques long employed by obstetric providers to aid the parturient during the labor and delivery process. These blocks aim to aid in delivery by providing relief in either the first, second, or third stage of labor (Table 14.1). These include paracervical block, pudendal block and perineal infiltration (Figure 14.1).

Paracervical Block

Clinical Indications

The paracervical block (PCB) provides analgesia for uterine contractions and cervical dilation in the first stage of labor.[1] The goal is to block the visceral pain fibers from the uterus and cervix in the lateral fornix of the upper vaginal canal near the cervix. PCB became popular in the United States in the early 1960s but was abandoned by some practitioners as early as 1963 due to case reports of fetal deaths and profound bradycardias (often secondary to direct fetal injection). Though routine use of the PCB in today's obstetric practice is sporadic, papers published in the past two decades compare PCB to subarachnoid block, highlight local anesthetic options, and give a historical perspective.[2-4]

Technique

The transvaginal PCB is a blind technique, and providers should employ needle guides to decrease self-needle-stick risk. A long 22-guage needle is inserted bilaterally at the 4 and 8 o'clock positions on the edge of the cervix and local anesthetic is injected in the submucosa (Figure 14.2). The simplicity, time of onset, practicality, and cost of PCB has kept it in the obstetric textbooks.[2]

Table 14.1 Comparison of the Use of Different Alternative Blocks for Labor

Type of Block	Stage of Labor	Nerve Roots Involved	Volume of Dilute Local Anesthetic*	Notes
Paracervical	First	T10, T11, T12, L1	5–10 mL (without epinephrine) on each side	3–7 mm depth watch for fetal bradycardia, do not use in cases of fetal distress
Pudendal	Second	S2, S3, S4	7–10 mL on each side, medial and posterior to each ischial spine	Does not treat contraction pain
Perineal Infiltration	Second (can give before episiotomy) or third (laceration/ episiotomy repair)	S2, S3, S4	Volume varies, *10 mL pre-delivery lidocaine and mepivacaine have led to fetal toxicity	Local anesthetic effect equivalent to saline placebo, take care not to inject fetal scalp

*Please note 2-chloroprocaine is likely the safest choice for all three blocks. Concentrated local anesthetics lead to toxicity and greater risk to the fetus.

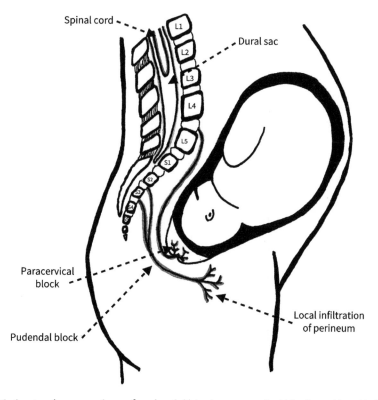

Figure 14.1 Anatomic comparison of pudendal block, paracervical block, and local infiltration of perineum.

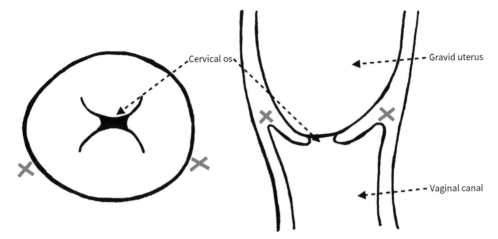

Figure 14.2 Location of paracervical block injections (red x): local anesthetic is injected in the submucosa at the 4 and 8 o'clock positions on the edge of the cervix.

Complications

Studies concerning paracervical blocks highlight the incidence of post-block fetal bradycardia. Fetal bradycardia is defined as change in FHR > 20% or an absolute FHR < 100. Recent evidence suggests the incidence of fetal bradycardia is around 15% after PCB, and fetal heart rate changes were short-lived and did not lead to immediate operative delivery. Of note, both a single-shot spinal and PCB cause fetal bradycardia. Fortunately, the incidence of maternal side effects such as sacral neuritis, hematoma, or peripheral vascular collapse is quite low with PCB. Though PCB is somewhat less efficacious than subarachnoid block, it still may be a consideration for obstetric patients when neuraxial analgesia is not available.[3]

Pudendal Block

Clinical Indications

The pudendal nerve block (PB) is indicated for pain relief during the second stage of labor. The pudendal nerve is the principal nerve of the perineum, receiving fibers from the second, third, and fourth sacral roots. PB provides analgesia to the lower vagina, vulva, and perineum as well as motor block to the external anal sphincter and perineal muscles.[4] PB is adequate for spontaneous vaginal delivery and may be suitable for low forceps, but it provides inadequate analgesia for mid-forceps delivery, upper vaginal, cervical, or uterine exploration postpartum.

Technique

PB can be performed via a transvaginal or transperineal approach, though the transvaginal approach is preferred. Obstetric providers typically inject 7–10 mL of dilute local anesthetic concentrations, such as 1% lidocaine and 2% 3-chloroprocaine, medial and posterior to each ischial spine. The right hand of the practitioner guides the needle to the patient's right side and the left hand to the left side. As with PCB, practitioners need to take care not to subject themselves to needle sticks during this relatively blind procedure.

Complications

Maternal complications of PB include local anesthetic systemic toxicity (LAST), hematoma, abscess, and damage to the adjacent structures/vaginal mucosa. Fetal complications include bradycardias and LAST. Most fetal complications are attributed to direct local anesthetic injection in the fetus.

Perineal Infiltration

Clinical Indications and Technique

Perineal infiltration (PI) is often employed for episiotomy or laceration repair and can be used to supplement pudendal block or neuraxial analgesia. Local anesthetic is injected directly into the perineal tissue with a small gauge needle along the track of a laceration or anticipated episiotomy. After delivery, PI with local anesthetic and vasoconstrictors can offer rapid pain relief for repairs, especially in the absence of a neuraxial block.[5]

Complications

Direct fetal injection of local anesthetic is again a complication of this technique. Both topical anesthetics applied to the perineum as well as injectable local has resulted in neonatal toxicity requiring intubation even without accidental fetal injection. Blood supply to the perineum is such that local anesthetic transfer from maternal to fetal circulation can be rapid; therefore, 2-chloroprocaine seems to have a safer neonatal side effect profile than longer-acting local anesthetics. LAST is a risk for the mother as well, while infection and hematoma at the site of injection appears rare.

Alternate Regional Techniques for Cesarean Delivery

Introduction

Although neuraxial anesthesia is most commonly used, alternative regional techniques can be used as part of a multimodal pain regimen following cesarean section. In patients who did not receive long-acting neuraxial opioids and/or received general anesthesia for cesarean section, these blocks and procedures can be effective interventions in helping to reduce acute postoperative pain. These procedures include truncal blocks—including the transversus abdominis plane (TAP) block and the quadratus lumborum block (QLB)—as well as wound infiltration catheters, the ilioinguinal-iliohypogastric (IIIH) block, and subcutaneous infiltration of local anesthetics.

Truncal Blocks

Setup

Equipment needed for a truncal block includes 2–3 20mL syringes for local anesthetic, a 21 or 22-gauge short-bevel needle with extension tubing (or an 18- to 21-gauge Tuohy needle with extension tubing and catheter for continuous infusions), antiseptic for skin disinfection, a linear high-frequency ultrasound transducer (10-5 MHz), and ultrasound gel (Figure 14.3).[6] Some providers may use a curved linear ultrasound transducer, particularly for the QLB. For high BMI patients, longer needles may be needed and imaging may be technically difficult. To prolong the block effect when catheters are not used, epinephrine may be added to the local anesthetic solution. Local anesthetic choice is provider dependent, with common choices including ropivacaine or bupivacaine 0.2–0.25% with 20–30 mL/side, and common infusion rates of 6–8 mL/hr/side of ropivacaine or

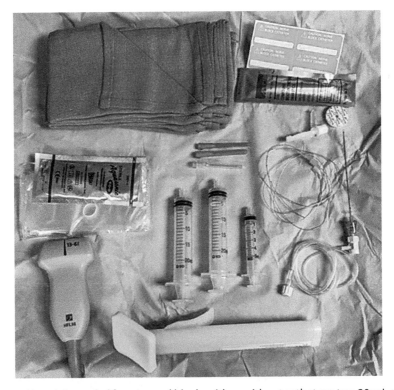

Figure 14.3 Materials needed for a truncal block, with or without catheters: two 20 mL syringes, a 19-gauge short-bevel needle with extension tubing, antiseptic, a linear high-frequency ultrasound transducer, ultrasound gel, and a catheter. Also pictured are blunt-tip needles for drawing up local anesthetic, a small-gauge needle for skin local if needed, compound benzoin tincture, a chlorhexidine impregnated disc, and a sterile cover for the ultrasound transducer.

bupivacaine 0.125–0.2%. The total local anesthetic dose needs to be considered in relation to the weight of the patient to ensure the maximum safe dosage is not exceeded.

Transversus Abdominis Plane Block

Clinical Indications

The TAP block has been effectively used for postoperative pain control for a variety of open abdominal surgeries and is a safe, technically simple procedure, especially under ultrasound guidance. The TAP block is performed by injecting local anesthetic between the internal oblique and transversus abdominis muscles of the abdominal wall, providing somatic coverage from about T6–T12 depending of the location of TAP block.[7] The lateral or midaxillary TAP block will provide coverage in the infraumbilical area from midline to the midclavicular line from T10–T12, covering the Pfannenstiel and low-midline vertical incisions for cesarean sections. The TAP block does not provide visceral coverage.

Step-by-Step Technique

With ASA standard monitors applied, the patient is placed in the supine position, and the abdominal area is prepped and draped. The ultrasound transducer is placed in the transverse plane between the lower costal margin and the iliac crest in the midaxillary line to visualize the three layers of abdominal wall muscles: external oblique, internal oblique, and transversus abdominis (Figure 14.4). Using in-plane technique, the needle is advanced in a posterolateral direction towards the fascial plane between the internal oblique and the transversus abdominis muscles (Figure 14.5). Once the needle reaches the aponeurosis

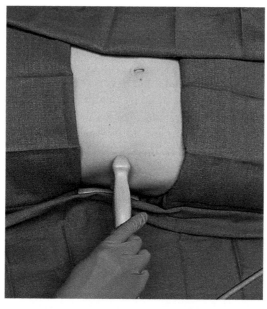

Figure 14.4 For both transversus abdominis plane and quadratus lumborum blocks, the ultrasound transducer is placed in the transverse plane between the lower costal margin and the iliac crest in the midaxillary line.

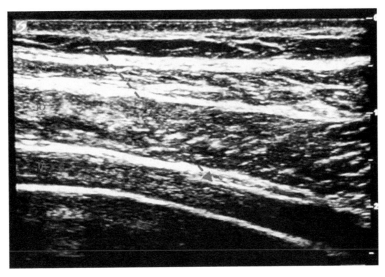

Figure 14.5 Transversus abdominis plane block: local anesthetic is injected once the needle (red arrow) reaches the aponeurosis of the internal oblique and transversus abdominis muscles. EO = external oblique muscle, IO = internal oblique muscle, TA = transversus abdominis muscle.

between the muscles, local anesthetic is injected with confirmed negative aspiration every 5 mL. The local anesthetic will be seen pushing the transversus abdominis down as it separates from the fascial layer. If needed, a catheter is placed through the needle and secured with sterile dressing.

Quadratus Lumborum Block

Clinical Indications
There are four main types of QLBs that differ in coverage area and are based on the location of local anesthetic administration: QLB1 (lateral), QLB2 (posterior), QLB3 (anterior/transmuscular), and QLB4 (intramuscular).[8] The QLB2 can be used for abdominal surgery either above or below the umbilicus and any type of operation that requires intra-abdominal visceral pain coverage; therefore, the QLB2 will cover Pfannenstiel, low-midline vertical, and classical-type incisions for cesarean section.[7] The QLB2 provides somatic and visceral coverage from T4 to L1 by injecting local anesthetic between the posterior aspect of the quadratus lumborum (QL) muscle and the middle layer of the thoracolumbar fascia, which separates QL muscle from the latissimus dorsi and erector spinae muscles.

Step-by-Step Technique
With ASA standard monitors applied, the patient is placed in the supine position and the abdominal area is prepped and draped. The ultrasound transducer is placed in the transverse plane between the lower costal margin and the iliac crest in the midaxillary line where the three layers of abdominal wall muscles are visualized, as in the TAP block (see "Transverse

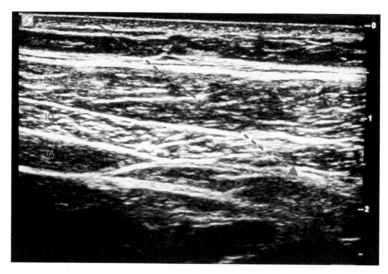

Figure 14.6 Quadratus lumborum block. Local anesthetic is injected once the needle (red arrow) is inside the middle layer of the thoracolumbar fascia on the posterior side of the QL muscle. Injection of local anesthetic will push the QL muscle down while spreading between the fascia and muscle. EO = external oblique muscle, IO = internal oblique muscle, TA = transversus abdominis muscle, QL = quadratus lumborum muscle.

Abdominis Plane Block," Figure 14.4). As the transducer is moved posteriorly, the transversus abdominis muscle tapers off and the fused aponeurosis of the internal oblique and transversus abdominis muscles is visualized near the QL muscle. The transducer is moved more posteriorly until the fused aponeurosis becomes the middle layer of the thoracolumbar fascia on the posterior side of the QL muscle (Figure 14.6). Using in-plane technique, the needle is advanced in a posterolateral direction until it is inside the middle layer of the thoracolumbar fascia and local anesthetic is injected with confirmed negative aspiration every 5 mL. The local anesthetic will push the QL muscle down as it separates from the fascia, with local anesthetic tracking posteriorly along the QL muscle. If needed, a catheter is placed through the needle and secured with sterile dressing.

Complications

Complications from truncal blocks are fortunately very rare, especially when performed under ultrasound guidance. LAST is possible due to the large volume of local anesthetic needed for these blocks and the vascularity of the area, particularly with the QLB (Table 14.2).[7] With landmark-based techniques, there are a few case reports of unintended puncture of visceral abdominal organs, such as kidney, liver, or spleen; however, with proper use of ultrasound this risk is significantly reduced.[9] Abdominal branches of lumbar arteries coarse in the fascial plane where the QLB is performed and hematoma from needle trauma is possible, especially in conjunction with anticoagulation use.[10] Spread of local anesthetic with QLB to the lumbar plexus and paravertebral space may cause lower-limb weakness and hypotension. With TAP blocks, spread of local anesthetic to the femoral

Table 14.2 Comparison of the Transversus Abdominis Plane (TAP) Block and Quadratus Lumborum 2 Block (QLB2) Indications, Coverage and Injection Areas, and Complications

Block	Clinical Indications	Dermatomes Covered	Injection Site	Potential Complications
Lateral TAP Block	Abdominal surgery around the infraumbilical area, with coverage from midline to midclavicular line	T6–T12	Between the internal oblique and transversus abdominis muscles	LAST, unintended puncture of visceral abdominal organs, lower extremity weakness (femoral nerve)
QLB2	Abdominal surgery either above or below the umbilicus, and any type of surgery needing intra-abdominal visceral pain coverage	T4–L1, plus visceral coverage	Posterior to the QL muscle, inside the middle layer of the thoracolumbar fascia	LAST, hematoma, unintended puncture of visceral abdominal organs, lower extremity weakness (lumbar plexus/paravertebral space), hypotension

nerve is possible as the fascial plane where the block is performed is continuous with the fascia iliaca.[9]

Wound Infiltration Catheter

Clinical Indications

Wound infiltration catheters are multi-orifice catheters that are placed in the surgical wound before closing. The administration of local anesthetic in wound infiltration catheters has been shown to reduce the amount of rescue morphine consumption and lower pain scores after obstetric surgery in some patients; however, they are not necessarily superior to other forms of pain control. They have been shown in some studies to provide equivalent pain relief when compared to TAP blocks and epidural analgesia.[11,12]

Technique

The infiltration catheter is frequently placed by the operating surgeon at the time of closure. It may be placed above or below the fascial layer, or intra-abdominally, and may be used for continuous infusion or intermittent injection of local anesthetics during the recovery period.[13] Studies indicate that catheters inserted below the fascia but pre-peritoneal resulted in better pain relief when compared to catheters placed subcutaneously.[14]

Complications

Possible complications cited in the literature include LAST and inhibition of the second stage in wound healing.[15] A meta-analysis of wound infiltration catheter studies by Gupta et al. did not find any increase in wound breakdown or infection rate or any difference in adverse side effects.[13]

Ilioinguinal-Iliohypogastric Block

Clinical Indications

The IIIH block is frequently used as an adjunct method of pain control in lower abdominal surgeries, both obstetric and nonobstetric. Since the ilioinguinal and iliohypogastric nerves supply the L1 and L2 dermatomes, the IIIH block can target the somatic pain generated at the site of Pfannenstiel incisions for cesarean section.[16] Postcesarean patients with an IIIH block demonstrate decrease in both pain scores and narcotic usage up to 24 hours postoperatively when compared to patients without the block.[16] Unfortunately, the literature also shows that the use of the IIIH block does not reduce opioid-related side effects such as nausea and itching.[17]

Technique

The IIIH block may be done using landmark techniques or with ultrasound guidance. The ilioinguinal and iliohypogastric nerves lie in the fascial plane between the internal oblique and transversus abdominis muscles. The technique begins with identifying the anterior superior iliac spine (ASIS).[18] The needle is inserted at a point 2 cm medial and 2 cm superior to the ASIS and advanced at an oblique angle toward the pubic symphysis until it is in the fascial plane between the two muscles (Figure 14.7). After confirming a negative aspiration test, 5 to 10 mL of local anesthetic in injected. Multiple injections along the nerve track may provide superior analgesia compared to single injections.[19]

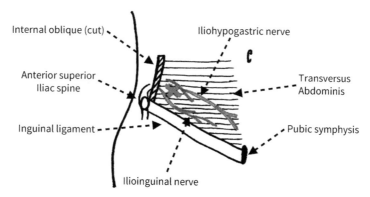

Figure 14.7 Ilioinguinal-iliohypogastric block. The needle is inserted at a point 2 cm medial and 2 cm superior to the ASIS (red x) and advanced at an oblique angle toward the pubic symphysis. Local anesthetic is injected in the fascial plane between the internal oblique muscle and transversus abdominis muscle.

Complications

The risks associated with this block include peritoneal cavity injection, bowel perforation, ecchymosis/hematoma, LAST, and femoral nerve blockade.[18] These can be minimized by using ultrasound guidance and applying a pressure to the injection site.

Subcutaneous Infiltration of Local Anesthetics

Clinical Applications

Subcutaneous local anesthetic infiltration is a single-dose injection around the wound incision at the conclusion of the surgery.[20] While it has been shown to reduce opioid consumption at 12 hours postcesarean section compared to placebo, it does not reduce pain scores or morphine requirements at 24 hours.[21] Compared with TAP blocks, local infiltration resulted in higher pain scores but similar total morphine requirements at 24 hours postcesarean section.[22] Despite its short duration, a single injection of local anesthetic into the surgical wound can be a simple and cheap component of multimodal analgesia when other regional techniques cannot be used.

References

1. Rosen MA. Paracervical block for labor analgesia: a brief historic review. *Am J Obstet Gynecol.* 2002;186(5 Suppl Nature):S127–S130.
2. Palomäki O, Huhtala H, Kirkinen P. What determines the analgesic effect of paracervical block? *Acta Obstet Gynecol Scand.* 2005;84(10):962–966.
3. Junttila EK, Karjalainen PK, Ohtonen PP, Raudaskoski TH, Ranta PO. A comparison of paracervical block with single-shot spinal for labour analgesia in multiparous women: a randomised controlled trial. *Int J Obstet Anesth.* 2009;18(1):15–21.
4. Chestnut D. Alternative regional analgesic techniques for labor and vaginal delivery. In: Chestnut D, Wong CA, Tsen LC, et al., eds. *Obstetric anesthesia principles and practice.* 6th ed. Philadelphia, PA: Elsevier; 2020: 540–552.
5. Colacioppo PM, Gonzalez Riesco ML. Effectiveness of local anaesthetics with and without vasoconstrictors for perineal repair during spontaneous delivery: double-blind randomised controlled trial. *Midwifery.* 2009;25(1):88–95.
6. Wiisanen MT, Hartwig JW. Transversus abdominis plane block technique: approach considerations. https://emedicine.medscape.com/article/2000944-technique. Published September 20, 2018. Accessed October 16, 2019.
7. Ultrasound-guided transversus abdominis plane and quadratus lumborum blocks—NYSORA. NYSORA. https://www.nysora.com/regional-anesthesia-for-specific-surgical-procedures/abdomen/ultrasound-guided-transversus-abdominis-plane-quadratus-lumborum-blocks/. Published September 15, 2018. Accessed October 16, 2019.
8. Akerman M, Pejčić N, Veličković I. A review of the quadratus lumborum block and ERAS. *Front Med.* 2018;5:44.

9. Young MJ, Gorlin AW, Modest VE, Quraishi SA. Clinical implications of the transversus abdominis plane block in adults. *Anesthesiol Res Pract.* 2012;2012:731645.

10. Elsharkawy H, El-Boghdadly K, Barrington M. Quadratus lumborum block: anatomical concepts, mechanisms, and techniques. *Anesthesiology.* 2019;130(2):322–335.

11. Klasen F, Bourgoin A, Antonini F, et al. Postoperative analgesia after caesarean section with transversus abdominis plane block or continuous infiltration wound catheter: A randomized clinical trial. TAP vs. infiltration after caesarean section. *Anaesth Crit Care Pain Med.* 2016;35(6):401–406.

12. Mungroop TH, Bond MJ, Lirk P, et al. Preperitoneal or subcutaneous wound catheters as alternative for epidural analgesia in abdominal surgery: a systematic review and meta-analysis. *Ann Surg.* 2019;269(2):252–260.

13. Rackelboom T, Le Strat S, Silvera S, et al. Improving continuous wound infusion effectiveness for postoperative analgesia after cesarean delivery: a randomized controlled trial. *Obstet Gynecol.* 2010;116(4):893–900.

14. Gupta A, Favaios S, Perniola A, Magnuson A, Berggren L. A meta-analysis of the efficacy of wound catheters for post-operative pain management. *Acta Anaesthesiol Scand.* 2011;55(7):785–796.

15. Brower MC, Johnson ME. Adverse effects of local anesthetic infiltration on wound healing. *Reg Anesth Pain Med.* 2003;28(3):233–240.

16. Naghshineh E, Shiari S, Jabalameli M. Preventive effect of ilioinguinal nerve block on postoperative pain after cesarean section. *Adv Biomed Res.* 2015;4:229.

17. Bell EA, Jones BP, Olufolabi AJ, et al. Iliohypogastric-ilioinguinal peripheral nerve block for post-Cesarean delivery analgesia decreases morphine use but not opioid-related side effects. *Can J Anaesth.* 2002;49(7):694–700.

18. Waldman SD. *Atlas of pain management injection techniques.* 4th ed. Philadelphia PA: Elsevier. 2015;86–87:431–440.

19. Wolfson A, Lee AJ, Wong RP, Arheart KL, Penning DH. Bilateral multi-injection iliohypogastric-ilioinguinal nerve block in conjunction with neuraxial morphine is superior to neuraxial morphine alone for postcesarean analgesia. *J Clin Anesth.* 2012;24(4):298–303.

20. Chestnut D. Postoperative analgesia. In: George RB, Carvalho B, Butwick A, Flood P, eds. *Chestnut's obstetric anesthesia principles and practice.* 6th ed. Philadelphia PA: Elsevier; 2020: 665–666.

21. Adesope O, Ituk U, Habib AS. Local anaesthetic wound infiltration for postcaesarean section analgesia: A systematic review and meta-analysis. *Eur J Anaesthesiol.* 2016;33(10):731–742.

22. Yu N, Long X, Lujan-Hernandez JR, Succar J, Xin X, Wang X. Transversus abdominis-plane block versus local anesthetic wound infiltration in lower abdominal surgery: a systematic review and meta-analysis of randomized controlled trials. *BMC Anesthesiol.* 2014;14:121.

15

Non-Opioid Analgesic Techniques for Labor and Vaginal Delivery

Anvinh Nguyen, Yi Deng, and Melissa A. Nikolaidis

Stages of Vaginal Delivery

Vaginal delivery is divided into three distinct stages. Stage one begins with the onset of true labor until full cervical dilation (of 10 cm) occurs. True labor can be differentiated from false labor by the presence of regular rhythmic contractions that gradually shorten as labor progresses. Cervical dilation of least 1.2 cm per hour for nulliparous patients and 1.5 cm per hour for multiparous patients is expected.[1] Moreover, true labor causes progressive cervical effacement and dilation while false labor does not.

The second stage of labor begins when the cervix is fully dilated until the delivery of the newborn occurs. Contractions during this stage push the fetus down the vaginal canal resulting in the parturient sensing strong pressure. This stage of labor can last anywhere between 20 minutes to 2 hours.

The third stage of labor includes the time period from delivery of the newborn through the delivery of the placenta. During this stage, the placenta is separated from the inner uterine wall and expelled through the vaginal canal.[1] Manual pulling of the umbilical cord to facilitate this separation can cause discomfort. Oxytocin, a medication that stimulates uterine contractions, may be administered to assist in this stage of labor.[2]

The first stage of labor is typically the longest and is further divided into three phases. The latent (early) labor phase begins with the start of true labor until the cervical dilation reaches 6 cm. This is followed by the active labor phase which begins when the cervix is 6 cm dilated until it achieves 8 cm dilation. The last phase is the transitional phase. This phase starts at 8 cm cervical dilation and ends when the cervix is fully dilated at 10 cm (see Table 15.1).[3]

The American College of Obstetricians and Gynecologists (ACOG) states that, "there are no other circumstances in which it is considered acceptable for an individual to experience untreated severe pain that is amenable to safe intervention while the individual is under a physician's care."[4] As such, appropriate analgesia should be provided for the laboring patient without causing harm to the mother or fetus. Epidural analgesia and opioids have been used for decades with significant reduction in labor pain. However, these treatments present their own set of accompanying side effects and adverse risks and therefore should be used with caution. Systemic opioids are associated with respiratory depression, sedation, nausea, vomiting, pruritis, and further impairment of gastric emptying. This class of medications also causes deleterious fetal effects such as neonatal respiratory depression, feeding issues, and fetal distress.[5] The remainder of this chapter will review non-opioid oral, intravenous,

Table 15.1 The Different Stages of Labor, Average Duration, and Associated Changes

Stage of Labor	Duration of Stage	Contraction Frequency	Contraction Duration	Cervical Dilation
First Stage: Latent (Early) Phase	8 to 12 hours	Every 5 to 10 minutes	20 to 30 seconds	0 to 6 cm
First Stage; Active Phase	4 to 8 hours	Every 3 to 5 minutes	40 to 50 seconds	6 to 8 cm
First Stage: Transitional Phase	Minutes to hours	Every 2 to 3 minutes	50 to 60 seconds	8 to 10 cm
Second Stage	< 3 hours for nulliparous, < 2 hours for multiparous	Every 2 to 3 minutes		10 cm to birth
Third Stage	5 to 30 minutes			

and inhalational analgesic medications for the management of pain during labor and vaginal delivery.

Labor Pain

Labor pain is complex and subjective, it varies significantly between each patient, and it can vary between separate pregnancies in the same patient. Pain is a perception and is multifaceted. It is influenced by the patient's environment, emotions, cognition, social circumstances, and culture.[6] Constant attention, assessment, and understanding of the laboring patient is required to reduce her pain.

As labor progresses through its predictable stages, different nerves are involved in the transmission of pain. The location of pain can be described by the spinal nerve roots that are carrying the noxious stimuli. For instance, during the first stage of labor, pain is diffuse and poorly localized. Pulling and stretching of the uterine segment, uterine muscle contractions, and initial cervical dilation result in a dull, colicky pain. The correlating spinal nerves associated with stage one labor pain include T10, T11, T12, and L1 nerves. These nerves are derived from the lumbar sympathetic chain. Pain during this stage of labor is mostly visceral in nature. First-stage labor pains often radiate to the abdomen and lower lumbar regions.[7] Length of contractions can vary between 20–60 seconds in duration.

The second stage of labor is associated with pain that is sharper and better localized. This correlates with perineal stretching caused by movement of the baby down the vaginal canal. This pain has both visceral and somatic components. Pain in the second stage of labor involves the S2, S3, and S4 spinal nerves, mediated by the pudendal nerve.[8] Patients will commonly experience the sensation of bearing down ("pushing") to further move the fetus down the vaginal canal which is associated with generalized pressure and/or pain that intensifies as labor progresses (see Table 15.2).

Severe pain can stimulate a neuroendocrine stress response that results in profound deleterious effects on multiple maternal organ systems. Maternal hyperventilation leads to

Table 15.2 Key Differences Between Stage 1 and Stage 2 Labor Pain

Stage of Labor	Pain type	Characteristic	Pain Transmission	Nerve block(s)
First Stage	Mostly visceral pain	Progressive cervical dilation Distension of lower uterine segment	T10 to L1 nerve roots	Epidural Paracervical nerve block
Second Stage	Mostly somatic pain	Involvement of pelvic floor, vaginal canal, and perineum	S2 to S4 nerve roots	Epidural Pudendal nerve block

hypocarbia and corresponding respiratory alkalosis. An increased sympathetic response can cause elevations in peripheral vascular resistance, blood pressure, and myocardial oxygen consumption. Pain can also result in decreased placental perfusion and uterine activity desynchrony. All laboring patients face an increased risk of aspiration of gastric contents; severe labor pain can further amplify the aspiration risk by causing gastric inhibition and increased gastric acidity. Severe, poorly controlled labor pain can also result in long-term consequences, such as adverse psychological effects including an increased risk of postpartum depression, PTSD, and increased severity of acute postpartum pain.[8,9]

Epidural and Regional Techniques

Conventional epidural analgesia provides a continuous treatment capable of covering all stages of labor. Pain control provided by an epidural is unparalleled. A long, thin and flexible catheter is placed in the epidural space by an anesthesia provider. This is typically done between the L3–L4 or L4–L5 vertebral spaces. A dilute local anesthetic medication with or without added opioids is commonly used for continuous infusion. The epidural coverage must include the T10 to L1 dermatomes for the first stage of labor and S2 to S4 for the second stage of labor. Contraindications to epidural placement include coagulopathy, thrombocytopenia, infection at the needle puncture site, elevated intracranial pressure, severe uncorrected maternal hypovolemia, and patient refusal. A conversation with the patient about the risks and benefits of this procedure is required, and informed consent should be obtained prior to performing epidural analgesia (see Table 15.3).[8]

Regional nerve blocks can also provide analgesia for labor pain. A paracervical block can be performed by injecting local anesthetic near the paracervical ganglion on both sides of the cervix. This would inhibit pain signals originating from the uterus and cervix which helps alleviate stage-one labor pain. A pudendal nerve block can be performed to cover pain associated with the second stage of labor. The pudendal nerve carries signals from the S2–S4 spinal nerves which innervates the perineum, vulva, and vagina. By performing both a paracervical block and a pudendal block, pain from the first and second stages of labor will be reduced.[8]

This section discusses non-opioid analgesic techniques for labor analgesia, including oral, intravenous, and inhalational medications. Further discussion about epidural and regional techniques for labor analgesia is beyond the scope of this chapter.

Table 15.3 Absolute and Relative Contraindications for Neuraxial Techniques During Labor

Absolute Contraindications	Patient refusal
	Severe coagulopathy (disseminated intravascular coagulation)
	Severe maternal hypovolemia
	Infection at needle insertion site
Relative Contraindications	Mild coagulopathy
	Central nervous system disorders (increased intracranial pressure, multiple sclerosis, etc.)
	Spinal deformities
	Severe cardiac disease
	Severe fetal depression
	Sepsis

Nonsteroidal Anti-Inflammatory Drugs

Although nonsteroidal anti-inflammatory drugs (NSAIDs) are prescribed in pregnancy for inflammatory diseases, fever, and pain, exposure to NSAIDs after 32 weeks gestation has been shown to increase the incidence of premature closure of the fetal ductus arteriosus.[10] Premature closure of the fetal ductus arteriosus could cause profound fetal right heart dysfunction, congestive heart failure, fetal hydrops, and intrauterine demise. There is also an association between NSAIDs use and a reduction in fetal urine output which increases the risk of oligohydramnios.[11] Because of these adverse effects NSAIDs have generally been avoided for labor analgesia. Examples of NSAIDs include aspirin, celecoxib, diclofenac, ibuprofen, indomethacin, ketorolac, and naproxen.

Acetaminophen

Acetaminophen has analgesic and antipyretic properties. It is well tolerated and does not have a significant side effect profile compared to opioid analgesics. Its mechanism of action is not completely understood. However, it is known to inhibit the cyclooxygenase (COX) enzyme in the central nervous system which contributes to its antipyretic properties. For a normal, healthy parturient, the maximum dose of acetaminophen should be limited to less than 4000 mg per day. As acetaminophen is hepatically metabolized, risks and benefits should be discussed before its administration to patients with liver disease. Acetaminophen can be administered via multiple routes including oral, suppository, and intravenous.

Oral is the most common route of administration. It has a relatively quick onset of action of about 30 minutes and attains peak concentrations in 1 hour. Oral acetaminophen is available in both tablet and capsule forms. It is also available as immediate-release or extended-release, in a range of dosage strengths.

Regarding the intravenous form of acetaminophen, the onset of action is approximately 15 minutes for analgesia and 30 minutes for antipyresis. It is hepatically metabolized with a

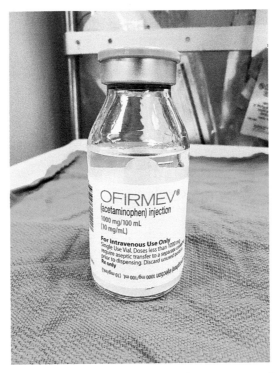

Figure 15.1 Intravenous acetaminophen (Ofirmev®) bottle in 10 mg per ml concentration.

duration of action of approximately 4 to 6 hours. Intravenous acetaminophen is manufactured in a 100 ml glass bottle containing 1000 mg of acetaminophen. Its side effect profile is minimal and it can safely be used for labor pain. Several small studies have shown that intravenous acetaminophen provides reduction in the visual analogue scale pain scores comparable with placebo (see Figure 15.1).[12]

Phenothiazines

Phenothiazines are sedative medications that may alleviate labor pain by reducing maternal anxiety, increasing relaxation, and potentiating the effects of opioids or other analgesics. They work by decreasing the reuptake of catecholamines such as norepinephrine and serotonin in the central nervous system. Phenothiazines also have antiemetic properties by virtue of their effects on the chemoreceptor trigger zone of the medulla. Caution must be used with its administration as phenothiazines can cross the placenta and reduce beat-to-beat variability of the fetus. Other side effects, although rare, include tardive dyskinesia (unwanted muscle movement disorders), neuroleptic malignant syndrome, confusion, tachycardia, hypertension, hypotension, changes in breathing pattern, muscle rigidity, and trembling.

The most common phenothiazine used for labor pain is promethazine. Promethazine has antihistamine properties as well. It is available for administration via oral, intramuscular, or intravenous routes. As an adjunct for labor analgesia, intramuscular or intravenous dosing is 50 mg for early labor and 25 to 75 mg in combination with another analgesic at reduced dose

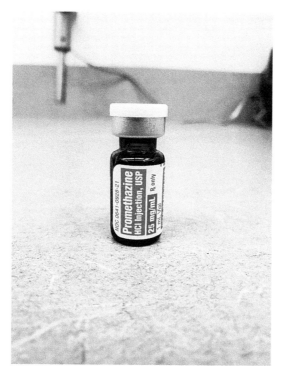

Figure 15.2 Intravenous promethazine vial in 25 mg per ml concentration.

for established labor. This dose can be repeated every 4 hours for up to two additional doses if necessary, with a maximum dose of 100 mg per day while in labor. Phenothiazines are less effective for pain relief than opioids if used alone, but multiple studies have shown their efficacy when used as an adjunct with other analgesics (see Figure 15.2).[13]

Ketamine

Ketamine is a dissociative anesthetic medication with profound analgesic properties. It works primarily as an N-Methyl-D-aspartate (NMDA) receptor antagonist, but is also thought to affect opioid receptors, dopamine receptors, serotonin receptors, and acetylcholine receptors as well. It was originally synthesized by American chemist Calvin Lee Stevens at the Parke-Davis Lab. Ketamine has indirect sympathomimetic properties, so it increases maternal blood pressure, heart rate, and uterine blood flow. This allows uterine perfusion to be maintained during its use. Another benefit is that ketamine preserves both maternal and fetal respiratory drive.[14] Common side effects include confusion, agitation, hallucinations, increased secretions, hypertension, tachycardia, and muscle tremors. Ketamine can be given via intravenous and intramuscular routes. Its onset of action is within 30–40 seconds if administered intravenously. The duration of action is 5–10 minutes unless a maintenance infusion is started. However, the patient's dissociative state may last greater than 30 minutes (see Figure 15.3).

For labor analgesia, an initial induction dose of 0.1 to 0.2 mg/kg over 30 minutes followed by a maintenance infusion of 0.2 mg/kg/hour is recommended. Several studies have

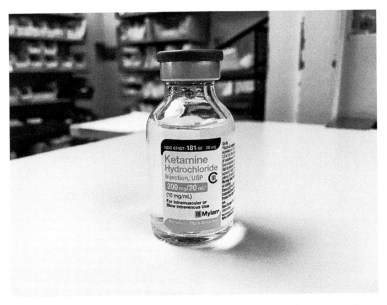

Figure 15.3 Intravenous ketamine hydrochloride vial in 10 mg per ml concentration.

concluded that even with higher doses of ketamine (2 mg/kg given as a single bolus induction dose) there are no detrimental effects on APGAR scores. It does not appear to prolong the duration of labor and does not appear to cause an increased incidence of caesarian or instrument-assisted deliveries.[15]

Nitrous Oxide

Nitrous oxide is a safe, odorless, tasteless inhalational medication used for labor analgesia and anxiolysis. Nitrous oxide is generally safe and must be delivered with oxygen. The use of nitrous oxide is common in the United Kingdom, Finland, Australia, and New Zealand.[16] At this time, the only FDA-approved nitrous oxide delivery system is Nitronox with a blend of 50% nitrous oxide and 50% oxygen. It is delivered via a face mask or a mouthpiece into which the patient is also instructed to exhale in order to facilitate gas wasting. The National Institute for Occupational Safety and Health (NIOSH) recommends an exposure limit of 25 ppm for nitrous oxide (see Figure 15.4).

Nitrous oxide has been shown to provide effective analgesia during all three stages of labor as well as for postvaginal delivery procedures. Onset of action is rapid, which allows it to be timed prior to each uterine contraction with appropriate patient instruction. It also has a rapid offset of action, within a few minutes after discontinuation.[16] Its mechanism of action is not well understood. It is thought that nitrous oxide works as an agonist at the mu-opioid receptors as well as an antagonist at the NMDA receptors to establish its effect.[17]

Side effects include maternal drowsiness, light-headedness, nausea, and vomiting. Because nitrous oxide is an anesthetic agent, the parturient patients are usually confined to the hospital bed as a fall precaution. Although widely utilized in European countries, nitrous oxide is rarely used for labor analgesia in the United States (see Figure 15.5).[16]

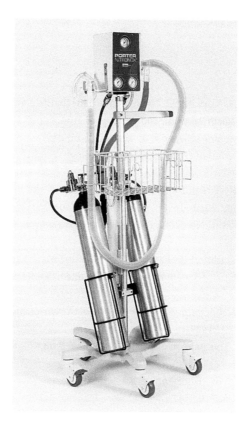

Figure 15.4 Porter Nitronox blend system with nitrous oxide and oxygen cylinders, circuit, and face mask. Photo provided by Porter Instrument, Parker Hannifin Corporation, Hatfield, PA.

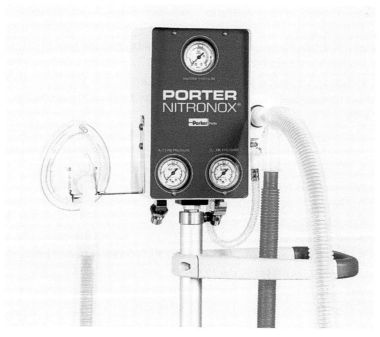

Figure 15.5 Close-up view of Porter Nitronox blend system showing pressure gauges for both nitrous oxide and oxygen. There is also a gauge for the mixture pressure. Photo provided by Porter Instrument, Parker Hannifin Corporation, Hatfield, PA.

References

1. Liao JB, Buhimschi CS, Norwitz ER. Normal labor: mechanism and duration. *Obstetrics and Gynecology Clinics of North America.* 2005;32(2):145–164. doi:10.1016/j.ogc.2005.01.001.

2. Shojai R, Dercole C, Boubli L. The use of oxytocin administration to manage the third stage of labor. *American Journal of Obstetrics and Gynecology.* 2002;187(2):516–517. doi:10.1067/mob.2002.125738.

3. Zhang J, Sundaram R, Troendle J. The natural history of the normal first stage of labor. *Obstetrics & Gynecology.* 2010;116(1):193. doi:10.1097/aog.0b013e3181e5b09a.

4. ACOG Practice Bulletin No. 209. *Obstetrics & Gynecology.* 2019;133(3). doi:10.1097/aog.0000000000003132.

5. Smith LA, Burns E, Cuthbert A. Parenteral opioids for maternal pain management in labour. *Cochrane Database of Systematic Reviews.* 2018;(6):CD007396. doi:10.1002/14651858.cd007396.pub3.

6. Lowe N. The nature of labor pain. *American Journal of Obstetrics and Gynecology.* 2002;186(5). doi:10.1067/mob.2002.121427

7. Labor S, Maguire S. The pain of labour. *Reviews in Pain.* 2008;2(2):15–19. doi:10.1177/204946370800200205.

8. Wong C. Advances in labor analgesia. *International Journal of Womens Health.* 2009;139(1):139–154. doi:10.2147/ijwh.s4553.

9. Brownridge P. The nature and consequences of childbirth pain. *European Journal of Obstetrics & Gynecology and Reproductive Biology.* 1995;59(1):S9–S15. doi:10.1016/0028-2243(95)02058-z.

10. Koren G, Florescu A, Costei AM, Boskovic R, Moretti ME. Nonsteroidal antiinflammatory drugs during third trimester and the risk of premature closure of the ductus arteriosus: a meta-analysis. *Annals of Pharmacotherapy.* 2006;40(5):824–829. doi:10.1345/aph.1g428.

11. Antonucci R, Zaffanello M, Puxeddu E, et al. Use of non-steroidal anti-inflammatory drugs in pregnancy: impact on the fetus and newborn. *Current Drug Metabolism.* 2012;13(4):474–490. doi:10.2174/138920012800166607.

12. Zutshi V. Efficacy of intravenous infusion of acetaminophen for intrapartum analgesia. *Journal of Clinical and Diagnostic Research.* 2016;10(8):18–21. doi:10.7860/jcdr/2016/19786.8375.

13. Jones L. Pain management for women in labour: an overview of systematic reviews. *Journal of Evidence-Based Medicine.* 2012;5(2):101–102. doi:10.1111/j.1756-5391.2012.01182.x.

14. Yuying T, Renyu L, Peishan Z. Ketamine: an update for obstetric anesthesia. *Translational Perioperative and Pain Medicine.* 2017;4(4). doi:10.31480/2330-4871/058.

15. Joselyn A, Cherian V, Nandhakumar A, Raju N, Kaliaperumal I, Joel S. Low-dose ketamine infusion for labor analgesia: A double-blind, randomized, placebo controlled clinical trial. *Saudi Journal of Anaesthesia.* 2014;8(1):6. doi:10.4103/1658-354x.125897.

16. Likis F, Andrews J, Collins M, et al. Nitrous oxide for the management of labor pain. *Obstetric Anesthesia Digest.* 2014;34(4):191. doi:10.1097/01.aoa.0000455280.68551.83.

17. Emmanouil DE, Quock RM. Advances in understanding the actions of nitrous oxide. *Anesthesia Progress.* 2007;54(1):9–18. doi:10.2344/0003-3006(2007)54[9:aiutao]2.0.co;2.

16

Non-pharmacologic Labor Analgesia

Michael Marotta and David Gutman

Introduction

Ideally, the birth of a child should be a memorable, happy, and emotionally fulfilling event. Many women, however, are terrified of giving birth due to the associated pain. The pain of labor is among the most intense forms of pain commonly experienced.[1] The individual experience of labor pain is multifactorial and has both physiologic and psychosocial components. Various approaches to labor analgesia target one or more of labor pain's contributing factors. Pharmacologic approaches to labor analgesia aim to relieve the pain of labor by blocking its well-defined physiologic sources. Non-pharmacologic labor analgesia, generally speaking, attempts to help women cope with or distract them from their labor pain by targeting less well-defined psychosocial and physiologic sources.[2]

Multiple studies have proven pharmacologic labor analgesia effective in managing the physiologic sources of labor pain. Labor pain is both visceral and somatic in nature. In the first stage of labor, uterine contractions and cervical dilation cause painful stimulation that is carried centrally by the T10–L1 nerve roots. In the second stage of labor, the trauma and stretching of the birth canal, pelvic floor, and perineum cause painful stimulation that is carried centrally by the S2–S4 nerve roots.[3]

Some women desire to avoid pharmacologic interventions for a variety of reasons including, but not limited to, cultural influences, fear, and/or personal goals and beliefs. Some of these include the fear of neurologic complications, fear of neonatal complications, value assigned to "natural childbirth," and associating pharmacologic intervention with feelings of inadequacy or "giving up." Additionally, the experience of labor and labor pain is not purely physiologic. Even in the presence of pharmacologic labor analgesia, psychosocial factors play a large role in the experience of labor, and these often do not get the attention they deserve.

Non-pharmacologic labor analgesia encompasses techniques that aim to treat psychosocial and/or secondary physiologic sources of pain. The psychosocial contributions to labor pain are not well understood but likely include tension, anxiety, and fear.[4] Their presence and impact vary greatly between individuals. As such, they are difficult to define, difficult to study, and difficult to treat. This has led to a paucity of high-quality data on the subject of non-pharmacologic labor analgesia.

Though the data are generally inconclusive and the subject matter foreign to traditional anesthesia providers, non-pharmacologic techniques are likely an important and useful component of labor analgesia. Various approaches to non-pharmacologic treatment include biofeedback, continuous labor support, hypnosis, relaxation, acupuncture, water immersion, manual methods, and sterile water injections. Other modalities not discussed here include TENS, aroma therapy, temperature therapy, and labor positioning. Generally speaking, these techniques have been shown to have questionable and variable efficacy but are noninvasive and overall appear to be safe.[2] In this chapter, we will discuss the definition, techniques, potential value, possible dangers, and how/when to incorporate some of these methods into peripartum labor analgesia. For a more detailed discussions, the Cochrane Library has conducted reviews on several topics in the field which have largely informed the material found here.

Biofeedback

Biofeedback is a therapist-guided, equipment-assisted treatment that attempts to teach individuals to control physiological responses by changing cognitive processes and engaging the relaxation response as an adaptive coping skill. Biofeedback can be used in an attempt to modulate the experience of pain.[5] In other words, it is an attempt to consciously and purposefully self-regulate physiology. The theory is that the ability to diminish the physiologic changes associated with labor pain along with a sense of control and autonomy may help parturients cope with pain in labor.

Techniques

There are various approaches to biofeedback in non-pharmacologic labor analgesia (Table 16.1). The biofeedback paradigm:

- An instrument sensitive for a specific physiologic parameter is attached to the patient.
- Physiologic changes (e.g., heart rate as related to the laboring parturient's experience of pain) are detected by the instrument.
- The instrument alerts the parturient to these changes via a continuous display (e.g., light, sound, graph, generated number).
- One or more cognitive or relaxation techniques are employed in an attempt to control these physiologic changes (e.g., visualization, deep breathing, muscle relaxation, etc.).
- The instrument detects if/when the physiologic changes diminish.
- Patients are able to see and experience that they can change their physiology, which helps them establish a sense of control and autonomy.
- The monitor will alert the patient if/when the physiologic change happens again.[6]

Table 16.1 Examples of Biofeedback Modalities

Modality	Parameter Measured
Electromyograph	Muscle Tension
Skin Thermometer	Temperature (Changes in Blood Flow)
Galvanic Skin Response	Sweat Production via Skin Conductivity
Electroencephalograph	Brain Waive Activity
Electrocardiograph	Hear Rate and Rhythm (in turn high blood pressure)
Respiration Feedback	Rate, Rhythm, Type of Breathing

Potential Value/Possible Dangers

- A small study demonstrated that biofeedback may be associated with lower reported pain scores, increased satisfaction with pain relief, and a sense of control in laboring women.[7]
- Biofeedback for Pain Management During Labor: 2011 Cochrane Review:
  - Overall there is not enough evidence to determine whether biofeedback is effective in reducing labor pain.
  - Biofeedback did not have a significant influence on rates of assisted vaginal delivery, cesarean section, labor augmentation, or the use of pharmacologic pain relief.
- Biofeedback is noninvasive and likely a safe approach as a component of labor analgesia, but its efficacy has not been proven.[8]

How/When to Incorporate Biofeedback

- Requires antenatal training and intrapartum application
- Generally requires some degree of guidance by a trained professional
- Minimum of 10 clustered training sessions (30–60 minutes each)
- Sessions may be during prenatal classes or given privately in the home by the pregnant woman herself.[8]

Hypnosis

Hypnosis has different definitions depending on the source. Most agree, however, that it is in some way a state of narrow focused attention, reduced awareness of external stimuli, increased responsiveness to hypnotic suggestions, and deep relaxation.[9] These hypnotic suggestions may be either verbal or nonverbal and are aimed at therapeutic goals.[10]

Hypnosis can attempt to modulate the experience of labor pain by focusing suggestions and concentration towards ideas or stimuli (e.g., feelings of safety, comfort, achievement) and/or away from them (e.g., pain, anxiety).[11] It is a tool to cope with pain in labor, not eliminate it.

Techniques

There are two main ways to administer hypnosis:

- In-person practitioner guided
- Self-hypnosis: requires initial in-person training or independent study

Patient willfully enters the aforementioned state of focus and decreased sensitivity to external stimuli through guidance or previous training and then responds to hypnotic suggestions generated by themselves or a hypnotherapist.

- Can use audiovisual supplementation/aides.[11]
- Neuroimaging suggests hypnosis suppresses specific neural activity that may inhibit the emotional interpretation pain.[10]

- Patients vary in susceptibility to hypnosis and hypnotic suggestion.
- Pregnancy may increase susceptibility.[12]

Potential Value/Possible Dangers

- Hypnosis for Pain Management During Labour and Childbirth: 2016 Cochrane Review.[11]
  - Low quality data suggests hypnosis may decrease the use of pharmacologic labor analgesia overall, but not epidural usage.
  - Overall evidence is inconsistent and not robust enough to determine whether hypnosis is efficacious in labor analgesia, increased satisfaction, or postpartum depression.
- There have been isolated case reports of antenatal and postnatal psychologic disturbances in women receiving hypnotherapy.[10]
- Hypnosis is noninvasive and likely a safe approach as a component of labor analgesia, but its efficacy has not been proven.[11]

How/When to Incorporate Hypnosis

- In-person practitioner guided:
  - Administration started intrapartum and/or antepartum
- Self-hypnosis: requires initial in-person training or independent study:
  - Generally requires intensive antepartum training (multiple sessions over multiple weeks, frequent self-study/practice).
  - Administered intrapartum and/or antepartum.
  - Can be taught privately or in groups.[11]

Acupuncture

Acupuncture is a technique in which practitioners stimulate specific points on the body, most often by inserting a thin needle through the skin. A similar technique, acupressure, involves the application of pressure at specific points without the insertion of needles. Several points theorized to reduce labor pains are located on the ears, hands, and feet. One proposal regarding the action of acupuncture is based on "The Gate Theory of Pain"[13] in which stimulation of certain nerve fibers prevents the conduction of painful stimuli along parallel tracts that pass through "gates," only allowing a certain amount of stimuli to pass at a given time. Another theory is that acupuncture stimulates the body to release endogenous opioids called endorphins,[14] thus decreasing labor pains.

Technique

- The part of the body that is painful and in need of pain relief is first identified.
- Acupuncture needles are inserted to various depths at specific points of the body which are thought to involve neural structures that modulate pain.

- The needles may be twirled or otherwise manipulated by the proceduralist, including the application of heat or electrical impulses.
- After a certain period, the needles are removed and the labor continues.
- Responses to the intervention are highly variable.

Potential Value/Possible Dangers

- Acupuncture for Pain Management During Labor: 2011 Cochrane Review:
  - Acupuncture and acupressure may have a role with reducing pain, increasing satisfaction with pain management, and reduced use of pharmacological management; however, there is need for further research.
  - Women reported less intense pain in both acupuncture and acupressure groups for these comparisons.
  - However, this evidence was generally limited to single studies.
  - The tools used to assess pain intensity or satisfaction with pain relief were not reported in the review.
- National Center for Complementary and Integrative Health:
  - Clinical practice guidelines are inconsistent in recommendations about acupuncture.
  - Many factors—like expectation and belief—may play important roles in the beneficial effects of acupuncture.
  - When not delivered properly, serious adverse side effects including infection, punctured organs, collapsed lungs, and central nervous system injury may occur.

How/When to Incorporate Acupuncture

- Antenatal coordination and intrapartum application.
- Requires an experienced and licensed acupuncture proceduralist.
- Unclear as to when, for how long, and at what intervals acupuncture is to be applied intrapartum.
- There is a paucity of randomized controlled studies and further research is necessary for this intervention.

Water Immersion

Water immersion involves the immersion of a parturient during the first or second stage of labor whereby the pregnant woman's abdomen is completely submerged. This can take place in a bath, pool, or any other body of water large enough to hold the parturient. Some theorize this aids in labor analgesia by facilitating the mother's mobility, improving uterine perfusion due to vasodilation, decreasing catecholamine release, increasing oxytocin release by relaxing the parturient, and stimulating the release of endogenous opioids. A major challenge in studying water immersion is that the definition and qualifications for it varies and it is referred to by many other names such as but not limited to water birth and hydrolabor.

Technique

- The decision and preparation for a water immersion delivery is discussed at length with the pregnant woman and her delivery facility and provider of choice well in advance.
- The delivery arena is arranged for and filled with typically warm water.
- The parturient is immerged in the water during the first or second stage of labor for variable amount of time.
- Mobility may be enhanced and the parturient is able to move around and also in-and-out of the delivery water arena as necessary for various interventions or fetal monitoring.

Potential Value/Possible Dangers

- Immersion in Water during labor and birth: 2018 Cochrane Review:
  - Immersion during labor and birth is becoming increasingly popular.
  - In the appropriately selected patient population, there is moderate to low-quality evidence that water immersion during stage 1 of labor has little effect on the birth but may reduce the use of regional anesthesia.
  - No clear difference in maternal or neonatal outcomes when water immersion is utilized during stage 2 of labor.
  - Evidence is limited by clinical variability and heterogeneity across trials.
- Committee Opinion on Immersion in Water During Labor and Delivery: 2016 American College of Obstetricians and Gynecologists (ACOG):
  - Water immersion during stage 1 of labor may be associated with shorter labor and decreased use of spinal and epidural analgesia between 37 and 41 weeks.
  - There is insufficient data on which to draw conclusions regarding water immersion during stage 1 of labor—thus it is recommended that birth occur on land, not water.
  - Risks and benefits have not been clearly studied or delineated.
  - Further prospective and controlled studies should be conducted.
  - Rigorous protocols and standard of care should be developed and implemented at centers that wish to offer and/or provide water immersion births to parturients.

How/When to Incorporate Water Immersion

- Requires antenatal preparation and intrapartum application.
- The delivery provider should be supporting and encouraging of this delivery modality.
- The site of delivery must have water immersion as an option with the appropriate resources.
- Risks, benefits, and alternatives must be thoroughly discussed and evaluated with the parturient.
- Contingency plans for fetal monitoring, maternal or fetal decompensation, and appropriate considerations for transfers must be worked out well in advance.

Subcutaneous or Intracutaneous Sterile Water Injection

- May possibly help relieve labor pains when injected over the sacrum.
- An option when neuraxial anesthesia is contraindicated, undesired, or unavailable.
- May work through endogenous opioid release and is based on gate theory of pain.
- There exists a paucity of clinically significant studies involving subcutaneous water injection.

Manual/Massage/Reflexology

- Manual and massage therapy techniques involve physical manipulation of bony joints or soft tissues of the body aimed at increasing relaxation.
- Reflexology proposes that manipulation and touch pressure points on the feet help provided anesthetizing effects on remote parts of the body which may aid in labor analgesia.
- Overall there is a paucity of clinically significant studies that implemented the scientific method in studying manual, massage, and reflexology in regards to labor analgesia.

Conclusion

The individual woman's experience of labor and associated labor pain is multifactorial. The physiologic components of the experience and their treatments are generally well understood by the western medical community. The psychosocial contributors to the labor experience and labor pain, however, are more enigmatic for most healthcare providers. Non-pharmacologic methods for treating labor pain largely address these psychosocial facets through coping mechanisms or distraction techniques. These methods and their intended targets are difficult to define, identify, measure, standardize, and therefore study. This has led to a scarcity of high-quality data on non-pharmacologic labor analgesia and its usefulness. Despite this, the psychosocial components of the labor experience and non-pharmacologic labor analgesia's aims of coping and distraction likely play a crucial role in labor experience and may even affect outcomes or satisfaction. Many women also desire to avoid pharmacologic interventions during labor, further highlighting the importance of non-pharmacologic approaches to labor analgesia. Though not well understood and of equivocal efficacy, many options exist. They include biofeedback, continuous labor support, sterile water injections, acupuncture, TENS, hypnosis, relaxation, water immersion, aroma therapy, manual methods, temperature therapy, and labor positioning. Of these techniques water immersion, acupuncture, and massage have the strongest (yet still weak) evidence for being effective in managing labor pain.[2]

References

1. Melzack, R. The myth of painless childbirth (the John J. Bonica lecture). *Pain.* 1984;19(4)321–337.
2. Jones L, Othman M, Dowswell T, Alfirevic Z, Gates S, Newburn M, Jordan S, Lavender T, Neilson JP. Pain management for women in labour: an overview of systematic reviews.

Cochrane Database of Systematic Reviews. 2012;(3):CD009234. doi:10.1002/14651858. CD009234.pub2.

3. Labor S, Maguire S. The Pain of Labour. *Rev Pain.* 2008;2(2):15–19. doi:10.1177/ 204946370800200205

4. Smith CA, Collins CT, Cyna AM, Crowther CA. Complementary and alternative therapies for pain management in labour. *Cochrane Database of Systematic Reviews.* 2006;(4):CD003521. doi:10.1002/14651858.CD003521.pub2.

5. Darnall BD, Sturgeon JA. Pain psychology for perioperative and chronic pain management. In: Longnecker DE, Mackey SC, Newman MF, Sandberg WS, Zapol WM, eds. *Anesthesiology.* 3rd ed. New York, NY: McGraw-Hill Education;2018. http://accessanesthesiology.mhmedical.com/content.aspx?bookid=2152&sectionid=164242672. Accessed October 20, 2019.

6. Rockers D. Mind/body interventions in the management of chronic pain. In: Bajwa ZH, Wootton R, Warfield CA, eds. *Principles and practice of pain medicine.* 3rd ed. New York, NY: McGraw-Hill Education; 2017. http://accessanesthesiology.mhmedical.com/content.aspx?bookid=1845&sectionid=133685637. Accessed October 20, 2019.

7. Duchene P. Biofeedback and childbirth. *International Journal of Childbirth Education.* 1988;3(1):12–13.

8. Barragán Loayza IM, Solà I, Juandó Prats C. Biofeedback for pain management during labour. *Cochrane Database of Systematic Reviews.* 2011;(6):CD006168. doi:10.1002/14651858. CD006168.pub2.

9. Gamsa, Ann. Hypnotic analgesia. *Handbook of pain management.* In: Melzack R, Wall P, eds. Churchill Livingstone, 2003:521–531.

10. Cyna AM, McAuliffe GL, Andrew MI. Hypnosis for pain relief in labour and childbirth: a systematic review. *BJA: British Journal of Anaesthesia.* 2004;93(4):505–511. https://doi.org/ 10.1093/bja/aeh225.

11. Madden K, Middleton P, Cyna AM, Matthewson M, Jones L. Hypnosis for pain management during labour and childbirth. *Cochrane Database of Systematic Reviews.* 2016(5):CD009356. doi:10.1002/14651858.CD009356.pub3.

12. Alexander B, Turnbull D, Cyna A. The effect of pregnancy on hypnotizability. *American Journal of Clinical Hypnosis.* 2009;52(1):13–22.

13. Melzack R, Wall PD. Pain mechanisms: A new theory. *Science.* 1965;3699:971–979.

14. Pomeranz B, Stux G. *Basics of Acupuncture.* 2nd ed. Springer-Verlag Berlin Heidelberg; 1991.

17

Neuraxial Techniques and Medications for Cesarean Delivery

Elvera L. Baron and Daniel Katz

Introduction

It is well established that neuraxial anesthesia is the preferred anesthetic for cesarean delivery. However, there are several options for mode of neuraxial anesthesia, which is further compounded by the choices and doses of medications that could be included. The main techniques that may be employed are epidural, spinal, and combined spinal-epidural (CSE). Each of these will be discussed in detail later in this section. Generally, the medication is injected either into the epidural space or into cerebral spinal fluid (CSF) surrounding the spinal cord (in the case of spinal or CSE).

There are several advantages to neuraxial anesthetic as compared to general anesthetic (GA):

- Relatively safe and reliable
- Avoidance of airway management
- Less impact on uterine tone
- Minimal risk of postoperative respiratory depression
- Less postoperative nausea and vomiting
- Ability to utilize neuraxial space for postoperative pain medications
- Early maternal/baby bonding
- Higher patient satisfaction[1]

Although neuraxial techniques are preferred,[2] in some patients these may be more dangerous than GA. See Table 17.1 for a summary of contraindications for placement of neuraxial anesthetic.

Furthermore, every anesthetic technique has its own risks. Table 17.2 lists the most common and dangerous complications that can occur after placement of neuraxial anesthesia, the patients who may be at increased risk of such complications, and some early management strategies.

One of the most common side effects from neuraxial anesthesia is maternal hypotension. This can result in fetal heart rate abnormalities because uterine/placental blood flow does not have autoregulatory mechanisms and is directly related to maternal cardiac output. Additionally, hypotension can cause maternal nausea and vomiting along with dysphoria. Preloading or co-loading parturients with crystalloid fluids, as a single intervention after spinal placement, was found to be ineffective in preventing hypotension.[3] Several drugs have been utilized to prevent maternal hypotension. Currently, phenylephrine is the drug of

Table 17.1 Contraindications for Placement of Neuraxial Anesthetic

Absolute	Relative
Patient refusal	Uncooperative patient
Sepsis	Infection near the site of needle insertion
Severe aortic stenosis or mitral stenosis	Mild to moderate aortic stenosis or mitral stenosis
Severe coagulopathy	Risk of bleeding
Known increased intracranial pressures (ICP)	Anticipated intraoperative major blood loss and fluid shifts
	Prior surgery at the site of injection
	Congenital abnormalities of spine or meninges
	Pre-existing neurological deficits or demyelinating disorders
	Hypovolemia

choice given its safety profile and favorable impact on neonatal blood gases when compared to ephedrine. Traditionally, boluses of medication were used; however, recent evidence has shown that infusions of vasopressors are superior to bolus administration at preventing hypotension, nausea, and vomiting surrounding placement of neuraxial anesthetic.[4] Finally, fluid co-loading together with phenylephrine infusion have recently gained popularity as measures to decrease severity of maternal hypotension after neuraxial anesthetic placement.[5] Table 17.3 summarizes common dosing for vasopressor administration used for mitigating post-neuraxial hypotension.

Choice of Technique

There are several choices of technique including traditional epidural, spinal, and combined spinal-epidural.

Epidural Anesthesia

Local anesthetic, with or without opioid, is injected into the epidural space to produce analgesia by blocking conduction at the intradural spinal nerve roots. This can be used as the main intraoperative anesthetic, as an analgesic adjuvant to GA, or as a postoperative analgesic. Epidural is preferred over spinal for surgical procedures of longer duration; unlike single-shot spinal administration, an epidural placement provides the anesthesiologist with an ability to maintain continuous anesthesia for the duration of the surgical intervention. Common medications for epidural administration include 2% lidocaine, 2% lidocaine with 1:200,000 μg epinephrine, 3% chroloprocaine, and others.

> *Note*: One advantage of the epidural as opposed to spinal anesthesia is the opportunity to slowly load the epidural to get less hypotension

Table 17.2 Complications, Their Mechanisms, and Suggested Management

Complication	Mechanism	Patients at Increased Risk	Suggested Management
Immediate/Intraoperative			
Hypotension	• Affects sympathetic chain T2–T10 • Creates "sympathectomy" • Leads to decreased venous return	• Young, skinny, pregnant • Dehydrated or hypovolemic perioperatively	• Co-load with intravenous (IV) fluids • Consider vasopressor bolus injections and/or continuous infusion (see Table 17.3)

Bradycardia	• Affects cardiac accelerator fibers T1–T4
	• Leads to decreased venous return with resultant reflex bradycardia via either
	  • paradoxical Bezold-Jarisch reflex pathway or
	  • low-pressure baroreceptors in the right atrium or
	  • pacemaker reflex
		• Recent administration of phenylephrine
		• Resting heart rate (HR) < 60 bpm (x5 ↑ risk)
		• ASA 1 (x3 ↑ risk)
		• Taking perioperative beta-blockers
		• Younger patients (< 50 yo)
		• Known prolonged PR interval on the EKG
		• Achieved sensory level above T6
			• Co-load with IV fluids
			• Consider vasopressor bolus injections and/or continuous infusion
			
			Note: If bradycardia is due to prior phenylephrine administration, consider discontinuing phenylephrine and/or using small dose ephedrine, epinephrine or atropine

Total Spinal	• High cephalad LA spread due to either
	  • medication administration intrathecally after already given epidurally or
	  • error in medication administration
		• Short stature	• Protect the airway: consider inducing GA with endotracheal tube (ETT) placement
			• Support hemodynamic instability with vasoactive medications, as needed
			• Consider placing patient in reverse Trendelenberg position to minimize cephalad spread
			• Consider CSF barbotage

Cauda Equina Syndrome	• Local anesthetic toxicity to the nerve roots		• Supportive treatment with IV fluid administration and vasoactive medications

(continued)

Table 17.2 Continued

Complication	Mechanism	Patients at Increased Risk	Suggested Management
Delayed/Postoperative			
Local site infection	• Break in sterile technique • Bacteremia surrounding labor and delivery	• Immunocompromised	• May necessitate antibiotic use • Requires keeping site clean and dry
Meningitis	• Break in sterile technique • L/D bacteremia	• Immunocompromised • Congenital abnormalities of meninges	• Requires antibiotics for treatment • Requires close monitoring of symptom resolution • Supportive measures, as needed
Epidural abscess	• Break in sterile technique • L/D bacteremia	• Immunocompromised • Spinal deformities	• Requires imaging for definitive diagnosis • Requires consultation with neurology and neurosurgical services, as needed • Requires antibiotics for treatment • Requires close monitoring of symptom resolution • Supportive measures, as needed
Backache	• Musculoskeletal / positioning	• Very skinny patients • Perioperative backache • Prolonged immobility	• Supportive measures • Consider heat pads • Patient reassurance after ruling out neurologic causes
Postdural puncture headache (PDPH)	• Unintended dural puncture with large bore needle	• Young, skinny • Difficult anatomic landmarks, necessitating multiple attempts at placement • Personal history of PDPH	• Supportive with IV fluids and/or caffeine administration • May consider blood patch placement if symptoms persist > 24 hours

Table 17.3 Vasopressor Strategies for Treatment of Hypotension
After Neuraxial Placement

Medication	Typical Doses: IV Boluses	Typical Doses: IV Infusions
Ephedrine	5–10 mg	n/a
Epinephrine	8–10 μg	10–20 ng/kg/min
Norepinephrine (NE)	6–8 μg	20–40 ng/kg/min
Phenylephrine	80–100 μg	80–100 μg /min

The dose of medication needed to bring up a surgical level varies greatly depending on whether the epidural has already been "activated," as is common for cases where the epidural is used for labor analgesia, unlike when a catheter is placed *de novo* for cesarean delivery. In cases where the epidural space is filled with medications for labor analgesia, often 5–10 mL of 2% lidocaine with 1:200,000 epinephrine is sufficient to bring the surgical level to T4. Much larger volumes (20+ mL) of the same local anesthetic (LA) mixture are required to raise a level in a new catheter.

In addition to LA, neuraxial preservative-free morphine is often added for postoperative pain control. Doses between 2–4 mg are commonly employed. Hydromorphone (0.6–1 mg) may be substituted when morphine is not available.

Spinal Anesthesia

A small amount LA with or without opioid is injected into the subarachnoid space to produce a reversible loss of sensation and motor function. There is much debate about the "optimal" spinal for cesarean delivery. See Table 17.4 for common medications and doses used to achieve adequate surgical anesthesia. Spinal anesthesia has the advantage over epidural anesthesia in terms of a faster onset and more reliable blockade, but it is associated with more hypotension than an epidural.

Table 17.4 Common Spinal Medications and Doses

Medication	Dose Range	Role in Anesthetic
0.75% bupivacaine with dextrose	1.2–1.5 mL	Produces surgical anesthesia
0.5 % bupivacaine	2–3 mL	Produces surgical anesthesia
fentanyl	12.5–25 μg	Additive for improved visceral analgesia[6]
sufentanil	2.5–10 μg	Additive for improved visceral analgesia[6]
hydromorphone	50–100 μg	Postoperative pain relief
preservative-free morphine	0.05–0.250 mg	Postoperative pain relief
epinephrine	100–200 μg	Prolonged duration of surgical block, improved quality of block
clonidine	75 μg	Postoperative pain relief[6,7]

Note: Single-shot spinal medications have a limited duration. Surgical levels of anesthetic may vary based on volumes and doses injected as well as the utility of adjunct medication.

A commonly used combination of medications would be 1.5 mL 0.75% bupivacaine with dextrose with 12.5 μg of fentanyl and 0.125 mg of preservative free morphine. This mixture of medication will reliably provide mid-thoracic sensory level for 1.5 hours; however, total duration of action may exceed 3 hours. We utilize this mixture at our institution for primary, secondary, and tertiary sections. For higher-order cesarean deliveries, or in deliveries where salpingectomy is also being performed, we would recommend either utilizing an epidural or CSE techniques.[8]

Note: Utilization of preservative-free morphine and hydromorphone may cause delayed respiratory depression up to 6–18 hours after administration. Although it is very rare, consider respiratory monitoring in these patients.

Combined Spinal-Epidural Anesthesia

In this technique, the epidural space is first identified with a Tuohy needle. Then a spinal needle is placed through the epidural needle and the IT space is accessed. Spinal medication is administered; the spinal needle is retracted followed by insertion of an epidural catheter prior to removal of the Tuohy needle. This technique is often utilized when the surgical duration may be prolonged and the spinal medication may not be of adequate duration, such as high-order cesarean delivery or combined cesarean delivery with bilateral salpingectomy.[9]

Relevant Anatomy and Placement

Detailed knowledge of vertebral anatomy is recommended prior to placement of neuraxial anesthetic.[10]

Vertebral Anatomy

Each lumbar vertebra consists of pedicle, transverse process, two superior and inferior articular processes (synovial joint), and spinous process. The vertebrae are connected by intervertebral disks (Figure 17.1).

Ligaments Supporting Vertebral Column

Ligaments include those on the ventral side (anterior and posterior longitudinal ligaments) and on the dorsal side (supraspinous ligament, interspinal ligament, ligamentum flavum). In order to access the epidural or subdural spaces for medication of administration, all dorsal side ligaments are traversed by the injection needle.

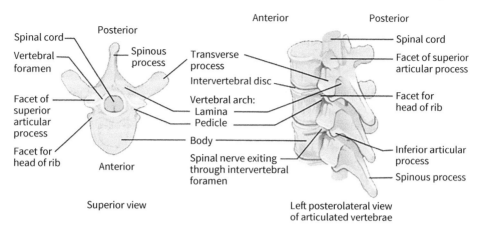

Superior view

Left posterolateral view
of articulated vertebrae

Figure 17.1 Diagram of vertebral anantomy.
Adopted with permission from Wikimedia.com.

Spinal Cord

The spinal cord terminates at different levels in adults compared to children. In newborns, spinal cord terminates at L3; in adults at L1. Additionally, conus medularis can be found at the terminal end of the spinal cord while filum terminale serves to anchor the cord in the sacral region (see Figure 17.2).[11,12]

Tip: In adults, it is safe to place spinal needle below L2 level.

Patient Positioning

The patient can be positioned either in a seated or decubitus position. If seated, the patient's legs should be supported by a smaller stool, so that hips are evenly flexed. Ideally, the patient should lean slightly forward while curving her lower back and bringing her head close to her abdomen. If the patient is laying on her side, she should be instructed to bring her knees as

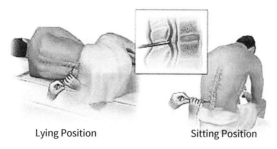

Lying Position   Sitting Position

Figure 17.2 Diagram of patient positioning for the placement of neuraxial anesthesia.
Adopted from Wikimedia with permission.

close to her abdomen as possible, while at the same time bringing her head to her knees as well ("fetal position;" see Figure 17.2).

> *Tip:* Guiding the patient to "hug a pillow" in front of them may help seated positioning.
> *Tip:* The landmark is iliac crest spinous process, which corresponds to about L4–L5 level in most people.
> *Tip:* The height of the table should be adjusted to the comfort level of the provider.

Approach to Epidural Placement

Midline: Needle entry is midline, between spinous processes
Paramedian: Needle entry is 1cm lateral and caudad, with goal to hit lamina and then "walk up" medially until "step off" is felt, which would result in entry into epidural space.

In the midline approach, the supraspinous ligament is entered followed by interspinous ligament, followed by ligamentum flavum. Once engaged in ligamentum flavum a syringe with either air or saline should be attached to the Tuohy needle and resistance should be felt. The Tuohy is then advanced until a "loss of resistance" is encountered. At this point the epidural space has likely been accessed.

In the paramedian approach, only paraspinous tissue is traversed prior to encountering ligamentum flavum. Checking for loss of resistance can be intermittent in between advancement (often with air) or can be checked by utilizing constant pressure on the syringe with advancement (often with saline). The epidural catheter is then threaded no more than 5 cm past the depth of the loss of resistance to avoid lateralized block.

> *Note*: There is no difference in accidental dural puncture rate comparing air to saline. In some studies, loss of resistance to saline is associated with a decrease in a lateralized or patchy block, but neither technique is recommended over the other.

Once the epidural catheter is in place, a test dose is performed to alert the anesthesiologist to either intrathecal or intravascular catheter placement. Common test doses are 3 mL of 1.5% lidocaine with 1:200,000 epinephrine. A heart rate increase of greater than 10 beats per minute or an increase in systolic blood pressure greater than 15 mm Hg is considered positive for intravascular injection, as are the signs of local anesthetic toxicity such a tinnitus and metallic taste. Intrathecal injection can be detected by the rapid onset of motor blockade.[11,12]

Approach to Spinal Placement

The approach to the placement of a spinal is like that of an epidural regarding patient positioning and preparation. Instead of inserting a Tuohy in the skin, however, an introducer is often utilized to aid in the insertion of a spinal needle. Most spinal needles for cesarean section are non-cutting needles 25-gauge or smaller, with many institutions utilizing 27-gauge needles to decrease post-dural puncture headache (PDPH) rate. Tactile feedback with needles this fine may be limited, and it is therefore prudent to check for entry into the intrathecal space at regular intervals as one may not feel a "pop." Once CSF has been encountered, the syringe with the spinal medication is attached and aspiration is performed to ensure good CSF flow. Once CSF flow is confirmed, the medication is administered at a slow steady pace. After injection, the patient should be positioned in left uterine displacement, especially if the spinal was placed in the seated position, to prevent the onset of a saddle block.

Equipment Needed

As shown in Figure 17.3, the following equipment is needed:

- Spinal or epidural kit
- Additional 3mL syringe and blunt needle to be opened sterilely
- Sterile gloves, mask, and hat
- Additional personnel to stand in front of the patient
- Alcohol or iodine-based prep sticks

Tip: Set up the tray consistently the same way each time—this will expedite the procedure completion and will help maintain sterility. Check the plunger of the glass syringe by breaking the seal before use.

Tip: Make sure all equipment is working properly. Read each kit prior to opening to ensure additional medications are available if the kit does not contain them. Common medication that may not be included in every kit is 2% lidocaine, to be used for skin infiltration. Additionally, if opioid use is planned intrathecally or epidurally, these medications should be available to be drawn up in a sterile manner. Prepare an extra syringe and blunt needle to draw these up.

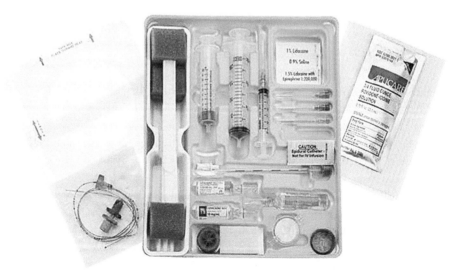

Figure 17.3 Example of a typical epidural tray.

Failed or Inadequate Neuraxial Block

Even in the most experienced hands, neuraxial anesthesia can fail. Depending on the route of prior administration, certain options are preferred:

- Failed Spinal Anesthesia
  - Wait up to 20 minutes for onset
    - Partial Block
      - Place an epidural
        - Repeat spinal in this case may lead to high spinal
    - No Block
      - Repeat spinal
      - Failed Epidural Anesthesia
        - Replace epidural and reload
        - Do NOT place a spinal, as high spinal may easily occur

In the case that neuraxial has failed and there is no time to follow the above plan, then a risk-benefit discussion should occur with the surgical team and the patient about conversion to general anesthesia.

Conclusion

There are a variety of options for neuraxial techniques for cesarean delivery. Each has their advantages and disadvantages. Knowledge of each method as well as comfort with different regimens will result in the best outcomes for patients. With constant equipment constraints, medication shortages, and logistical challenges, flexibility in technique for cesarean delivery is important.

References

1. Guglielminotti, J., Landau, R., Li, G. *Anesthesiology*. 2019;130(6):912.
2. Bucklin, B. A., Hawkins, J. L., Anderson, J. R., Ullrich, F. A. Obstetric anesthesia workforce survey: twenty-year update. *Anesthesiology*. 2005;103(3):645.
3. Siddik-Sayyid, S. M., Nasr, V. G., Taha, S. K., Zbeide, R. A., Shehade, J. M, et al. A randomized trial comparing colloid preload to coload during spinal anesthesia for effective cesarean delivery. *Anesth Analg*. 2009;109(4):1219–1224.
4. Heesen, M., Kolhr, S., Rossaint, R., Straube, S. Prophylactic phenylephrine for caesarean section under spinal anaesthesia: systematic review and meta-analysis. *Anaesthesia*. 2014;69(2):143.
5. Staikou, C., Paraskeva, A., Karmaniolou, I., Mani, A., Chondrogiannis, K. Current practice in obstetric anesthesia: a 2012 European survey. *Minerva Anesthesiol*. 2014;80(3):347–354.
6. Khezri, M. B., Rezaei, M., Delkhosh, R. M., Haji S. J. E. Comparison of postoperative analgesic effect of intrathecal clonidine and fentanyl added to bupivacaine in patients undergoing cesarean section: a prospective randomized double-blind study. *Pain Res Treat*. 2014;513628.

7. Crespo, S., Dangelser, G., Haller, G. Intrathecal clonidine as an adjuvant for neuraxial anaesthesia during caesarean delivery: a systematic review and meta-analysis of randomised trials. *Int J Obstet Anesth*. 2017;32:64.

8. Katz, D., Hamburger, J., Gutman, D., Wang, R., Lin, H.-M., Marotta, M., Zahn, J., Beilin, Y. The effect of adding subarachnoic epinephrine to hyperbaric bupivacaine and morphine for repeat cesarean delivery: a double-blind prospective randomized control trial. *Anesthesia & Analgesia*. 2018;127(1):171–178.

9. Lee, S., Lew, E., Lim, Y., Sia, A. T. Failure of augmentation of labor epidural analgesia for intrapartum cesarean delivery: a retrospective review. *Anesth Analg*. 2009;108(1):252–254.

10. Atashkhoei, S., Samudi, S., Abedini, N., Khoshmaram, N., Minayi, M. Anatomical predicting factors of difficult spinal anesthesia in patients undergoing cesarean section: An observational study. *Pak J Med Sci*. 2019;35(6):1707–1711. doi:10.12669/pjms.35.6.1276.

11. Barash, P. G. *Clinical anesthesia*, 6th ed. Philadelphia, PA: LWW. 2009;929–930.

12. Miller, R. D. *Miller's anesthesia*, 7th ed. New York: Elsevier. 2009;1613–1616, 2519–2521.

18

Airway Management

Joel Sirianni and Robert Mester

Airway Management Overview

Obstetric airway management provides challenges unseen in other areas of anesthesia. There are major changes in maternal anatomy and physiology that anesthesia providers must take into consideration before airway management. Prophylactic medications are a mainstay, aspiration concerns are high, and potential failed intubations and the difficult airway must be anticipated. Failed intubation in the parturient is roughly 8 times higher, quoted as 1 in 224 to 1 in 390 compared to 1 in 2,230 in nonpregnant patients undergoing surgery.[1] Aspiration and airway-related complications have historically negatively affected maternal outcomes. Maternal mortality is greater with general anesthesia compared to neuraxial anesthesia, although there has been significant improvement over the last 30 years.[2] Airway management for elective cesarean cases remains limited at 3–4% compared to neuraxial, but general anesthesia and airway management occur in roughly 20% of emergency cases.[3-4] Neuraxial alternatives to general anesthesia and airway manipulation include spinal, epidural, combined spinal-epidural, continuous spinal catheter, or even local infiltration and abdominal wall blocks. Neuraxial anesthesia remains the gold standard despite improving outcomes with general anesthesia.

Airway Changes of Pregnancy

Physiologic and Anatomic Changes

Anesthesia providers must be aware of numerous physiologic adaptations in the parturient's respiratory system. Oxygen consumption increases by 30–40% due to increasing fetal requirements and increased cardiac and respiratory effort. As seen in Table 18.1, lung volumes and capacities are altered with a notable decrease in functional residual capacity (FRC) to 80% of baseline at term with another 10% decrease seen in the supine position.[5] Minute ventilation also increases throughout pregnancy, leading to alterations in blood gas parameters including decreases in $PaCO_2$ and bicarb levels and increases in PaO_2 and pH (Table 18.2). Up to 75% of pregnant women complain of shortness of breath secondary to a combination of nasal congestion, increased oxygen consumption, increased minute ventilation, anemia, and increasing size of uterus with upward displacement of the diaphragm.[6]

Table 18.1 Respiratory Physiology Changes at Term Gestation

Parameter	Change
Inspiratory Reserve Volume	+5%
Tidal Volume	+45%
Expiratory Reserve Volume	−25%
Residual Volume	−15%
Inspiratory Capacity	+15%
Functional Residual Capacity	−20%
Vital Capacity	No Change
Total Lung Capacity	−5%
Minute Ventilation	+45%
Alveolar Ventilation	+45%

Capillary engorgement is common early in pregnancy, leading to tissue edema throughout pregnancy, particularly in the oropharynx, larynx, and intranasally. Nasal airway manipulation must be attempted with caution, as epistaxis may occur easily. Mallampati scores can increase several levels throughout pregnancy and may deteriorate quickly during labor (Figure 18.1). There is a 34% increase of women who have a Mallampati IV airway by 38 weeks gestation.[7] The mean weight gain in pregnancy is roughly 26 lbs. or 17% of the prepregnant weight due to growth of the uterus and its contents, blood and interstitial volume, and body tissues.[8] All of these changes lead to important anesthetic implications to consider, as shown in Box 18.1.

Gastrointestinal Changes of Pregnancy

Physiologic and Anatomic Changes

Although the incidence of maternal aspiration has declined dramatically in recent decades to an estimated case fatality rate of 6.5 per million anesthetics in the United

Table 18.2 Blood Gas Parameters during Pregnancy

Parameter	Non-pregnant	1st Trimester	2nd Trimester	3rd Trimester
$PaCO_2$ (mmHg)	40	30	30	30
PaO_2 (mmHg)	100	107	105	103
pH	7.4	7.44	7.44	7.44
Bicarbonate (mEq/L)	24	21	20	20

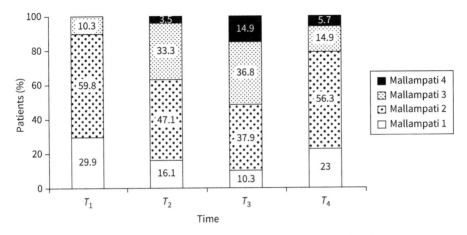

Figure 18.1 The Mallampati classes at different time points. T1, 8 months of pregnancy; T2, during labor; T3, 20 min after delivery; T4, 48 h after delivery. The percentages of patients with Mallampati class 3 or 4 changed significantly: T1 vs. T2, P=0.0000; T2 vs. T3, P=0.0005; T3 vs. T4, P=0.0000; T4 vs. T1, P=0.0062.

Reproduced with permission from Boutonnet M, Faitot V, Katz A, Salomon L, Keita H. Mallampati class changes during pregnancy, labour, and after delivery: can these be predicted? *British Journal of Anaesthesia.* 2010;104:67–70.

States, it still remains an important factor during induction of anesthesia.[9] The physiologic and anatomic changes of pregnancy on the gastrointestinal (GI) tract increase the risk of aspiration to levels higher than the general population. Cephalad displacement of the stomach and esophagus occur during pregnancy, as seen in Figure 18.2. This displacement, progesterone induced effects, and slowed esophageal peristalsis lead to a reduction in lower esophageal sphincter tone by up to 50%.[9] Unsurprisingly, up to half of women experience gastroesophageal reflux disease (GERD) during pregnancy. Intestinal transit is slowed but there is no alteration of gastric emptying during pregnancy until labor advances. Nausea and vomiting are prevalent early in pregnancy but can persist and become a severe condition called hyperemesis gravidarum. These changes and patient comorbidities are important to understand and consider, as they place the parturient at risk for aspiration.

Box 18.1 Anesthetic Implications of Parturient Airway Changes

- Elevated risk of nasal and oropharyngeal bleeding
- Less space for airway manipulation secondary to tissue edema
- Smaller endotracheal tube (ETT) recommended secondary to laryngeal edema
- Quicker desaturation due to less reserve (decreased FRC/increased O_2 consumption, more atelectasis as FRC < closing capacity, supine position, +/-GA)
- PaO_2 decreases twice as rapidly during apnea in pregnancy
- Preoxygenation and denitrogenation is faster because of elevated minute ventilation and a decreased FRC

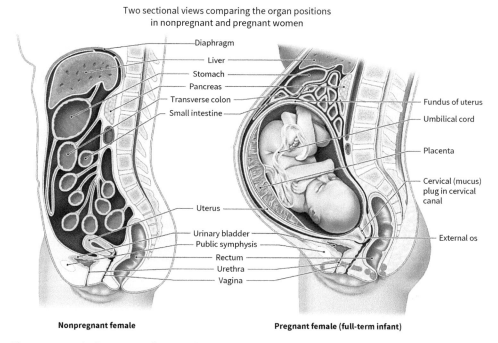

Two sectional views comparing the organ positions
in nonpregnant and pregnant women

Diaphragm
Liver
Stomach
Pancreas
Transverse colon
Small intestine
Fundus of uterus
Umbilical cord
Placenta
Cervical (mucus) plug in cervical canal
Uterus
Urinary bladder
Public symphysis
Rectum
Urethra
Vagina
External os

Nonpregnant female   **Pregnant female (full-term infant)**

Figure 18.2 Displacement of stomach cephalad during pregnancy.

Aspiration

Aspiration can lead to pneumonitis and rapid clinical decline. A higher volume and lower pH of gastric contents increase the chance of pneumonitis. Increased aspiration risks are seen with physiologic and anatomic GI changes, patient comorbidities (e.g., GERD, obesity, and diabetes), and patients with a higher chance for difficult airway.

Prophylaxis

The best way to avoid aspiration is to proceed with neuraxial anesthesia, thus avoiding the ablation of airway reflexes and decreased lower esophageal sphincter tone encountered during induction of general anesthesia. Aspiration rates have declined thanks to significant improvements in education and avoidance of general anesthesia, strictly following nil per os (NPO) guidelines, prophylactic medications, rapid sequence inductions, and improved airway training. The American Society of Anesthesiologists (ASA) Guidelines for Obstetric Anesthesia state that "the uncomplicated patient undergoing elective surgery may have moderate amounts of clear liquids up to 2 h before induction of anesthesia," 6–8 hour fasting depending on type of food, further restrictions on a case-by-case basis for patients with additional risk factors for aspiration, and that solid foods should be avoided in laboring patients altogether.[10] Prophylactic medications, as seen in Table 18.3, include timely administration of a nonparticulate antacid for gastric acidity, H2 antagonist for gastric acidity and volume reduction, and metoclopramide for volume reduction

Table 18.3 Aspiration Prophylaxis Options

Agent	Example	Dose/Route	Administration Time Prior to Airway Manipulation
Nonparticulate antacid	Sodium citrate	30 ml PO	Immediately
Dopamine antagonist, anticholinergic	Metoclopramide	10 mg IV	15 minutes
H2 Receptor Antagonist	Famotidine	20–40 mg IV	30 minutes

and increased lower esophageal sphincter tone. In an emergency, a nonparticulate antacid should be given at minimum prior to induction. The additional prophylactic agents should still be given after induction to prevent aspiration on emergence and gastric suctioning performed prior to extubation, as aspiration risk is nearly as high during emergence as induction. Cricoid pressure during induction can be considered but its utility has been questioned.

Treatment

Following witnessed aspiration, the provider should immediately perform tracheal suctioning and consider intubation or reintubation, treatment of hypoxemia, lung protective ventilation including continuous positive airway pressure/positive end-expiration pressure (CPAP/PEEP). Rigid bronchoscopy for large food particles should be considered as well as closer observation in recovery or an intensive care unit (ICU). In addition to hypoxemia and pulmonary shunting, aspiration can lead to laryngospasm, bronchospasm, acute lung injury, and acute respiratory distress syndrome (ARDS) but it does not necessarily lead to infection. Radiographic abnormalities occur in up to 90% of postaspiration imaging within 24 hours.[11] Therefore antibiotics should be based on clinical signs of infection but are not indicated for prophylaxis, as bacterial infections occur in less than 35% of aspiration events.[12] Saline or bicarbonate lavage are not proven to be useful and are potentially harmful. Steroids should not be routinely used, as they may increase infection risk, but a low-dose short-course therapy may have an impact on ARDS survival.[12]

Difficult Airway in Pregnancy

As mentioned previously, there are numerous physiologic and anatomic changes in pregnancy that require a vigilant anesthesiologist to ensure patient safety. Even the healthy parturient will have increased weight gain, breast enlargement, vascular engorgement and edema in the upper airway, decreased FRC with faster desaturation, a presumed full stomach with high risk for aspiration, and a progressively more unfavorable airway exam. Add in common comorbidities such as obesity, obstructive sleep apnea (OSA), diabetes, GERD, or preeclampsia and these patients become even more challenging. The ASA Task Force on Management of a Difficult Airway defines a difficult airway as a situation when a "conventionally trained anesthesiologist experiences difficulty with face mask ventilation of the upper airway, difficulty with tracheal intubation, or both."[13] The ASA difficult airway algorithm (as seen in Figure 18.3) is well known to anesthesia providers. However, Figure 18.4 is an example of an algorithm specific to the obstetric difficult airway.

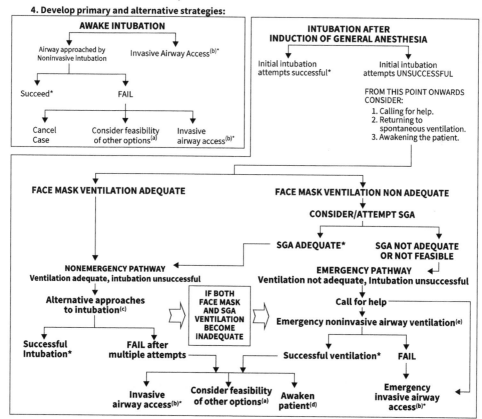

Figure 18.3 ASA difficult airway algorithm.

Reproduced with permission from Apfelbaum JL, Hagberg CA, Caplan RA, et al. Practice guidelines for management of the difficult airway: an updated report by the American Society of Anesthesiologists Task Force on Management of the Difficult Airway. *Anesthesiology.* 2013;118:251.

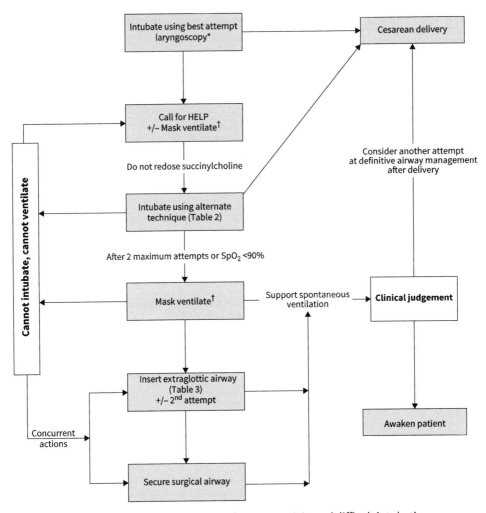

Figure 18.4 Suggested obstetrics algorithm for an unanticipated difficult intubation.

*Adjust cricoid pressure; backward, upward, rightward pressure (BURP); bougie; minor position adjustments.

†Oral airway, jaw thrust, adjust cricoid pressure, 2-handed technique.

Reproduced with permission from Wolters Kluwer Health. Mhyre JM, Healy D. The unanticipated difficult intubation in obstetrics. *Anesthesia & Analgesia*. 2011;112(3):648–652.

Preparation

If time allows, a thorough history and physical should be completed as soon as possible after a patient arrives on the labor and delivery floor. The history should include any past anesthetics with difficult masking or intubation, known airway or ear, nose, and throat (ENT) problems, recent colds or upper respiratory infections (URIs), recent nausea/vomiting, NPO time, and a review of the patient chart for airway records if available. Preeclampsia or obesity should raise a high suspicion for a difficult maternal airway. Gestation is important, as patients greater than 16–18 weeks must be considered a full stomach, but earlier than this a laryngeal mask airway (LMA) would be reasonable if no other contraindications preclude its use. At minimum, the airway exam should include thyromental distance, mouth opening, neck extension, and Mallampati score. Other difficult airway predictors such as incisor distance, neck circumference, body mass

---

Box 18.2 Airway Checklist

- NPO times must be strictly followed for elective cases
- Aspiration prophylaxis (nonparticulate antacid at minimum)
- Optimal patient positioning (see Figure 18.5): ramped, sniffing, breast retraction
- Adequate preoxygenation performed (3 minutes passively or 8VC breaths[14])
- Suction and intubation equipment at head of bed
- Extra anesthesia personnel and difficult airway equipment on standby
- Rapid-sequence intubation or awake intubation
- Avoid excessive cricoid pressure or eliminate completely
- Familiarity with the OB Difficult Airway Algorithm
- Extubate awake

---

index, lack of teeth, and history of snoring should be considered jointly, as there is no consensus on the best predictor of a truly difficult airway. Airway exams change rapidly during pregnancy and especially during labor so repeat exams are necessary immediately before instrumentation. The anesthesiologist should be prepared with a mental airway checklist (see Box 18.2) and have difficult airway essentials (see Box 18.3) nearby in case of an emergency.

Difficult Airway Management

Prophylactic epidurals should be placed in any laboring patient with an anticipated difficult airway to avoid emergent cesarean requiring airway placement. If an airway is required and a difficult airway is anticipated, then the decision must be made whether to proceed with asleep or awake airway placement (see Table 18.4). This discussion should be made jointly with the obstetrical team if obtaining an airway will delay delivery of a compromised fetus but ultimately maternal safety is the primary concern. Ultrasound can be used to mark the cricothyroid membrane in case there is need of an emergency surgical airway; however, one might argue that awake intubation is the better option if there is that level of concern. Fiberoptic intubation is most common, but awake direct laryngoscopy or video laryngoscopy are also options. Awake intubation can be performed quickly and safely with patient

---

Box 18.3 Difficult Airway Essentials

- Second anesthesia provider
- Multiple working laryngoscope blades, 6.0–7.0 ETTs
- Video laryngoscope
- Flexible fiberoptic
- LMAs size 3–5 and Intubating LMAs
- Gum elastic bougie
- Needle cricothyrotomy kit and jet ventilator
- Trauma or ENT (ear, nose, throat) surgeon

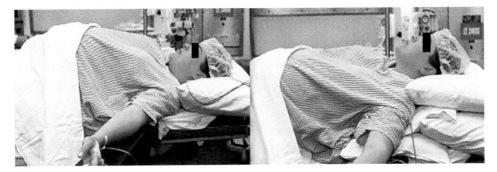

Figure 18.5 Head elevated "ramped" position.
Reproduced with permission from Elsevier. Rucklidge M, Hinton C. Difficult and failed intubation in obstetrics. *Contin Educ Anaesth Crit Care Pain*. 2012;12:86–91.

reassurance and proper airway anesthesia with either nerve blocks or topical anesthesia. Topicalization is more common and user friendly with many options including lidocaine gargle, nebulized lidocaine, spray as you go techniques, and atomized lidocaine to name a few. Difficult airways following induction may be unexpected or occur despite excellent planning. The Obstetric Anaesthetists' Association and Difficult Airway Society has several easy-to-follow, stepwise difficult-airway algorithms specifically for obstetrics to help with planning, when encountering a difficult airway (Figure 18.6), and after failed tracheal intubation (Box 18.4).[15] Clear communication, planning, and execution is critical to prevent devastating injury to the mother and fetus.

Emergence

The anesthesiologist must also be mindful of potential morbidity and mortality during and after extubation. Reports from Michigan during an 18-year period showed eight parturients died following surgery potentially as a result of anesthesia.[16] Diseases like preeclampsia can progress during surgery, fluid shifts and massive transfusion can occur, and patients may be obese or have OSA, which can lead to hypercarbia or hypoxemia in recovery. Rates of death and brain injury following extubation and recovery have remained fairly constant compared to improvement with intubation.[17]

Postpartum Airway

Return to Prenatal Baseline

It is imperative that anesthesia providers remain vigilant during postpartum airway manipulation. An important question is when do physiologic and anatomic changes of pregnancy return to prepregnant baseline? FRC returns to normal in 2–3 weeks whereas oxygen consumption, $PaCO_2$, tidal volume, and minute ventilation all take 6–8 weeks. Difficult airway concerns from anatomic changes, including Mallampati score and airway edema, have been shown to regress significantly by 24 hours after delivery.[18] Gastric emptying time, volume,

Table 18.4 Proceed with Surgery

Factors to consider		WAKE	→		PROCEED
Before induction	Maternal condition	• No compromise	• Mild acute compromise	• Haemorrhage responsive to resuscitation	• Hypovolaemia requiring corrective surgery • Critical cardiac or respiratory compromise, cardiac arrest
	Fetal condition	• No compromise	• Compromise corrected with intrauterine resuscitation, pH <7.2 but >7.15	• Continuing fetal heart rate abnormality despite intrauterine resuscitation, pH <7.15	• Sustained bradycardia • Fetal haemorrhage • Suspected uterine rupture
	Anaesthetist	• Novice	• Junior trainee	• Senior trainee	• Consultant/specialist
	Obesity	• Supermorbid	• Morbid	• Obese	• Normal
	Surgical factors	• Complex surgery or major haemorrhage anticipated	• Multiple uterine scars • Some surgical difficulties expected	• Single uterine scar	• No risk factors
	Aspiration risk	• Recent food	• No recent food • In labour • Opioids given • Antacids not given	• No recent food • In labour • Opioids not given • Antacids given	• Fasted • Not in labour • Antacids given
	Alternative anaesthesia • regional • securing airway awake	• No anticipated difficulty	• Predicted difficulty	• Relatively contraindicated	• Absolutely contraindicated or has failed • Surgery started
After failed intubation	Airway device/ventilation	• Difficult facemask ventilation • Front-of-neck	• Adequate facemask ventilation	• First generation supraglottic airway device	• Second generation supraglottic airway device
	Airway hazards	• Laryngeal oedema • Stridor	• Bleeding • Trauma	• Secretions	• None evident

Criteria to be used in the decision to wake or proceed following failed tracheal intubation. In any individual patient, some factors may suggest waking and others proceeding. The final decision will depend on the anaesthetist's clinical judgement.

© Obstetric Anaesthetists' Association/Difficult Airway Society (2015).

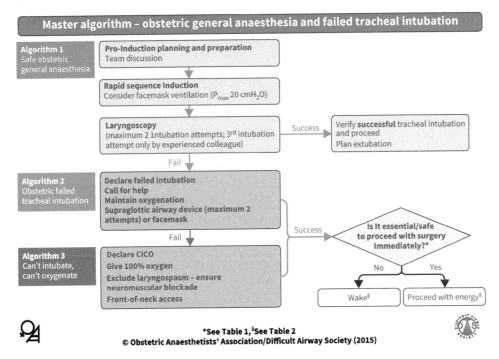

Figure 18.6 Master algorithm—obstetric general anaesthesia and failed tracheal intubation.

Reproduced with permission from Obstetric Anaesthetists' Association/Difficult Airway Society. Mushambi MC, Kinsella SM, Popat M, Swales H, Ramaswamy KK, Winton AL, Quinn AC. Obstetric Anaesthetists' Association and Difficult Airway Society guidelines for the management of difficult and failed tracheal intubation in obstetrics. *Anaesthesia* 2015;70:1286–1306.

Box 18.4 Management After Failed Tracheal Intubation

Wake
- Maintain oxygenation
- Maintain cricoid pressure if not impeding ventilation
- Either maintain head-up position or turn left lateral recumbent
- If rocuronium used, reverse with sugammadex
- Assess neuromuscular blockade and manage awareness if paralysis is prolonged
- Anticipate laryngospasm/can't intubate, can't oxygenate

After waking
- Review urgency of surgery with obstetric team
- Intrauterine fetal resuscitation as appropriate
- For repeat anaesthesia, manage with two anaesthetists
- Anaesthetic options:
  - Regional anaesthesia preferably inserted in lateral position
  - Secure airway awake before repeat general anaesthesia

> **Proceed with surgery**
> - Maintain anaesthesia
> - Maintain ventilation—consider merits of:
>   - controlled or spontaneous ventilation
>   - paralysis with rocuronium if sugammadex available
> - Anticipate laryngospasm/can't intubate, can't oxygenate
> - Minimise aspiration risk:
>   - maintain cricoid pressure until delivery (if not impeding ventilation)
>   - after delivery maintain vigilance and reapply cricoid pressure if signs of regurgitation
>   - empty stomach with gastric drain tube if using second-generation supraglottic airway device
>   - minimise fundal pressure
>   - administer H_2 receptor blocker i.v. if not already given
> - Senior obstetrician to operate
> - Inform neonatal team about failed intubation
> - Consider total intravenous anaesthesia
>
> © Obstetric Anaesthetists' Association/Difficult Airway Society (2015).

and pH have been shown to drastically change to near baseline levels by 18 hours postpartum per the Society for Obstetric Anesthesia and Perinatology (SOAP) continuing-education NPO guidelines.

Further Reading

Chestnut DH, Wong CA, Tsen LC, et al., eds. *Chestnut's obstetric anesthesia: principles and practice*. 6th ed. Philadelphia, PA: Elsevier; 2020.

References

1. Obstetric analgesia and anesthesia. ACOG Practice Bulletin No. 209. American College of Obstetricians and Gynecologists. *Obstet Gynecol*. 2019;133:e208–25.
2. Hawkins JL, Chang J, Palmer SK, et al. Anesthesia-related maternal mortality in the United States: 1979–2002. *Obstet Gynecol*. 2011;117:69–74.
3. Traynor AJ, Aragon M, Ghosh D, et al. Obstetric anesthesia workforce survey: a 30-year update. *Anesth Analg*. 2016;122:1939–1946.
4. Mcquaid E, Leffert L, Bateman B. The Role of the Anesthesiologist in Preventing Severe Maternal Morbidity and Mortalilty. *Clin Obstet Gynecol*. 2018;61(2):372–386.
5. Conklin KA. Maternal physiological adaptations during gestation, labor and the puerperium. *Semin Anesth*. 1991;10:221–234.
6. Jensen D, Webb KA, Davies GA, O'Donnell DE. Mechanisms of activity-related breathlessness in healthy human pregnancy. *Eur J Appl Physiol*. 2009;106:253–265.

7. Pilkington S, Carli F, Dakin MJ, et al. Increase in Mallampati score during pregnancy. *Br J Anaesth.* 1995;74:638–642.

8. Spatling L, Fallenstein F, Huch A, et al. The variability of cardiopulmonary adaptation to pregnancy at rest and during exercise. *Br J Obstet Gynaecol.* 1992;99(suppl 8):1–40.

9. Lim et al. A review of the impact of obstetric anesthesia on maternal and neonatal outcomes. *Anesthesiology.* 2018;129:192–215.

10. American Society of Anesthesiologists. Practice Guidelines for Obstetric Anesthesia: an updated report by the American Society of Anesthesiologists Task Force on Obstetric Anesthesia and the Society for Obstetric Anesthesia and Perinatology. *Anesthesiology.* 2016;124:270–300.

11. Landay MJ, Christensen EE, Bynum LJ. Pulmonary manifestations of acute aspiration of gastric contents. *AJR Am J Roentgenol.* 1978;131:587–592.

12. Marik PE. Pulmonary aspiration syndromes. *Curr Opin Pulm Med.* 2011;17:148–154.

13. American Society of Anesthesiologists. Practice guidelines for management of the difficult airway: an updated report by the American Society of Anesthesiologists Task Force on Management of the Difficult Airway. *Anesthesiology.* 2013;118:251–270.

14. Chiron B, Laffon M, Ferrandiere M, et al. Standard preoxygenation technique versus two rapid techniques in pregnant patients. *Int J Obstet Anesth.* 2004;13:11–14.

15. Mushambi MC, Kinsella SM, Popat M, et al. Obstetric Anaesthetists' Association and Difficult Airway Society guidelines for the management of difficult and failed tracheal intubation in obstetrics. *Anaesthesia.* 2015;70:1286–1306.

16. Mhyre JM, Riesner MN, Polley LS, Naughton NN. A series of anesthesia-related maternal deaths in Michigan, 1985–2003. *Anesthesiology.* 2007;106:1096–1104.

17. Peterson GN, Domino KB, Caplan RA, et al. Management of the difficult airway: a closed claims analysis. *Anesthesiology.* 2005;103:33–39.

18. Aydas AD, Basaranoglu G, Saidoglu L, et al. Airway changes in pregnant women before and after delivery. *Ir J Med Sci.* 2015;184:431–433

19
General Anesthesia for Cesarean Delivery

Lacey E. Straube

Introduction

When neuraxial anesthesia is contraindicated or otherwise inappropriate (see Box 19.1), general anesthesia can be safely administered to facilitate cesarean delivery. Given the altered anatomy and unique physiology of the parturient, there are inherent risks to general anesthesia in this population that must be carefully considered (see Table 19.1).[1,2] For a schematic representation of the perioperative sequence of events for providing general anesthesia for cesarean delivery, see Figure 19.1.[2]

Preoperative Preparation, Management, and Evaluation

Parturients undergoing cesarean delivery with general anesthesia may be scheduled for surgery, have an emergent indication, or have failed an attempt at vaginal delivery. A focused preoperative history and physical examination should be performed in each patient if feasible given the acuity of the delivery. In addition to the routine assessment, special attention must be paid to the airway examination and nil per os (NPO) status, as difficult airway and aspiration are known risk factors in this population that contribute to anesthesia-related maternal morbidity and mortality.[3] In emergency settings, the preoperative evaluation must often be abbreviated. In fact, the anesthesia provider must sometimes efficiently induce general anesthesia with limited knowledge of the patient, prioritizing maternal safety and rapid fetal delivery.

Aspiration Risk and NPO Guidelines

Standard NPO guidelines should be followed by all patients undergoing scheduled cesarean delivery, and patients at particularly high risk for aspiration may benefit from even more conservative fasting intervals.[1] Patients may consume clear liquids until two hours prior to their scheduled surgery. In fact, many Enhanced Recovery After Surgery (ERAS) pathways for cesarean delivery are beginning to incorporate the consumption of nonparticulate carbohydrate-containing liquids two hours preoperatively in nondiabetic women to limit hypoglycemia before scheduled cesarean delivery. Given the risk of pulmonary aspiration and its morbid sequela, prophylactic use of a nonparticulate antacid (sodium citrate 30 mL orally), histamine-2-receptor antagonist (famotidine 20 mg/ranitidine 50 mg intravenously),

---

Box 19.1 Indications for General Anesthesia for Cesarean Delivery

---

1. Contraindication to neuraxial anesthesia
   - Recent administration of anticoagulation
   - Coagulopathy
   - Sepsis/bacteremia
   - Focal infection over procedure site
   - Patient refusal or lack of patient cooperation
   - Hypovolemia/hemodynamic instability
   - Allergy to local anesthetic
   - Certain intracranial pathologies
2. Failed neuraxial anesthesia
   - Inability to successfully accomplish procedure
   - Failed/inadequate surgical blockade
   - Inability to achieve surgical anesthesia from an existing labor epidural
3. Conversion from a neuraxial anesthetic to a general anesthetic
   - High/total spinal anesthetic
   - Intraoperative hemodynamic instability
   - Persistent pain/patient intolerance of surgery
   - Surgical time required exceeding longevity of spinal anesthetic
4. Anatomic barriers
   - Postsurgical interruption of epidural or intrathecal space
   - Severe scoliosis or other spinal dysraphism
5. Fetal indications
   - Planned ex utero intrapartum treatment (EXIT) procedure
6. Any maternal or fetal emergency

---

and a dopamine-receptor antagonist (metoclopramide 10 mg intravenously) should be considered, individually or in combination, before induction if time permits.[1] Sodium citrate has a rapid onset, so it should be administered before induction, even in an emergency. Metoclopramide also takes effect within minutes. However, histamine-2-receptor antagonists can take 30 minutes to take effect. If given in close proximity to induction, they will not yet be protective during induction and intubation. However, they can be effective in time for extubation depending on the length of the procedure.

Preparation for Airway Management

A thorough examination of the airway can facilitate detection of and preparation for a difficult airway in the parturient. A comprehensive airway exam should include the Mallampati score, thyromental distance, neck extension and thickness, mouth opening, interincisor distance, and upper lip bite. The airway exam can deteriorate significantly during labor, so a

Table 19.1 Risks of General Anesthesia for Cesarean Delivery

Risk	Reasons	Prevention
Awareness	Often emergent nature of surgery Immediate incision after induction Use of low concentration of volatile agent because of atony, hypotension, hemorrhage, or decreased requirements in pregnancy Avoidance of preoperative sedatives Use of NMBAs	Maintain adequate depth of anesthesia, utilizing IV agents and N_2O when decreasing volatile anesthetic Administer opioids & benzodiazepines after delivery Avoid long-acting NMBAs if possible Consider BIS monitor
Aspiration/aspiration pneumonitis	Possible recent oral intake Decreased gastric transit time in labor Decreased LES tone	Avoid solid food in labor[a] Aspiration prophylaxis RSI OG suction before extubation Extubate awake
Hemorrhage	Impairment of uterine contractility by volatile anesthetics	Decrease volatile agent after delivery TIVA for persistent atony
Difficult/failed airway	Airway edema Increased breast mass Weight gain in pregnancy	Ramped, sniffing position Immediate availability of emergency airway supplies Consider awake intubation for anticipated difficult airway Know airway algorithm Call for help early
Rapid desaturation during apnea	Decreased FRC Increased oxygen consumption	Preoxygenate with 3 minutes of TV breaths or 8 deep breaths of 100% FiO_2[b]
Fetal exposure to anesthetic agents	Placental transfer	Facilitate efficient delivery Administer IV anesthetics after delivery if appropriate to wait
Postoperative pain	Absence of neuraxial opioids	Consider pre-emptive truncal block or wound infiltration Multimodal analgesia

NMBAs = neuromuscular blocking agents; IV = intravenous; N_2O = nitrous oxide; BIS = bispectral index; LES = lower esophageal sphincter; RSI = rapid-sequence induction; OG = orogastric; TIVA = total intravenous anesthesia; FRC = functional residual capacity; TV = tidal volume; FiO_2 = fraction of inspired oxygen

[a]American Society of Anesthesiologists, Society for Obstetric Anesthesia and Perinatology. Practice guidelines for obstetric anesthesia; an updated report by the American Society of Anesthesiologists Task Force on Obstetric Anesthesia and the Society for Obstetric Anesthesia and Perinatology. *Anesthesiology.* 2016;124:270–300.

[b]Chiron B, Laffon M, Ferrandiere M, Pittet J, Marret H, Mercier C. Standard preoxygenation technique versus two rapid techniques in pregnant patients. *Int J Obstet Anesth.* 2004;13:11–14.

recent exam prior to induction is pertinent if the patient has been laboring.[4] Along with routine airway management supplies, emergency airway equipment should be readily available at all times, as the difficult airway encounter can be unpredictable (see Box 19.2). If a difficult airway is anticipated for a cesarean delivery requiring general anesthesia, consideration should be given to awake fiberoptic intubation. Finally, knowing how and whom to call for help before it is needed is critical.

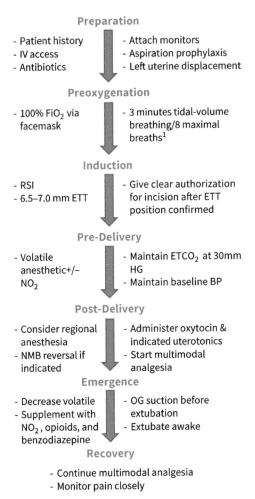

Figure 19.1 Sequence of events for providing general anesthesia for cesarean delivery. IV = intravenous; FiO_2 = fraction of inspired oxygen; RSI = rapid sequence induction; ETT = endotracheal tube; NO_2 = nitrous oxide; $ETCO_2$ = end-tidal carbon dioxide; BP = blood pressure; NMB = neuromuscular blockade; OG = orogastric suction.

1. Chiron B, Laffon M, Ferrandiere M, Pittet J, Marret H, Mercier C. Standard preoxygenation technique versus two rapid techniques in pregnant patients. *Int J Obstet Anesth*. 2004; 13:11–14.

Management in the Operating Room

Preparation for Induction

Prior to induction, the patient must be properly positioned and adequately preoxygenated. In the emergent setting, anesthesia providers must multitask to efficiently ensure appropriate intravenous access, administer a nonparticulate antacid and appropriate antibiotics, and properly position and preoxygenate the patient.

Box 19.2 Suggested Available Equipment for Airway Management

---

1. Ramp for proper positioning
   - Commercially available ramp or one built with pillows/blankets
2. Face mask
3. Head strap for face mask
4. Oral airways
5. Oxygen source
6. Appropriate monitors: pulse oximetry, capnography, pressure alarms
7. Self-inflating bag for positive-pressure ventilation
8. Functioning laryngoscopes
   - Consider having a laryngoscope with a short handle
9. Various blades for laryngoscope (Macintosh and Miller types)
10. Endotracheal tubes with stylet (size 6.5–7.0 mm)
11. Endotracheal tube guides (e.g., light wand, forceps to guide endotracheal tube)
12. Suction
13. Video laryngoscope
14. Flexible fiberoptic scope
15. Bougie
16. Laryngeal mask airway
    - Consider intubating laryngeal mask airway
17. Jet ventilation equipment
18. Topical anesthetics
19. Equipment for surgical airway
20. Stethoscope

Modified from: American Society of Anesthesiologists, Society for Obstetric Anesthesia and Perinatology. Practice guidelines for obstetric anesthesia; an updated report by the American Society of Anesthesiologists Task Force on Obstetric Anesthesia and the Society for Obstetric Anesthesia and Perinatology. *Anesthesiology.* 2016;124:270–300.

Positioning and Monitors

To avoid aortocaval compression and subsequent supine hypotension and placental malperfusion, the patient should be placed in left uterine displacement and maintained in this position until delivery. This can be accomplished by either tilting the entire bed to the left or placing a wedge under the patient's right hip.

Positioning should be optimized for intubation prior to induction, with the external auditory meatus at the level of the suprasternal notch. As illustrated in (see Figure 18.5) a ramp facilitates proper sniffing position for successful laryngoscopy and intubation and is of particular importance in the morbidly obese population.[5] Such a ramp can be constructed with pillows or blankets, but the commercially available option may provide faster achievement of correct positioning in an emergency situation.

Standard monitors, including a pulse oximeter, electrocardiogram, and noninvasive blood pressure cuff, should be applied to the patient prior to induction. Prophylactic antibiotics should be administered within the hour prior to incision to decrease the risk of surgical site infection.[6] Given that incision immediately follows induction of general anesthesia, antibiotics should be infused prior to induction.

Preoxygenation

Preoxygenation is of particular importance for the parturient, whose physiologic and anatomic changes of pregnancy result in a significant risk of rapid desaturation (see Table 19.1). Three minutes of tidal volume breathing or 8 maximum-volume breaths of 100% oxygen through a tight-fitting face mask protects best against desaturation.[2] Attaching a head strap to the face mask frees the provider's hands to facilitate multitasking while still providing effective preoxygenation. This is especially useful when preparing for an emergency cesarean delivery.

Induction

To reduce exposure time of the fetus to anesthetic agents, the patient is prepped and draped for surgery, the urinary catheter is placed, and the obstetricians are gowned and prepared for incision prior to induction of general anesthesia. After effective preoxygenation, a rapid-sequence induction is performed to decrease the risk of aspiration during induction and intubation. Pregnant patients are at particularly high risk of aspiration (see Table 19.1) because of the decreased lower esophageal sphincter tone created by the upper displacement of the stomach during pregnancy. Use of cricoid pressure remains controversial, but if used it should be released if compromising the laryngoscopic view. To prevent insufflation of the stomach, mask ventilation is avoided for the routine induction.

The rapid unconsciousness and muscle relaxation provided by the administration of propofol (2–2.5 mg/kg) and succinylcholine (1–1.5 mg/kg) respectively have made this combination the standard for induction of general anesthesia in the parturient. Propofol-induced hypotension and decreased cardiac output are countered by the sympathetic response to laryngoscopy. However, blood pressure should be carefully monitored and any hypotension briskly corrected to avoid placental hypoperfusion and maternal morbidity. Etomidate (0.3 mg/kg) and ketamine (1–1.5 mg/kg) are viable alternatives for the hemodynamically unstable patient who may not tolerate propofol-induced hypotension.

The young, healthy parturient can typically tolerate hypertension and tachycardia that may result from laryngoscopy. However, the sympathetic response to laryngoscopy should be pharmacologically blunted with short-acting agents like esmolol, nitroglycerin, or remifentanil in patients with certain pathologies. In preeclampsia, especially with severe features, blunting the response to laryngoscopy can decrease the risk of severe hypertension and its morbid sequela such as stroke and eclampsia. Laryngoscopy is also a high-risk period for patients with increased intracranial pressure (ICP), as further increases in ICP can potentially provoke brainstem herniation.

Intubation

Airway edema and friability from mucosal capillary engorgement can provoke difficult and traumatic laryngoscopy and intubation in the parturient. For this reason, a smaller-sized endotracheal tube (6.5–7.0 mm) should be utilized. Prior to intubating a pregnant patient, a video laryngoscope should be prepared and within arm's reach to use if a difficult or failed direct laryngoscopy is encountered. Suction should be readily available for managing secretions (saliva, blood, or emesis) that hinder the laryngoscopist's view.

If a challenging airway is encountered after induction, the difficult-airway algorithm should be followed, and assistance should be sought early (see Figure 19.2)[7]. If intubation fails, emergent cesarean delivery can be completed with a supraglottic airway or even mask ventilation with cricoid pressure, if necessary[7]. However, in a nonemergent setting, awakening the patient and proceeding with an awake fiberoptic intubation decreases the risk of intraoperative aspiration and loss of ability to ventilate. As in the nonpregnant patient, a surgical airway should be placed when both ventilation and intubation fail.

The obstetrician makes incision once proper endotracheal tube positioning is confirmed with end-tidal carbon dioxide. Bilateral breath sounds on auscultation and continuous end-tidal carbon dioxide monitoring prevent unrecognized esophageal or endobronchial intubation and should be utilized for every patient.

Awake Tracheal Intubation

When neuraxial anesthesia is contraindicated, awake tracheal intubation should be considered for the parturient with a suspected difficult airway. Engorged nasal capillaries may bleed with minimal manipulation, so the oral route is preferred for fiberoptic intubation. As in the nonpregnant population, the airway should be adequately topicalized to maximize patient tolerance. Notably, progesterone-induced increased nerve tissue sensitivity to local anesthetics reduces the dose requirements in pregnancy.[8] The total dose of local anesthetics used should be carefully monitored to avoid local anesthesia systemic toxicity (LAST), especially if the patient has already been exposed to local anesthetics through a labor epidural infusion.

Maintenance of General Anesthesia

Predelivery

After intubation and confirmation of correct endotracheal tube position, the anesthesia provider gives the obstetrician clear authorization to make incision. The depth of anesthesia is immediately increased with volatile anesthetic. Adding nitrous oxide can expedite this process, but 100% FiO_2 should be administered during fetal compromise or maternal desaturation. The minimum alveolar concentration (MAC) requirement in pregnancy is decreased compared to the nonpregnant population,[9] but the provider must ensure an adequate depth of anesthesia to avoid the known risk of intraoperative awareness during cesarean delivery (see Table 19.1). Although less studied in the pregnant population, a bispectral index (BIS) monitor can be a useful adjunct for assessment of anesthetic depth. Long-acting neuromuscular blockade is seldom necessary during cesarean delivery, and its avoidance may further decrease the risk of intraoperative awareness. After delivery and clamping of the umbilical cord, opioids and a benzodiazepine can be administered for analgesia and amnesia respectively. Predelivery sedative medications are typically avoided to reduce further fetal exposure to anesthetics. However, small doses of opioids and benzodiazepines have not been shown to negatively impact neonatal well-being,[10] so administration prior to delivery is appropriate with a clear maternal indication.

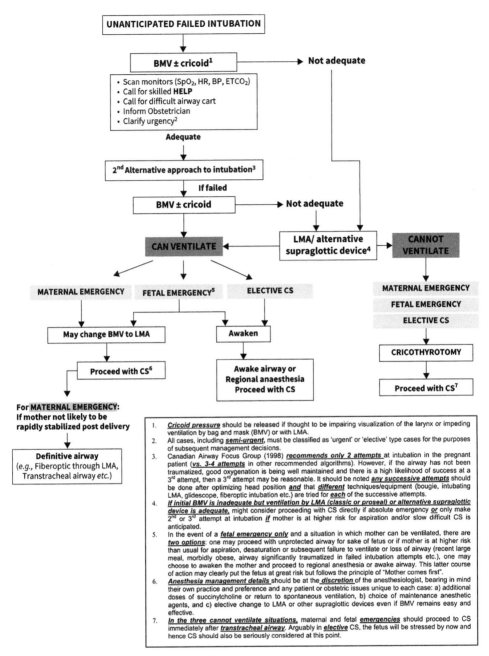

Figure 19.2 Algorithm for unanticipated difficult airway in obstetric patients. BP = blood pressure; BMV = bag and mask ventilation; CS = cesarean section; ETCO$_2$ = end-tidal carbon dioxide; HR = heart rate; LMA = laryngeal mask airway; SpO$_2$ = oxygen saturation.

Reproduced with permission from Balki M, Cooke M, Dunington S, Salman A, Goldszmidt E. Unanticipated difficult airway in obstetric patients. Development of a new algorithm for formative assessment in high-fidelity simulation. *Anesthesiology*. 2012;117:883–897. (Figure 1).

Placental Perfusion and Fetal Well-Being

When anesthetizing the parturient, the provider must also carefully consider placental perfusion and fetal well-being. Maternal blood pressure should be maintained at or near baseline to optimize placental perfusion. Increased alveolar ventilation in pregnancy results in a relative hypocapnia that should be maintained during general anesthesia, with an end-tidal carbon dioxide goal of around 30 mmHg. Hyperventilation can result in fetal acidosis via umbilical artery constriction. Likewise, maternal hypercapnia can also lead to fetal acidosis, as carbon dioxide readily crosses the placenta.

Postdelivery

Uterine Atony

Volatile anesthetics contribute to uterine atony in a dose-dependent fashion by inhibiting uterine contraction. The concentration administered should be decreased to about 0.5–0.75 MAC immediately after delivery and supplemented with nitrous oxide, opioids, a benzodiazepine, and other IV anesthetics as needed. Oxytocin should be administered prophylactically, and second-line uterotonic medications should be readily available. If uterine atony persists beyond uterotonic medication administration, the volatile anesthetic can be completely replaced by a total intravenous anesthetic (TIVA) technique. The anesthesia provider should also be prepared for the tocolytic potential of magnesium and its contribution to uterine atony for patients receiving an infusion perioperatively.

Intraoperative Analgesia

Especially in the absence of neuraxial anesthesia, postoperative pain can substantially decelerate recovery. Pain management should be addressed starting in the operating room. If long-acting neuromuscular blockade is not administered, opioids can be tailored to respiratory rate. Acetaminophen and nonsteroidal anti-inflammatory drugs (NSAIDs) provide excellent multimodal analgesia and should be administered in the operating room or recovery room if no contraindications exist. Pre-emptive or rescue regional truncal blocks can also be utilized for postoperative pain control. If time permits preoperatively, the patient can be consented for a truncal block under general anesthesia after the cesarean delivery is completed. Alternatively, the obstetrician can infiltrate the incision with local anesthesia. The total amount of local anesthesia administered, accounting for any given through an epidural catheter, should be tabulated to avoid LAST.

Emergence

Neuromuscular Blockade Reversal

Cesarean delivery under general anesthesia can be safely and successfully completed without long-acting neuromuscular blocking agents (NMBAs). However, if one is administered, special consideration should be given to its reversal. There is currently insufficient evidence to determine the impact of Sugammadex on lactation and fetal exposure. A recent statement released by the Society for Obstetric Anesthesia and Perinatology (SOAP) recommends against the administration of sugammadex in this patient population but, if given, the patient should be counseled that its use in lactation is not yet well understood[11]. However, this an evolving subject, and recommendations may change as new research surfaces. For now, the combination of a cholinesterase inhibitor with an anticholinesterase (neostigmine and glycopyrrolate respectively) is the preferred mechanism for NMBA reversal. Neuromuscular blockade status should be carefully followed with a twitch monitor in all patients who have received a NMBA. This is especially true for patients who have received a perioperative magnesium infusion, as magnesium is known to prolong the effect of nondepolarizing muscle relaxants.

Extubation

As with during induction, extubation is a high-risk period for aspiration. Orogastric suction should be performed prior to emergence. The patient should be fully awake and following commands prior to extubation to ensure adequate airway protection.

Postoperative Care

Multimodal Analgesia

In the absence of neuraxial opioids, effective postcesarean pain control can be challenging to achieve. As illustrated in Table 19.2, multimodal analgesia should be implemented and pre-emptive or rescue truncal blocks considered. Codeine and tramadol should be avoided

Table 19.2 Postcesarean Analgesia in the Absence of Neuraxial Anesthesia

Multimodal Analgesics	Examples

NSAIDs	• Ketorolac IV 15-30 mg in OR[a]/PACU followed by either:
	  • Motrin PO 600 mg q6H scheduled
	  • Naproxen PO 500 mg q12H scheduled

Acetaminophen	• Acetaminophen IV in OR or IV/PO in PACU followed by: • Tylenol PO 650–1000 mg q6H scheduled

Opioids	• Oxycodone PO 2.5–5 mg q4–6H PRN
	  • Consider 5–10 mg for severe pain
	  • Consider IV Morphine/Dilaudid for uncontrolled breakthrough pain
	• Avoid tramadol and codeine in breastfeeding patients because of neonatal adverse events in CYP_2D6 ultra-rapid metabolizers[b]

Supplemental Analgesia	• Lidocaine Patches • Gabapentinoids
Regional Anesthesia	• Pre-emptive or rescue truncal blocks: TAP, ESP, QLB • Wound infiltration

NSAIDs = Nonsteroidal anti-inflammatory drugs; IV = intravenous; OR = operating room; PACU = postanesthesia care unit; PO = per os; q = every; H = hours; PRN = as needed; CYP_2D6 = Cytochrome P_{450} isoenzyme $_2D6$; TAP = transversus abdominis plane; ESP = erector spinae plane; QLB = quadratus lumborum block.

[a]If given in the operating room, it should be administered after neonate delivery and cord clamping.

[b]US Food and Drug Administration. FDA drug safety communications: FDA restricts use of prescription codeine pain and cough medicines and tramadol pain medicines in children; recommends against use in breastfeeding women. 2018. Available at https://www.fda.gov/media/104268/download.

in breastfeeding women, as neonatal respiratory depression can occur if the mother is a cytochrome P_{450} isoenzyme $_2D6$ (CYP_2D6) ultra-rapid metabolizer.[12] Scheduled acetaminophen and NSAIDs provide excellent opioid-sparing postoperative analgesia and should be administered to every patient after cesarean delivery unless contraindicated. Oral opioids should be available as needed, and intravenous opioids may become necessary if effective pain control is difficult to achieve.

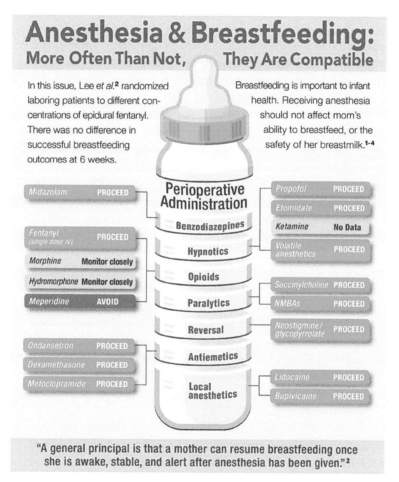

Figure 19.3 Anesthesia and breastfeeding: More often than not, they are compatible. IV = intravenous; NMBAs = neuromuscular blocking agents.

1. Lee A, McCarthy R, Toledo P, Jones M, White N, et al. Epidural labor analgesia—fentanyl dose and breastfeeding success: A randomized controlled trial. *Anesthesiology.* 2017;127:614-624.

2. Cobb B, Liu R, Valentine E, Onuoha O. Breastfeeding after anesthesia: A review for anesthesia providers regarding the transfer of medications into breast milk. *Transl Perioper Pain Med.* 2015;1:1-7.

3. Dalal P, Bosak J, Berlin C. Safety of the breast-feeding infant after maternal anesthesia. *Paediatr Anaesth.* 2014;24:359-371.

4. Drugs and Lactation Database (LactMed), United States National Library of Medicine, National Institutes of Health, Department of Health and Human Services. Available at: https://toxnet.nlm.nih.gov/newtoxnet/lactmed.htm.

Breastfeeding After General Anesthesia

Once the patient is awake, alert, and able to hold her baby, she can safely breastfeed.[13] As shown in Figure 19.3, almost all of the medications administered during general anesthesia for cesarean delivery are safe in breastfeeding.[13–16]

References

1. American Society of Anesthesiologists, Society for Obstetric Anesthesia and Perinatology. Practice guidelines for obstetric anesthesia; an updated report by the American Society of Anesthesiologists Task Force on Obstetric Anesthesia and the Society for Obstetric Anesthesia and Perinatology. *Anesthesiology*. 2016;124:270–300.
2. Chiron B, Laffon M, Ferrandiere M, Pittet J, Marret H, Mercier C. Standard preoxygenation technique versus two rapid techniques in pregnant patients. *Int J Obstet Anesth*. 2004;13:11–14.
3. Cantwell R, Clutton-Brock T, Cooper G, Dawson A, Drife J, et al. Saving mothers' lives: reviewing maternal deaths to make motherhood safer: 2006–2008. The eighth report of the confidential enquires into maternal deaths in the United Kingdom. *BJOG*. 2011;118:1–203.
4. Kodali B, Chandrasekhar S, Bulich L, Topulos G, Datta S. Airway changes during labor and delivery. *Anesthesiology*. 2008;108:357–62.
5. Rucklidge M, Hinton C. Difficult and failed intubation in obstetrics. *Continuing Education in Anaesthesia, Critical Care & Pain*. 2012;12:86–91.
6. American College of Obstetricians and Gynecologists. ACOG Practice Bulletin No. 199: Use of Prophylactic Antibiotics in Labor and Delivery. *Obstet Gynecol*. 2018;132:103–119.
7. Balki M, Cooke M, Dunington S, Salman A, Goldszmidt E. Unanticipated difficult airway in obstetric patients. Development of a new algorithm for formative assessment in high-fidelity simulation. *Anesthesiology*. 2012;117:883–897.
8. Datta S, Lambert D, Gregus J, Gissen A, Covino B. Differential sensitivities of mammalian nerve fibers during pregnancy. *Anesth Analg*. 1983;62:1070–1072.
9. Gin T, Chan M. Decreased minimum alveolar concentration of isoflurane in pregnant humans. *Anesthesiology*. 1994;81:829–832.
10. Frölich M, Burchfield D, Euliano T, Caton D. A single dose of fentanyl and midazolam prior to cesarean section have no adverse neonatal effects. *Can J Anaesth*. 2006;53:79–85.
11. Willett A, Butwick A, Togioka B, Bensadigh B, J Hofer, et al. Society for Obstetric Anesthesia and Perinatology. Statement on Sugammadex during pregnancy and lactation. 2019. Available at https://soap.org/wp-content/uploads/2019/06/SOAP_Statement_Sugammadex_During_Pregnancy_Lactation_APPROVED.pdf.
12. US Food and Drug Administration. FDA drug safety communications: FDA restricts use of prescription codeine pain and cough medicines and tramadol pain medicines in children; recommends against use in breastfeeding women. 2018. Available at https://www.fda.gov/media/104268/download.
13. Cobb, B, Liu, R, Valentine, E, Onuoha, O. Breastfeeding after anesthesia: A review for anesthesia providers regarding the transfer of medications into breast milk. *Transl Perioper Pain Med* 2015;1:1–7.

14. Lee A, McCarthy R, Toledo P, Jones, M, White N, Wong C. Epidural labor analgesia—fentanyl dose and breastfeeding success: A randomized controlled trial. *Anesthesiology.* 2017;127:614–624

15. Dalal P, Bosak J, Berlin C. Safety of the breast-feeding infant after maternal anesthesia. *Paediatr Anaesth.* 2014;24:359–371

16. Drugs and Lactation Database (LactMed), United States National Library of Medicine, National Institutes of Health, Department of Health and Human Services. Available at: https://www.ncbi.nlm.nih.gov/books/NBK501922/.

20

Obstetric Hemorrhage

Faiza A. Khan and Jill M. Mhyre

Overview

Obstetric hemorrhage is a major cause of maternal morbidity and mortality. Effective management requires a multidisciplinary approach. In this chapter, we review the general management plan, different types of obstetric hemorrhage, and specific considerations for each cause.

Preanesthestic Evaluation

Planning for obstetric hemorrhage is part of any obstetric preanesthetic evaluation. Specifically, evaluations in the antenatal period or upon hospital admission should identify risk factors for bleeding, consider the patient-specific consequences of bleeding, and ascertain patient characteristics that will influence the resuscitation plan. The evaluation provides an opportunity to explain the role of the anesthesiologist as an expert in resuscitation, allowing the obstetrician to focus on delivery and controlling the source of bleeding.

Risk Assessment

Risk assessment should be conducted by all providers who assess the patient, including obstetricians, anesthesiologists, and nurses. Association of Women's Health, Obstetric and Neonatal Nurses (AWHONN) advises obstetric nurses to screen for hemorrhage risk on admission, upon entry to the second stage of labor or transfer to the operating room for cesarean delivery, and prior to discharge from intrapartum care. The following checklist may be used:

1. Prenatal → Referral as needed
2. On admission
   a. Moderate Risk
      [ ] Prior uterine surgery or CD
      [ ] Multiple gestation
      [ ] > 4 prior births
      [ ] Prior OB hemorrhage
      [ ] Large fibroid
      [ ] EFW > 4000 g
   b. High Risk
      [ ] Previa
      [ ] Accreta/percreta
      [ ] Platelets < 100k/mm^3

[ ] bleeding disorder or anticoagulant medication
3. Intrapartum/Postpartum
   a. Moderate Risk
      [ ] Chorio
      [ ] Prolonged oxytocin > 24hr
      [ ] Prolonged second stage
      [ ] Magnesium sulfate
   b. **High Risk**
      [ ] Active bleeding
      [ ] > 2 medium-risk factors

Consequences of Bleeding

Women with smaller weights and those with anemia are more vulnerable to the consequences of hemorrhage.

$$\text{Allowable blood loss} = \left[\frac{\text{starting hot} - \text{target hot}}{\text{starting hot}}\right] * \left[\text{blood volume}\left(\frac{mL}{kg}\right) * \text{body weight } (kg)\right]$$

In normal-weight pregnant women, blood volume at the end of pregnancy is 95 mL/kg (identical to a term fetus), representing a 45% increase in blood volume from the nonpregnant state (65 mL/kg). For obese women, the blood volume of excess adipose tissue does not increase with pregnancy.

Women who refuse blood products and those with medical conditions that would exacerbate the consequences of anemia or hemorrhage (e.g., cardiac disease, sickle cell anemia) require tailored peripartum plans to minimize risk of bleeding and to address its consequence. Women with blood antibodies or known difficult cross match require a lower threshold for blood product preparation.

Resuscitation Planning

Resuscitation planning may include the following considerations:
1. Airway evaluation
   a. Large volume resuscitation can lead to airway and pulmonary edema.
2. Venous and arterial access
   a. Central venous access is best for potent vasopressors and calcium chloride.
   b. Peripheral intravenous catheters are shorter and allow for faster blood transfusion when an identical bore cannula is used.
   c. For antepartum patients, it may be best to avoid cannulation in order to preserve venous targets in the event of bleeding.
3. Obstetric management plan
   a. Multidisciplinary contingency plans for out-of-hours bleeding or non-reassuring fetal heart rate (NRFHR) are recommended.

4. Neuraxial anesthesia considerations
   a. Hypovolemia and severe cardiac disease (e.g., aortic stenosis) increase risk for hemodynamic collapse with induction of neuraxial anesthesia.
   b. Coagulopathy (e.g., abruption, anticoagulants) increases risk for epidural hematoma.

Hemorrhagic Response

The American Committee of Obstetrics and Gynecology (ACOG) guidelines recommend a team-based response to effectively manage hemorrhage at every stage of the peripartum period. This is presented by the National Partnership for Maternal Safety in terms of readiness, recognition, response, and reporting and systems learning. Key elements of obstetric hemorrhage management are outlined below.

Key Elements of Obstetric Hemorrhage Management: ACOG

Recognition and Prevention (every patient)

- Risk assessment
    1. Prenatal → transfer to higher level of care
    2. On admission → transfusion preparedness, large bore IV, resuscitation as needed
    3. Intrapartum/Postpartum →transfusion preparedness, mobilize team response
- Universal active management of 3rd stage of labor (AMTSL)
    1. Uterotonic within 1 min (oxytocin 10–40 U/1000 ml titrated)
    2. Controlled cord traction
    3. Fundal massage after delivery of placenta

Readiness (every unit)

- Blood bank (massive transfusion protocol)
- Hemorrhage cart & medication kit
- Hemorrhage team with education & drills for all stakeholders

Response (every hemorrhage)

- Checklist
- Support for patients/families/staff for all significant hemorrhages

Reporting/Systems Learning (every unit)

- Culture of huddles & debrief
- Multidisciplinary review of serious hemorrhages
- Monitor outcomes & processes metrics

Adapted from ACOG bulletin, November 2015.

Diagnosis of Hemorrhage

Hemorrhage is defined as cumulative blood loss greater than 1000 mL, regardless of mode of delivery. Bleeding more than 500 mL after vaginal birth is abnormal and should prompt escalation of care. Bleeding is frequently underestimated. Expired blood from the blood bank may be used to facilitate training in visual blood loss estimation (see Figure 20.1). It is also possible to weigh all absorbent materials and convert 1 gram of wet weight to 1 mL of blood.

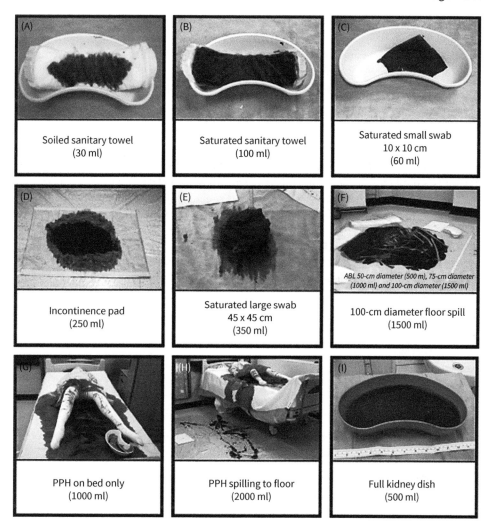

Figure 20.1 Quantification by visual blood loss estimation.

Reproduced with permission from: Hezelgrave N, Abbott D, Shennan A. Challenging concepts in obstetrics and gynaecology: cases with expert commentary. Chapter 19: Forewarned is forearmed in massive obstetric heamorrhage. Oxford University Press, 1st Edition, New York, 2015.

Hemorrhagic Shock

Hemorrhagic shock develops when oxygen delivery is insufficient to meet the metabolic needs of the tissues (e.g., maternal or fetal heart, kidneys and brain).

In the pregnant patient, blood loss may be underestimated if bleeding is concealed, especially if maternal vasoconstriction preserves blood pressure and heart rate. Tachycardia and hypotension are *late signs* of impending maternal collapse. The shock index (SI = HR/SBP) may be an early indicator of hemorrhage. Whereas SI > 1.0 increases the likelihood of acute blood loss, SI > 1.4 is associated with hypovolemic shock. Fibrinogen < 2 g/L identifies women with concealed hemorrhage, consumptive coagulopathy, or both.

Hypovolemic shock can be classified as follows:

- 15–20% blood loss: mild hypotension or HR < 100

- 20–25% blood loss: mild shock: HR>100, SBP 80–100 mm Hg, peripheral vasoconstriction, restlessness
- 25–30% blood loss: moderate shock: HR > 120, SBP < 60 mm Hg, decreased urine output, altered mental consciousness
- 35–40% blood loss: severe shock: anuria

Management of Hemorrhage

Rapid diagnosis and intervention can reduce cumulative blood loss and risk of coagulopathy. Systems solutions that improve the timeliness and reliability of response to obstetric hemorrhage include a hemorrhage cart, medication kit, response team, and unit-standard stage-based emergency hemorrhage management plan (Box 20.1, Figure 20.2).

Box 20.1 OB Hemorrhage: Carts, Kits and Trays

OB Hemorrhage Cart: Recommended Instruments
- Set of vaginal retractors (long right angle); long weighted speculum
- Sponge forceps (minimum: 2)
- Sutures (for cervical laceration repair and B-Lynch)
- Vaginal packs
- Uterine balloon
- Banjo curettes, several sizes
- Long needle holder
- Uterine forceps
- Bright task light on wheels; behind ultrasound machine diagrams depicting various procedures (e.g., B-Lynch, uterine artery ligation, balloon placement)

OB Hemorrhage Medication Kit: Available in L&D and Postpartum Floor PYXIS/refrigerator
- Pitocin 20 units per liter NS 1 bag
- Hemabate 250 mcg/ml 1 ampule
- Cytotec 200mg tablets 5 tabs
- Methergine 0.2 mg/ml 1 ampule

OB Hemorrhage Tray: Available on Postpartum Floor
- IV start kit
- 18 gauge angiocath
- 1 liter bag lactated Ringers
- IV tubing
- Sterile Speculum
- Urinary catheter kit with urimeter
- Flash light
- Lubricating jelly
- Assorted sizes sterile gloves

California Maternal Quality Care Collaborative. Leslie Casper, MD, San Diego Medical Center, Southern California Permanente Medical Group; Richard Lee, MD, Los Angeles County and University of Southern California Medical Center.

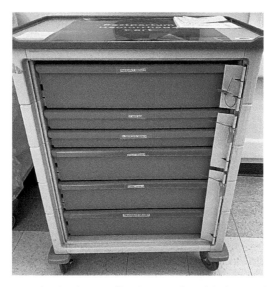

Figure 20.2 PPH cart at our institution. Medications can be added to top drawer according to institutional pharmacy guidelines.

A unit-standard, stage-based obstetric hemorrhage emergency management plan with checklists ensures that all members of the team escalate interventions as the severity of hemorrhage increases.

Hemorrhage Stages

Pre-admit	Up to time of admission
Stage 0	A ll Births
Stage 1	• >500mL VD or >1000mL CD **AND** <1500 mL • Brisk bleeding, large gush, large or multiple clots • Boggy uterus • Vital sign triggers—tachycardia, hypotension, hypoxemia
Stage 2	• Continued bleeding or VS instability or symptomatic **AND** <1500 mL cumulative blood loss
Stage 3	• Cumulative blood loss > 1500 mL • ≥2 units PRBCs given • Coagulopathy suspected
Stage 4	• Hypovolemic shock or AFE suspected

Stage 1 hemorrhage reflects the first signs of abnormal blood loss. Early involvement of the anesthesia team allows the obstetric provider to focus on obstetric management. For the anesthesiologist, attention is focused on volume resuscitation, administration of uterotonics, securing additional venous access, obtaining baseline labs, analgesia to facilitate obstetric interventions (e.g., manual evacuation of the uterus, laceration repair), and emotional support.

Stage 2 hemorrhage is diagnosed when bleeding continues despite secondary uterotonics and initial obstetric interventions, with less than 1500 mL cumulative blood loss. These patients require continued uterotonic therapy, volume resuscitation, hemodynamic support, hemostatic monitoring, blood product preparation, and anesthesia for progressively invasive obstetric interventions to control the source of bleeding.

Stage 3 hemorrhage is declared when bleeding exceeds 1500 mL and the patient requires blood products or demonstrates evidence of coagulopathy. Anesthesiology teams should continue all stage 2 interventions (e.g., uterotonic therapy) while addressing needs for hemodynamic and hemostatic resuscitation, thermoregulation, end-organ perfusion, and serial laboratory testing to detect and treat coagulopathy and electrolyte derangements. At this time, consider conversion to general anesthesia if bleeding is severe, patient is coagulopathic, or advanced surgical procedures are needed to control bleeding (e.g., hysterectomy).

Although crystalloids are appropriate for initial volume resuscitation, dilutional anemia and coagulopathy may develop. **Blood transfusion,** aiming for hemoglobin levels over 7 g/dL during hemorrhage, is indicated for any patient with active bleeding who develops signs of impaired oxygen delivery, hemodynamic instability, myocardial ischemia, and/or confusion. Urine output of at least 0.5 mL/kg/hour confirms adequate fluid resuscitation.

Massive blood transfusion (MBT) reflects the administration of 10 or more units of red blood cells within 24 hours, or more than 5 units in 4 hours. At this rate of blood loss, special MBT preparation and delivery protocols are needed to deliver large volumes of blood products to the bedside, including erythrocytes, plasma, cryoprecipitate and platelets.

With MBT, risk of **electrolyte** derangements increase. In particular, hypokalemia (< 2.5 mEq/L) may develop if high concentrations of endogenous catecholamine drive potassium into cells. Conversely, hemolysis of transfused blood may cause hyperkalemia. Citrate in erythrocytes, plasma, and platelets chelates calcium, leading to hypocalcemia, which can impair hemostasis and impede myocardial contractility. Calcium citrate or calcium chloride may be administered to maintain levels > 1.5 mEq/L.

Fibrinogen is the most frequently depleted coagulation protein in obstetric hemorrhage and should be maintained above 200 mg/dL during active bleeding. Ideally, the Clauss fibrinogen assay or viscoelastic monitoring (with thromboelastography or rotational thromboelastometry), allow for targeted replacement. Plasma contains approximately 400 mg fibrinogen per unit, along with other coagulation proteins. Fixed-ratio transfusion of plasma and erythrocytes (1:1 or 1:2 ratio) is appropriate to limit the risk of hypofibrinogenemia during large volume blood transfusion when fibrinogen cannot be measured quickly. For patients with severe hypofibrinogenemia (< 100 mg/dL) or signs of volume overload, lyophilized fibrinogen concentrate or cryoprecipitate are appropriate.

Thrombocytopenia is unusual during obstetric hemorrhage, presenting only in patients with antenatal thrombocytopenia (e.g., preeclampsia), abruption, amniotic fluid embolism, or more than 5 L of blood loss. Therefore, for obstetric hemorrhage fixed-ratio transfusion rarely requires platelet administration. Instead, goal-directed platelet transfusion is indicated to maintain the platelet concentration above 50×10^9/L during active bleeding.

Disseminated intravascular coagulation (DIC) includes a sequence of coagulation, microvascular thrombosis, fibrinolysis, and degradation of additional clotting factors. Obstetric conditions that most commonly trigger DIC include abruption, gram-negative sepsis, and amniotic fluid embolism. Treatment requires sequential monitoring and treatment with blood products (erythrocytes, platelets, plasma, cryoprecipitate).

Fibrinolysis is unusual during obstetric hemorrhage. Nevertheless, tranexamic acid appears to reduce blood loss.

Causes of Obstetric Hemorrhage

a. Antepartum:	b. Postpartum
Placenta previa	Uterine atony
Placental abruption	Genital trauma
Uterine rupture	Retained placenta
Vasa previa	Uterine inversion
	Placenta accreta

Antepartum hemorrhage: After 20 weeks' gestation, placenta previa or abruption are the most likely causes of bleeding. Uterine rupture and vasa previa are rare. Placental abruption and preeclampsia are most likely associated with coagulopathy (Figure 20.3).

Placenta Previa: Painless vaginal bleeding after 20 weeks' gestational age indicates placenta previa until proven otherwise. Transvaginal ultrasound is the best imaging modality to confirm the presence of previa and to measure its extent:

1. Total: completely covers the os
2. Partial: covers part, but not all, of the os
3. Marginal: lies within 2 cm of, but does not cover, the os

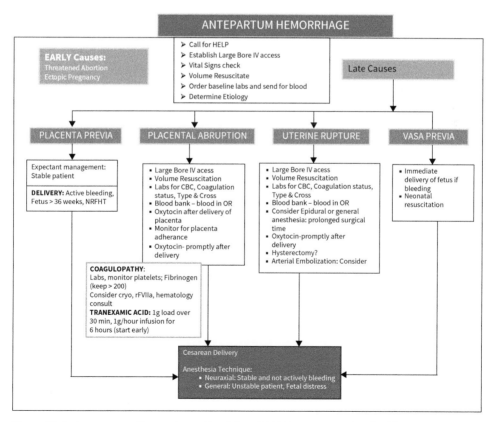

Figure 20.3 Antepartum Hemorrhage Algorithm. NRFHT, nonreassuring fetal heart rate tracing; CBC, complete blood count; IV, intravenous.

Once confirmed, placenta previa should always prompt assessment for coexisting accreta, which may also be evaluated with transabdominal ultrasound and/or MRI.

Conservative management is appropriate when bleeding is limited and the patient is pre-term; however, antenatal patients with placenta previa are at increased risk for preterm labor and emergency delivery. Cesarean delivery is indicated for patients with total previa or marginal previa within 1 cm of the cervical os. Regular review of all known inpatient and outpatient previa patients will help ensure continual preparation for emergency cesarean in the event of preterm labor, non-reassuring fetal status, and/or large volume blood loss. During active bleeding, previa patients need immediate large-bore venous access, preparation of blood products, and emergency cesarean to deliver the fetus and placenta. During antenatal observation, it may be appropriate to avoid large-bore venous access in order to preserve venous targets in the event of emergency.

Placental abruption reflects complete or partial separation of the placenta from the uterine wall before delivery of fetus. It can present with vaginal bleeding, concealed bleeding, preterm labor, non-reassuring fetal heart tones, uterine tenderness, and/or tetany. Bleeding is frequently concealed, and patients classically present with severe uterine tenderness and tetany. Fetal assessment determines the urgency and mode of delivery. Maternal assessment determines the intensity of resuscitation and anesthetic care.

Abruption occurs in < 1.0% pregnancies, with higher risk in women with advanced maternal age, African-American race, preeclampsia, hypertension, and substance abuse (e.g., cocaine, methamphetamine, tobacco use). Trauma or rapid uterine decompression (e.g., rupture of membranes with polyhydramnios) may cause shearing force through the placental bed, resulting in abruption.

Complications include maternal hemorrhage, coagulopathy, hypovolemic shock, acute kidney injury and intrauterine fetal demise. The combination of fetal death and maternal oliguria/anuria suggests abruption with concealed hemorrhage and should prompt aggressive fluid resuscitation and evaluation for maternal hypovolemia and coagulopathy.

Obstetric management depends on the maternal and fetal condition. Antenatal observation may be indicated if bleeding is limited and remote from term, and if both the mother and fetus are stable. Emergency cesarean delivery is indicated for non-reassuring fetal condition or active maternal bleeding. Abruption is a frequent cause of fetal demise; for women who develop severe coagulopathy, the safest route of delivery may be vaginal despite profuse bleeding and the need for ongoing blood product transfusion throughout labor and the stillbirth.

a. Maternal and fetal condition	Obstetric management
Stable with limited bleeding remote from term	Antenatal observation
Fetal nonreassuring cardiotography or maternal hemodynamic instability	Urgent or emergent cesarean delivery
Fetal death	Vaginal delivery
Reassuring maternal and fetal status at term	Vaginal delivery

With suspected abruption, concern for coagulopathy may mandate general anesthesia for cesarean delivery, regardless of the urgency of the delivery. Neuraxial analgesia or anesthesia may be appropriate as long as hemodynamic and hemostatic assessments are complete and reassuring. Regardless, maternal patients with suspected abruption need large-bore IV access, activation of blood transfusion, and laboratory evaluation for coagulopathy (e.g., platelet count, fibrinogen levels, and/or viscoelastic monitoring with Thromboelastography (TEG) or Rotational thromboelastography (ROTEM)).

Uterine rupture: Rupture of the uterus is a catastrophic emergency for both the mother and fetus necessitating an emergency surgery.

- *Uterine scar dehiscence* is defined as a uterine wall defect that does not result in excessive hemorrhage or FHR abnormalities.
- *Uterine rupture* refers to a uterine wall defect with maternal hemorrhage and/or fetal compromise requiring emergency surgery. Rupture of a classical uterine incision scar is associated with greater mortality as compared to a transverse incision. If lateral extension occurs, the hematoma can dissect into the broad ligament, uterine vessels, and retroperitoneal space, resulting in severe hemorrhage.
- The most common sign of uterine rupture is non-reassuring fetal cardiotocography.
- Other signs include abdominal tenderness or pain, breakthrough pain with neuraxial analgesia, uterine bleeding, uterine hypertonus, cessation of labor, or change in fetal presentation or station.

Uterine rupture: associated risk factors	
Excessive fundal pressure	Direct trauma to uterus
Grand multipara (distended uterus)	Uterine congenital anomalies
Forceps manipulation	Morbidly adherent placenta
Induction of labor or use of high dose oxytocin	Maternal connective tissue disorders; Ehlers-Danlos syndrome
Internal podalic version	

Vasa Previa is the velamentous insertion of the fetal vessels in the amniotic membranes near the internal cervical os. The fetal vessels are not protected and prone to rupture at the time of amniotic membrane rupture. Ruptured vasa previa is rare (1 in 2500 deliveries) but leads to fetal exsanguination.

- Risk factors: placenta previa, low-lying placenta, multiple gestation, or in vitro fertilization.
- It is diagnosed with ultrasound or on digital exam or when bleeding occurs with rupture of membranes.
- Although maternal health is rarely in jeopardy, rapid delivery is essential for fetal survival.

Postpartum hemorrhage can be due to genital trauma, retained placenta, uterine inversion, or adherent placenta (Figure 20.4).

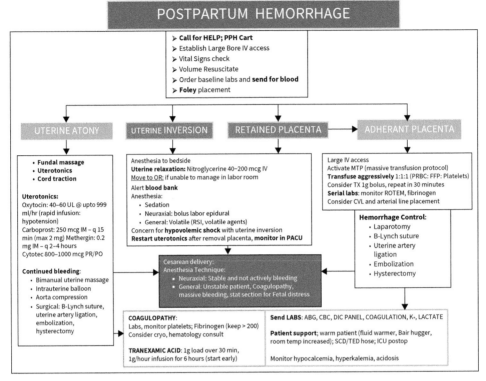

Figure 20.4 Postpartum Hemorrhage Algorithm. PPH, postpartum hemorrhage; IM, intramuscular; PACU, post-anesthesia care unit; CBC, complete blood count; SCD, sequential compression device; TED, thrombo-embolus deterrent; ICU, intensive care unit; DIC, disseminated intravascular coagulation; PR, per rectum; PO, by mouth.

Risk factors for postpartum hemorrhage include:

- Uterine atony (80%)
- Increased rates of cesarean section
- Adherent placenta
- Induction/augmentation of labor
- Multiple gestation
- Hypertensive diseases of pregnancy
- Advanced maternal age
- Obesity

Uterine Atony is the most common cause of postpartum hemorrhage, contributing to 80% of all cases. Factors that can worsen postpartum uterine atony include antenatal uterine distension (multiple gestation, macrosomia, polyhydramnios), myometrial dysfunction (e.g., precipitous labor, chorioamnionitis, funisitis, induced or augmented labor), residual intrauterine contents (e.g., retained placenta, placenta accreta), or pharmacologic impairment (e.g., tocolytics, volatile anesthetics).

Prophylactic oxytocin (0.3–0.6 IU/min IV) is the most effective intervention to both prevent and treat uterine atony and bleeding. Side effects predominate as the infusion rate (or bolus dose) increase. Instead, when atony continues, it is appropriate to increase the oxytocin infusion and add secondary uterotonics, such as methergine or prostaglandin F2α.

Uterotonics:

Medication	Dose	Side effects
Oxytocin	0.3–0.6 IU/min IV	Tachycardia, hypotension, water retention, cardiac ischemia
Methergine	0.2 mg IM (can repeat once in 2 hours)	Hypertension, nausea or vomiting, arteriolar constriction. (Preeclampsia and cardiac disease are relative contraindications.)
Hebamate (15-methyl prostaglandin F2 α)	0.25 mg IM (can repeat every 20 min, to 2 mg max)	Bronchospasm, fever, chills, nausea or vomiting, diarrhea. (Asthma is a relative contraindication.)
Misoprostol PgE	1000 mcg per rectal/ sublingual	Fever, chills, nausea or vomiting, diarrhea. No evidence of efficacy when added to oxytocin.

It is important to follow uterotonic protocols, and to alert the obstetricians when bleeding continues despite maximal uterotonic therapy. Unrelenting uterine atony can cause massive bleeding that requires escalating surgical interventions (e.g., intrauterine Bakri balloon, uterine curettage, uterine compression sutures, uterine artery embolization, hypogastric artery ligation, and/or hysterectomy).

Genital Trauma

Lacerations of perineum, vagina, or cervix should be suspected in any woman with vaginal bleeding despite a firm, contracted uterus. Transfer to the operating room may be needed to optimize visualization and repair. Depending on the extent of the laceration and bleeding, repair may be accomplished with intravenous or neuraxial analgesia, or neuraxial or general anesthesia.

Vaginal hematoma results from laceration of the descending branch of the uterine artery. It is most common with instrumental vaginal delivery. Other risk factors include nulliparous women, advanced maternal age, neonatal birth weight > 4000 g, prolonged second stage of labor, multiple gestation, preeclampsia, or vulvovaginal varicosities.

Vulvar hematoma develops when branches of the pudendal artery are torn. It is diagnosed by either extreme perineal pain, or hypovolemia in absence of bleeding. Conservative treatment may include ice packs and oral analgesics. Severe cases require volume resuscitation and either surgical intervention to ligate bleeding vessels or arterial embolization.

Cervical laceration and **retroperitoneal hematoma** are the most serious causes of genital tract trauma. Both can involve massive bleeding with injury to the uterine and/or hypogastric arteries. Particularly during cesarean delivery for arrest of descent, the lower uterine segment and cervix may be extremely thin, and obstetric attempts to free the fetal head can lacerate the cervix and extend the transverse incision into the broad ligament.

Hemorrhage may be evident and immediately repaired. It may also track through the broad ligament, leading to concealed hemorrhage into the retroperitoneal space.

With retroperitoneal hematoma, bleeding is typically concealed, and progressive tachycardia and hypotension may be the only presenting signs. Associated symptoms include lower abdominal pain, or a tender mass above inguinal ligament that displaces firm contracted uterus to contralateral side. Uterine ultrasound is not likely to demonstrate an intrauterine stripe as long as bleeding is entirely extrauterine. A strong index of suspicion for retroperitoneal hematoma is needed in post-cesarean delivery patients with evidence of hypovolemic shock. Return to the operating room is necessary for exploratory laparotomy.

Retained placenta is failure to deliver the placenta completely within 30 minutes of delivery. Ultrasound imaging of an intrauterine stripe confirms retained intrauterine contents. With vaginal delivery, rapid uterine contraction may trap the placenta behind a closing cervix; nitroglycerin (20–400 mcg IV) may facilitate manual evacuation of the placenta. Following cesarean delivery, retained placental fragments may not be visible. Manual removal of the placenta can occur in the delivery room or postoperative care unit (PACU)) with epidural or intravenous analgesia (e.g., fentanyl 1 mcg/kg or ketamine 0.1 mg/kg). If bedside obstetric maneuvers do not control the bleeding, then it is best to transfer to the operating room for uterine curettage or exploratory laparotomy under neuraxial or general anesthesia. After delivery of the placenta, prompt oxytocin administration will limit atonic bleeding.

Uterine inversion: The uterus can turn inside out after delivery, leading to risk of severe hemorrhage. Partial inversion may be visible only on ultrasound, appearing as a donut sign when the dome of the uterus inverts into the uterine cavity. Risk factors include uterine atony, short umbilical cord, uterine anomalies, and aggressive cord traction during the third stage of labor. Immediate replacement requires uterine relaxation with either nitroglycerin 20–400 mcg IV or induction of general anesthesia with 2–3 MAC (minimum alveolar concentration) of volatile anesthesia; this facilitates relaxation of the uterus. Blood loss can be extremely rapid with uterine inversion, so caution is advised when inducing general anesthesia. Once the uterus is reverted, oxytocin treatment will prevent uterine atony.

Placenta accreta spectrum (PAS) was previously known as morbidly adherent placenta, and encompasses placenta (1) accreta: adherence of the basal plate of the placenta to the uterine myometrium; (2) increta: chorionic villi invade the myometrium; and (3) percreta: invasion through the myometrium into the serosa (Figures 20.5, 20.6).

The population-level incidence of placenta accreta increases with the prevalence of women with prior cesarean deliveries (0, 1, 2, 3 and > 4 deliveries associated with an increased risk to 3%, 11%, 40%, 61% and 67% respectively). For individual patients, placental location (previa/overlying the uterine scar) is a more important predictor than the total number of prior cesarean deliveries. For women with placental previa, coexisting placenta accreta should always be suspected and is present in the majority of such patients with three or more prior cesarean deliveries.

Patients with suspected placenta accreta should only be delivered in accreta centers by teams who are prepared for cesarean hysterectomy and massive volume resuscitation. Usually placenta accreta spectrum is diagnosed antepartum, allowing for appropriate referrals and

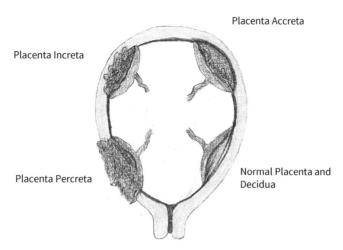

Figure 20.5 Abnormal placentation.

delivery planning. Occasionally, it is diagnosed at the time of cesarean delivery when unexpected placental varicosities are found on the serosal surface of the uterus prior to uterine incision (see Figure 20.7). In such cases, it may be appropriate to close the maternal abdominal wall without delivering the fetus and defer surgery until the team is fully prepared.

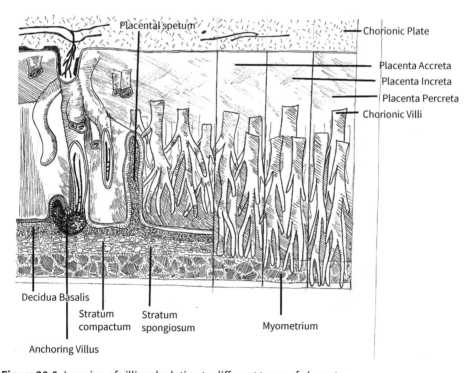

Figure 20.6 Invasion of villi and relation to different types of placenta.

Modified from Chapter 4; The placenta: anatomy, physiology and transfer of drugs; Chestnut's, fifth edition; *by Zoya Khan (9th grade, Central High School, Little Rock).*

Table 20.1 Algorithm of Management of Unanticipated Postpartum Hemorrhage and Anesthetic Considerations

	Assessment	Meds/Procedure/Blood bank	Anesthesia Considerations
Stage 0 Risk assessment Active management of 3rd stage of labor	Every woman in labor **Assess for risk factors** • **Evaluate for ongoing blood loss** • Serial assessment: fundal height and uterine tone • Normal postpartum monitoring: continue oxytocin	**Active management of 3rd stage (AMSTL)** 1. Fundal massage 2. Oxytocin IV infusion 3. Cord traction **Blood bank:** • T & S for patients with alloantibodies • High risk: T & C	**Antenatal preparation:** Correct iron deficiency anemia Jehovah's witness: Identify **Postpartum: concealed bleeding:** lightheadedness, shortness of breath, diaphoresis, hypotension or tachycardia
Stage 1 Activate PPH protocol Call for help	Blood loss: > 500 ml vaginal or > 1000 ml Cesarean or uterine atony or abnormal vital signs		
	Monitor vital signs **Begin volume resuscitation** **Quantification** of blood loss: weigh **Inspect** vaginal walls, cervix, uterine cavity, placenta Consider baseline labs	Large-bore IV access **Fluid bolus** **Fundal Massage** **Oxytocin:** increase rate Methergin 0.2 mg IM or Hebamate 0.25 mg IM Foley placement **Blood bank:** send for blood (T & C if not already done)	Monitor baseline labs Ensure blood bank has blood available Analgesia: sedation or bolus of epidural for any surgical stimulus (retained placenta, uterine inversion, lacerations repair)
Stage 2 Advance through protocol Reassess	Continued bleeding with total blood loss under 1500 ml		
	OB and anesthesia at bedside Monitor vital signs **Reassess/evaluate** Vaginal birth: • **Other causes:** AFE, inversion, retained placenta • Consider moving to OR	**Uterotonics:** Methergin 0.2 mg IM (repeat dose in 2 hours) or Hebamate 0.25 mg IM (every 20 min, max 2mg) **2nd IV access** (or Intraosseous) Call for blood to room/OR **Bimanual uterus massage** **Vaginal birth:** • Move to OR • Repair any lacerations • Rule out retained placenta • Place intrauterine balloon • Selective embolization (IR) **Cesarean birth:** • Inspect broad ligaments, retained placenta • B-Lynch suture • Place intrauterine balloon	Serial labs: ROTEM, ABG **Goal Directed Therapy:** • Hematocrit > 21–24 g/dL • Platelets > 50,000 • Fibrinogen > 200 mg/dL **Anesthesia plan:** • Spinal: select circumstances • Neuraxial: labor epidural catheter can be used

	Assessment	Meds/Procedure/Blood bank	Anesthesia Considerations
Stage 3	Total blood loss over 1500 ml, or > 2 units PRBCs given or VS unstable or suspicion of DIC		
Begin Massive Transfusion Protocol	**Team response:** Obstetrics; anesthesia; pediatrics OR staff; ICU staff: postpartum Repeat labs Consider CVL/arterial line Family support: social worker	**Activate Massive Transfusion Protocol** (MTP) **Hemorrhage Control:** if not done • Laparotomy • B-Lynch suture • Uterine artery ligation • Hysterectomy Patient support: keep patient warm; TED/hose	**Aggressive Transfusion: 1:1:1** **Coagulopathy** (rFVIIa, PCC) Consider TXA: 1 g bolus, repeat after 30 min (WHO) Monitor serial labs and electrolytes Anesthesia plan: • **General:** preferred if severe bleeding or coagulopathy

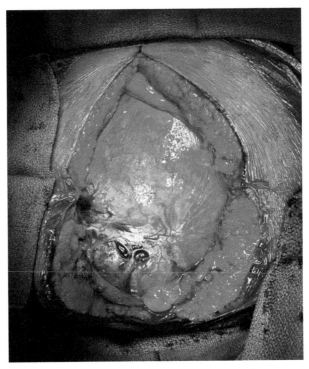

Figure 20.7 Image of placenta accreta at time of delivery showing placental varicosities on uterine serosal surface.

Image with permission from Dr. Adam Sandlin, M.D.

Frequently, controlled cesarean hysterectomy may be completed under epidural or combined spinal-epidural anesthesia. The fetus is typically delivered through a fundal incision to avoid the placenta, followed by uterine closure and hysterectomy. If the placenta is disturbed, then massive bleeding may commence, and immediate induction of general anesthesia is appropriate, before the patient develops profound hypovolemia, coagulopathy, pulmonary edema, or airway edema. Prompt recognition and coordinated management is essential for effective patient outcomes (Table 20.1).

21

Cesarean Delivery

Postoperative Management

Thais Franklin dos Santos, Arina Ghosh, and Reine Zbeidy

Introduction

The last Centers for Disease Control and Prevention (CDC) report indicates that nearly 1.3 million cesarean deliveries are performed every year in the United States, which makes it one of the most common surgical procedures.[1] Cesarean deliveries comprise more than 30% of all deliveries, and approximately 20% of the patients who undergo a cesarean delivery report severe pain in the initial postoperative period. Inadequately treated pain is associated with increased risk of developing chronic pain, postpartum depression, difficulty with breastfeeding, increased healthcare cost, and other complications.[2] Providing good postoperative pain management improves patient satisfaction, promotes early ambulation with less risk of thromboembolic events, and faster functional recovery in general.[3] The neurophysiology of pain is complex, and a multimodal approach leads to better postoperative analgesia.[4]

Postcesarean Delivery Pain Pathways

Postcesarean delivery pain has two main components: somatic and visceral. Somatic pain is related to stimulation of nociceptors in the abdominal wall, which leads to transmission of pain signals to the anterior rami of spinal nerves at T10 to L1. These nerves enter the abdominal wall between the internal oblique and the transverse abdominis muscles.[5]

Visceral pain from cesarean delivery arises from nociceptive stimuli of the afferent fibers in the inferior hypogastric plexus that mediates pain via sympathetic chain of the pelvic and lower abdominal viscera and enters the cord between T10 and L1.[6]

Neuraxial Opioids for Cesarean Delivery

Benefits of Neuraxial Opioids

Neuraxial anesthesia is the preferred anesthetic technique for most cesarean deliveries by the American Society of Pain and by the American Society of Anesthesiologists. Randomized control trials also indicate higher Apgar scores at 1 and 5 minutes with neuraxial anesthesia in comparison with general anesthesia.[7] Multimodal regimens should be used for postoperative pain management[4] and neuraxial opioids are considered the main component of multimodal analgesia after cesarean since they provide better pain control than systemic opioids, non-neuraxial regional techniques, and oral analgesics.[8] Neuraxial morphine is the gold-standard option for postcesarean analgesia.[9]

Other benefits of neuraxial opioids are less sedation and lower early postoperative total opioid consumption compared with systemic opioids. Effective postoperative analgesia is associated with earlier ambulation and return of gastrointestinal function, lower incidence of deep venous thrombosis and pulmonary embolism, less cardiovascular complications and pulmonary infections, and reduction in response to surgical stress and inflammation. Reduction is these perioperative morbidity factors are even more important in high-risk patients.[10-12] Pruritus, nausea, and vomiting are the most common side effects of neuraxial opioids that can negatively impact maternal satisfaction.

Pharmacology

When administered in the neuraxis, opioids selectively produce analgesia without impairing sympathetic tone, motor function, or proprioception.[13] When given in the epidural space, opioids must cross the meninges in order to reach the dorsal horn of the spinal cord where opioid receptors are located. Opioids can facilitate or inhibit synaptic transmission via G-protein coupled receptors. Mu opioid receptors can inhibit the voltage-gated calcium channel opening and can cause neuronal hyperpolarization, thus decreasing the conduction of pain signals.[14,15] The degree of uptake of a certain opioid from the cerebrospinal fluid (CSF) to the dorsal horn is determined by its lipid solubility.

Lipophilic drugs such as fentanyl and sufentanil have fast onset of action due to rapid uptake in the dorsal horn but have short duration of action. They also have rapid uptake by epidural veins and more absorption by epidural fat, thus they have lower CSF bioavailability and higher systemic absorption. The analgesia from all intrathecal opioids is in part due to spinal effects. Neuraxial doses of lipophilic opioid required to produce postoperative analgesia produce plasma concentrations within the minimal effective analgesic concentration (MEAC).[16]

Hydrophilic drugs such as morphine have slower onset of action but longer duration. They are retained in the CSF for a longer time, they have more CSF bioavailability with less systemic absorption, and they have greater rostral spread.[17]

Epidural Opioids

Epidural Morphine

Preservative-free epidural morphine is most commonly administered as a single bolus at a concentration of 0.5 mg/mL. Epidural morphine provides better postcesarean analgesia, increases the time to request the first postoperative analgesic, and decreases overall requests of postoperative analgesics during the first 24 hours when compared with systemic opioids, but it is associated with an increase in side effects such as nausea and pruritus.[8] Its onset time is between 30 and 60 minutes and the peak of analgesia occurs in 60 to 90 minutes. [18]It is usually administered after the delivery of the baby and it provides good analgesia for approximately 24 hours.

Epidural morphine has a ceiling effect with analgesia improving with increased doses until approximately 3.74 mg, after which further increases in dosage will increase the risk of side effects with no difference in analgesia. Doses between 2 and 4 mg are commonly used. Less effective analgesia is observed with doses lower than 2 mg and higher incidence of side effects with no improvement in analgesia is observed with doses higher than 4 mg.[19] A randomized trial by Singh et al. showed that, combined with ketorolac and acetaminophen, 1.5 mg of epidural morphine provided noninferior analgesia after cesarean delivery and it caused less side effects compared with 3 mg.[20] This suggests that, if it is part of a multimodal analgesia regimen, lower doses of epidural morphine can be appropriate when reducing risk of side effects is a priority. Epidural and intrathecal administration of morphine have similar analgesic efficacy but the intrathecal route has faster onset, less systemic absorption, and less potential for fetal exposure to the drug.[21]

Fentanyl

Commonly 50 to 100 micrograms of epidural fentanyl is given alone or in combination with morphine for cesarean deliveries. The commercial presentations are preservative free. Epidural fentanyl has less side effects than epidural morphine and it has faster onset, so it is often used to supplement intraoperative analgesia but it doesn't provide clinically significant pain relief beyond 4 hours of administration.[22] When combined, local anesthetics and fentanyl have synergistic effects, and the dose of epidural fentanyl required after a cesarean delivery is reduced.[23] In theory, a highly lipophilic opioid combined with morphine should provide fast onset and prolonged duration of analgesia.

Earlier studies suggest that there is no advantage in epidural fentanyl compared with intravenous. Later studies indicate that, when given as a bolus or combined with local anesthetics, epidural fentanyl has more spinal effects since it is associated with better analgesia and less supplemental analgesics despite lower plasma levels.[24,25] In the bolus group this effect may be due to concentration gradient between the epidural and the intrathecal spaces after the bolus. Epidural fentanyl combined with local anesthetic and epinephrine has spinal effects, and these effects are enhanced by synergism among these drugs.[26]

Sufentanil

Epidural sufentanil has a 5:1 potency ratio in relation to epidural fentanyl.[27] It has rapid onset and short duration of analgesia, and this effect is dose dependent.[28] It can provide pain relief within 15 minutes but its epidural use for postoperative pain is limited because it only provides analgesia for up to 4 hours.[22] The dose required to produce an effect in 95% (ED95) of epidural sufentanil is approximately 20 mcg and it is comparable to 100 mcg of epidural fentanyl with similar onset time, quality, and duration of analgesia and side-effect profile.[29]

Hydromorphone

Hydromorphone has lipophilicity, analgesic efficacy, and a side-effect profile similar to morphine when given via epidural and it has faster onset and shorter duration compared to morphine. A potency ratio of 3:1 for continuous infusions and 5:1 for bolus doses is suggested between epidural morphine and epidural hydromorphone.[30] In a study by Chestnut et al., the mean time to request supplemental analgesia after receiving 1 mg of hydromorphone for postcesarean analgesia was 13 hours.[31] There is evidence that analgesia duration can be prolonged with the addition of epinephrine.[32]

Extended-Release Epidural Morphine

Extended-release epidural morphine (EREM; Depodur®) delivers morphine sulfate encapsulated in multivesicular lipid particles. These particles are broken down by erosion and reorganization, which results in up to 48 hours of sustained release of morphine after a single shot epidural injection.[33]

Patients who received 10 mg of epidural EREM consumed 60% less supplemental analgesia than patients who received 4 mg of standard epidural morphine, with no significant difference in the incidence of side effects.[34]

Epidural EREM administration requires 48 hours of monitoring for respiratory depression, whereas standard epidural morphine requires 24 hours.[35] There are no studies evaluating the clinical safety of intrathecal administration of EREM, and there are cases of reported prolonged respiratory depression requiring ventilatory support or naloxone after accidental intrathecal injection of EREM.[36]

Epidural local anesthetics should not be coadministered with EREM because they can accelerate the release of the drug from the liposomes, increasing the risk of opioid toxicity. After a local anesthetic test dose, the catheter should be flushed and EREM administration should be delayed for 15 minutes. It also recommended that no epidural local anesthetic should be given for 48 hours following EREM administration. EREM should be drawn up with or given though a filter needle.[37]

Other Epidural Opioids

Epidural diamorphine (heroin) is very commonly used in the United Kingdom for postoperative analgesia but its use is not FDA approved in the United States. It has high lipid solubility, thus rapid onset of action, and its main metabolite is morphine which provides prolonged duration of analgesia. Doses between 2.5 and 5 mg are used[38] with duration lasting from 5 to 15 hours. Higher doses are associated with more prolonged duration whereas lower doses are associated with less nausea and vomiting.[39]

Patient-Controlled Epidural Analgesia

Single-shot morphine is used much more frequently than continuous epidural infusions for postcesarean analgesia, but patient-controlled epidural analgesia (PCEA) and continuous epidural infusion (CEI) are commonly used for pain management after thoracic and major upper abdominal surgery in nonobstetric patients. Epidural morphine is less ideal for a continuous infusion due to risk for delayed respiratory depression and prolonged latency compared with opioids such as fentanyl and hydromorphone, which are less hydrophilic. Lower pain scores and less side effects are observed in patients receiving fentanyl PCEA than in patients receiving respective intravenous PCA regimens.[40,41] A combination of epidural local anesthetic in low dose and opioid can provide better analgesia at rest and lower total drug requirements than epidural opioid or local anesthetic alone.[42] Adding epinephrine to the infusion can enhance analgesia, reducing the infusion rate and the total amount of opioid administered.[43] PCEA and CEI may decrease maternal satisfaction due to the potential for some degree of motor block from local anesthetics and decreased mobility from being connected to a pump. It can also increase cost, delay pharmacological thromboprophylaxis, and increase potential risks of catheter-related complications,[44,45] but it can be considered in special situations such as a history of chronic pain.

Intrathecal Opioids

Morphine

Spinal morphine is the gold-standard single-shot drug for pain management after cesarean delivery. Epidural morphine of 2 to 3 mg is equivalent to 0.075 to 0.2 mg of intrathecal morphine. Intrathecal morphine may have earlier onset of analgesia than epidural morphine but the time for peak effect, duration of effect, efficacy of analgesia, and the side-effect profile of intrathecal and epidural morphine are similar.[21] The duration of analgesia is dose dependent.

The ideal dose is between 0.1 and 0.2 mg with analgesia lasting from 14 to 36 hours.[46] Intrathecal morphine doses of 0.1 mg and 0.2 mg produce similar postcesarean analgesia, with 0.1 mg being associated with less side effects.[47-49] Intrathecal morphine of 0.2 mg can increase the duration of analgesia but it is associated with an increase in side effects with no improvement in quality of analgesia.[50] Although using a high dose of intrathecal morphine may be appropriate in patients at risk for severe postcesarean pain, the use of low-dose intrathecal morphine in a multimodal analgesic regimen is the standard of care for an optimal balance of analgesia after cesarean delivery and risk of side effects.

Fentanyl

Intrathecal fentanyl has rapid onset, improves intraoperative analgesia, reduces intraoperative local anesthetic requirements, and reduces intraoperative nausea and vomiting.[51] Pruritus is a frequent side effect but it rarely requires treatment. Intrathecal fentanyl has short duration of action which limits its use in the late postoperative period analgesic[52] but it provides immediate postoperative analgesia, optimizing pain control during the transition to the effect of neuraxial morphine. The degree and duration of analgesia and the side effects are dose related.[51,52] Doses of approximately 15 mcg combined with local anesthetic are associated with better analgesia intraoperatively and with increase in duration of analgesia.[53,54]

Sufentanil

Similar to fentanyl, intrathecal sufentanil enhances anesthesia intraoperatively and it decreases the total local anesthetic requirement.[55] They also have similar side-effect profiles with pruritus being a frequent side effect. If combined with local anesthetic doses of 5 mcg of intrathecal, sufentanil provides 3 to 6 hours of analgesia after cesarean delivery.[56] It provides effective analgesia at doses between 2.5 and 5 mcg.[57,58] A ceiling effect is observed at 5 mcg, and the incidence of pruritus increases with higher doses.[59]

Hydromorphone

Hydromorphone is a reasonable option for long-acting postoperative analgesia for cesarean delivery especially in situations where the use of morphine is not feasible, such as morphine allergy and morphine shortage. The ED90 for intrathecal hydromorphone is 75 mcg and a 2:1 ratio of intrathecal morphine to hydromorphone.[46] Duration of analgesia is approximately 12 to 15 hours. Intrathecal and epidural morphine provide better analgesia with longer duration of action and lower opioid consumption in the first 24 hours compared with hydromorphone, but the side-effect profiles are similar.[60]

Onset, duration, and doses of the neuraxial opioids most commonly used for analgesia after cesarean delivery are summarized in Table 21.1.

Table 21.1 Summary of Neuraxial Opioids

Drug	Onset	Duration	Commonly Used Doses	Comments
Morphine	30–60 min	12–24 h	E: 2–4 mg IT: 0.1–0.2 mg	Ceiling effect for analgesia. Duration of analgesia is dose dependent. Monitor for delayed respiratory depression.
Fentanyl	5–10 min	2–4 h	E: 50–100 mcg IT: 15 mcg	Synergistic effect with local anesthetics. Useful for pain control during transition to effect of neuraxial morphine.
Sufentanil			E: 20 mcg (5:1 ratio to epidural fentanyl) IT: 2.5–5 mcg	
Hydromorphone	5–10 min	Mean of 13 h	E: 0.6–1 mg (infusion 3:1 ratio to epidural morphine / bolus 5:1 ratio to epidural morphine) IT: 75 mcg (2:1 ratio to morphine)	Side effect profile similar to morphine.
EREM	30–60 min	Up to 48 h	E: < 15 mg (recommended dose) Not for IT use	Monitor for respiratory depression for 48h. Not to be drawn with filter. Not to be coadministered with local anesthetics. No study validating clinical safety of intrathecal administration.

E = epidural, IT = intrathecal, EREM = extended release epidural morphine

Other Intrathecal Opioids

Meperidine is a mu opioid receptor agonist, and unlike other opioids it has local anesthetic qualities. Intrathecal meperidine at 7.5 mg combined with bupivacaine prolongs the duration of analgesia and reduces pain intensity after regression of spinal block, but it is associated with increased incidence of nausea and vomiting.[61] Diamorphine has rapid onset due to its lipophilicity and long duration due its metabolism to morphine. The ED95 of intrathecal diamorphine[62] is 0.4 mg but doses of 0.25 and 0.3 provide effective analgesia. Duration of analgesia and side effects are dose related.[63] Diamorphine is not approved for clinical use in the United States.

Opioid Combinations

Both intrathecal and epidural opioids are often administered combined. A standard regimen of drugs in a single shot spinal block would be a local anesthetic such as 10.5 to 12 mg of 0.75% bupivacaine combined with 15 mcg of fentanyl and 0.1 mg of morphine. Addition of intrathecal lipophilic opioids such as fentanyl and sufentanil to morphine decreases visceral pain and nausea during surgery, decreases pain scores during regression of spinal anesthesia, and does not significantly impact the clinical effect of morphine in postoperative analgesia. Epidural lidocaine, bupivacaine, ropivacaine and chlorprocaine are commonly used in combination with 100 mcg of fentanyl and 2 to 3 mg of morphine for cesarean anesthesia and for postcesarean analgesia when no intrathecal morphine is given. Chlorprocaine may decrease the efficacy of neuraxial morphine.

Nonopioid Neuraxial Analgesics and Adjuvants

Clonidine can have an adjunct analgesic effect when given via epidural or spinal injection, likely due to activation of α-adrenergic receptors in the descending inhibitory pathways. It can augment the effect of intrathecal morphine in postcesarean analgesia. It can also increase analgesia from local anesthetics. The ideal dose is controversial, with studies suggesting use of 30 mcg, 75 mcg, and even higher doses.[64–66] Higher doses are usually associated with more side effects. Continuous infusion is preferred for postoperative analgesia due to its short duration of action. Routine use in obstetric patients is not recommended due to risk of sedation and decrease in blood pressure, but its use can be considered in patients at risk for severe pain after cesarean delivery.

Epinephrine can be used via intrathecal and epidural with the goal of prolonging analgesia from short-acting opioids and decreasing total dose and systemic uptake of local anesthetics. The addition of epinephrine does not increase effect or duration of neuraxial morphine and it does not decrease supplemental analgesic requirements after cesarean delivery.

Other drugs such as dexmedetomidine, ketamine, magnesium, and neostigmine have been used as neuraxial adjuvants for postcesarean analgesia.

Side Effects

Neuraxial morphine at the doses commonly used in practice have minimal neonatal effects due its slow absorption from the epidural space and low placental transfer.[67] Intrathecal opioids in small doses have less neonatal transfer than epidural or intravenous opioids. Intrathecal lipophilic opioids in low doses do not appear to affect neonatal outcome, but these drugs should be used in the lowest necessary dose.[68]

Pruritus is a common side effect of neuraxial opioids with incidence reports as high as 90% but it is usually mild, and patients who receive intrathecal opioids for cesarean delivery rank pain, nausea, and vomiting as more undesirable than pruritus.[69] The causative mechanism is unclear, but it is not secondary to histamine release. There is no consensus regarding prophylaxis and management of neuraxial-opioid induced pruritus. A 5-HT$_3$ antagonist such as ondansetron is used to reduce risk of pruritus.[70] Propofol in low doses may have antipruritic effect. Nalbuphine is an opioid antagonist used in doses from 2 to 5 mg to treat pruritus induced by neuraxial morphine.[71]

Neuraxial opioids increase the risk for nausea and vomiting from rostral spread in the CSF and by systemic absorption and stimulation of the chemoreceptor trigger zone. Treatment options include ondansentron, metoclopramide, and dexamethasone. Combination antiemetic regimens with drugs that act in different receptor sites may have better efficacy due to additive or synergistic effect.[72] Prophylactic phenylephrine infusion can be useful to manage spinal anesthesia-induced hypotension with the goal of maintaining systolic blood pressure above 90 mm Hg or within 20% of baseline.

Neuraxial opioids can cause direct and indirect depression of the respiratory center in the brainstem. Respiratory depression after neuraxial morphine is biphasic, with early depression occurring from 30 to 90 minutes due to systemic absorption from epidural veins, and late depression occurring from 6 to 18 hours due to rostral spread in the CSF and penetration into the brainstem.[73] The incidence of respiratory depression following neuraxial morphine in obstetric patients may be approximately 0.9%.[74] Neuraxial lipophilic opioids only cause early respiratory depression. It usually occurs within 30 minutes and it is uncommon. The Society of Obstetric Anesthesia and Perinatology (SOAP) tracked complications related to obstetric anesthesia from 2004 to 2009, and there were no cases of respiratory arrest secondary to neuraxial opioids.[75] Respiratory depression was more common in the past because patients used to receive higher doses of neuraxial opioids. After receiving neuraxial opioids patients should be monitored for adequacy of ventilation, oxygenation, and level of consciousness. The duration of monitoring should reflect the duration of action of the opioid administered. Patients with increased risk of respiratory depression such as those with morbid obesity, obstructive sleep apnea, cardiopulmonary conditions, and neurologic conditions, and those with coadministration of intravenous opioids, hypnotics, and magnesium, may need increased duration and other modalities of monitoring. Ventilatory support and reversal with naloxone may be necessary. The consensus by the SOAP published in 2019[76] provides monitoring recommendations for prevention and detection of respiratory depression associated with neuraxial morphine administration for cesarean delivery analgesia. Some of the recommendations are summarized in Figure 21.1.

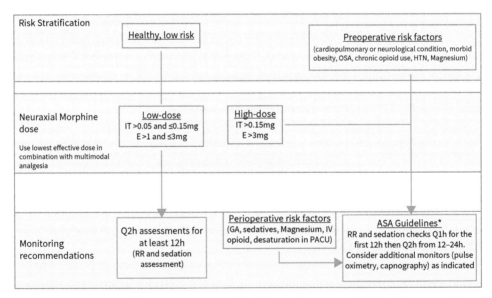

Figure 21.1 Summary of SOAP recommendations for respiratory monitoring after neuraxial morphine administration for analgesia after cesarean delivery. OSA = obstructive sleep apnea, IT = intrathecal, E = epidural, RR = respiratory rate, GA = general anesthesia, PACU = postrecovery anesthesia unit, ASA = American Society of Anesthesiologists.

* ASA Guidelines for respiratory monitoring.[35]

Table 21.2 Side Effects of Neuraxial Morphine

Side Effects of Neuraxial Morphine	Incidence	Treatment Options	Comments
Pruritus	As high as 90%	Ondansentron, nalbuphine, low dose propofol	Usually mild
Nausea/Vomiting	10–30%	Ondansentron, metoclopramide, droperidol, dexamethasone, combination regimen	Combination regimen may provide additive or synergistic effect
Respiratory depression	Approximately 0.9%	Assisted ventilation and naloxone in severe cases	Very rare in low-risk obstetric population

Urinary retention can be associated with neuraxial opioids; the mechanism is not fully understood and it can also be associated with neuraxial local anesthetics. Parturients who receive neuraxial anesthesia routinely receive a urinary catheter to avoid bladder distension and to avoid loss of bladder and detrusor function.[77] In problematic cases, opioid reversal with intravenous naloxone may be considered.

The side effects of neuraxial morphine are summarized in Table 21.2.

Systemic Opioid Analgesia

Systemic opioids are commonly used for postcesarean analgesia, either as an adjuvant agent to neuraxial or as a primary method of analgesia. Due to the opioid epidemic, drug overdose is the leading cause of injury-related deaths. Following cesarean delivery, 1 in 300 opioid-naive women become addicted to opioids.[78] While it is important to not undertreat pain, physicians should carefully evaluate a patient in the postdelivery period to determine if a patient should be treated with opioids.

Patient-Controlled Analgesia

Studies show that intravenous patient-controlled analgesia (PCA) provides better patient satisfaction and pain control when compared to standard nurse-administered analgesia.[79] The PCA can deliver fentanyl, morphine, or hydromorphone, each with its own risk and benefits. The side effects as well as the safety profile of the drug must be considered for the choice of the opioid. Patients with comorbidities such as renal dysfunction, hepatic dysfunction, and obstructive sleep apnea are at increased risk for respiratory depression.[80] Per the MD Anderson Post Operative Pain Management guidelines, patients should be alert and demonstrate ability to deliver demand dose for pain.[81] Examples of PCA settings are showed in Table 21.3. A basal dose can be considered 12 to 24 hours after surgery if pain continues to be uncontrolled. The American College of Obstetricians and Gynecologists (ACOG) recommends initiating a PCA when a patient's pain remains uncontrolled after several doses of intravenous opioid analgesia.[82]

Table 21.3 Examples of PCA Settings

	Example of PCA settings in opioid-naive patients		
	Hydromorphone	Morphine	Fentanyl
Drug presentation	1 mg/mL	1 mg/mL	10 mcg/mL
Bolus dose	0.2 mg	1–1.5 mg	20 mcg
Lockout	5–10 min	5–10 min	5 min
Rescue doses	0.3 mg IV Q5min (max. 3 doses)	2 mg IV Q5min (max. 3 doses)	25 mcg IV Q5min (max. 3 doses)

Common Oral Opioids

Oral opioids continue to have an important role in postoperative analgesia. Current recommendations include neuraxial morphine with continuous nonsteroidal anti-inflammatory drugs (NSAIDs) and acetaminophen postoperatively, while oral opioids should only be prescribed for breakthrough pain and when multimodal analgesics are ineffective.[82,83] The use of codeine and hydrocodone are cautioned, due to the reduced clearance of hydrocodone in neonates and possible infant mortality in mothers with ultra-rapid metabolism.[84] Oxycodone is the oral opioid of choice for postoperative pain due to its high and predictable oral bioavailability.[85] Oxycodone can provide equivalent analgesia to morphine PCA with less side effects.[86,87] In fact, oxycodone was also found to be comparable to intrathecal morphine.[88] However, oxycodone use should be discouraged due to high amounts of drug excreted in breastmilk.[84] If oral opioid is necessary for management of postoperative pain, physicians should prescribe the lowest dose with the shortest duration.

The major downside of opioids is their side-effect profile. Patients placed on opioids postoperatively should be counseled on the side effects, such as nausea, vomiting, respiratory depression, lethargy, and urinary retention.[89] New mothers should also be counseled about drug transfer into breast milk and the subsequent possibility of central nervous system (CNS) depression in the infant.[82,83]

Nonopioid Adjuvants

The exposure of opioids to opioid-naive patients can lead to addiction and abuse, further contributing to the opioid crisis.[78] Thus, the ACOG recommends a stepwise analgesic ladder for postpartum pain management, with nonopioid analgesia as step one.[82] Multimodal analgesia is a pain regimen that combines multiple classes of drugs to create a synergistic effect. Multimodal analgesia is associated with decreased opioid use.[90] The benefits of multimodal analgesia for postpartum pain include decreased sedation, minimal drug transfer to breast milk, early ambulation, and less disruption with mother-baby bonding.[82,91] Common agents include acetaminophen, NSAIDs, gabapentin, ketamine, and magnesium.

Acetaminophen

Acetaminophen is commonly a part of a multimodal postcesarean analgesia regimen due to its safety profile, minimal transfer to breast milk, and effective analgesia. The exact mechanism of action has not been established, but is known to have analgesic and antipyretic effects. Intravenous acetaminophen has been shown to be superior to oral acetaminophen in terms of lowering opioid consumption and decreasing length of stay.[91,92] However, when compared to NSAIDs, acetaminophen was found to be less effective than NSAIDs in relieving pain after cesarean delivery and decreasing postoperative opioid consumption.[93,94] However in combination, acetaminophen and NSAIDs have been shown to decrease morphine consumption and provide superior analgesia than either alone.[93,95] Although some studies recommend pre-emptive analgesia to reduce intraoperative nociception to the CNS,[96] preincisional acetaminophen is not beneficial. One must be careful not to exceed the daily maximum dosage of acetaminophen of 3–4 grams as it often is available in combination with opioids.

Nonsteroidal Anti-inflammatory Drugs

NSAIDs are also commonly used in multimodal analgesic regimens and work by the inhibition of cyclooxygenase (COX)-1 and COX-2 enzymes. They have been proven to be effective in decreasing postoperative pain, and reportedly have a 30–50% opioid sparing effect.[83] More importantly, they are analgesics ruled to be safe in breastfeeding postpartum patients.[84,94] Studies have shown that NSAIDs are minimally excreted into breast milk as they are highly protein bound.[83,84] It is important to identify patients who are breastfeeding infants born with ductal-dependent cardiac lesion, and avoid NSAIDs in this subgroup of patients.

Celecoxib

Celecoxib is a COX-2 inhibitor, which specifically targets inflammation. COX-2 inhibitors were found to have equipotent analgesia and opioid-sparing effect when compared to NSAIDs in nonobstetrical surgeries.[90] When compared to NSAIDs, celecoxib's side-effect profile seem to be more favorable as there is less inhibition of platelet aggregation. However, this may be of concern in the obstetric population who are already at increased risk for thrombosis. Cox-2 inhibitors should be reserved for patients who are unable to receive nonselective NSAIDs.[83]

Ketolorac

Ketolorac is a unique NSAID that is available in intravenous, intramuscular, and oral forms. According to the product label, ketolorac is contraindicated in labor and delivery due to the effect on fetal circulation. However, the ACOG recommends that ketorolac can be used in the immediate postpartum period due to the low infant dose after intravenous administration.[82,84,97] The postsurgical use of ketorolac is also safe in regards to postoperative bleeding and it is not associated with an increase in postoperative blood loss.[93] Like with other NSAIDs, ketorolac has shown to decrease opioid requirements, but there is conflicting evidence on the effect of ketorolac on the quality of analgesia.[93,98]

Gabapentin

Gabapentin is a neurotropic drug that mimics the neurotransmitter GABA and binds to presynaptic voltage-gated calcium channels in the dorsal root ganglion. It is an anticonvulsant with analgesic effects, primarily in neuropathic and chronic pain. Gabapentin's role in postcesarean analgesia remains controversial and unclear. Felder et al. conducted a systematic review and meta-analysis including popular studies looking at perioperative gabapentin use in cesarean deliveries. The authors found that a single preoperative 600mg dose of gabapentin significantly decreases postoperative pain and increases patient satisfaction at 24 hours in healthy patients undergoing spinal anesthesia.[99] However, the ACOG does not recommend gabapentin for routine postcesarean analgesia due to lack of evidence, side-effect profile, and limited data on neonatal safety profile.[82] Breast milk transfer is relatively high for gabapentin,[83] and thus physicians must continue to weigh risk versus benefit.

Ketamine

Ketamine is a selective N-methyl-D-aspartate (NMDA) receptor antagonist that binds to the phencyclidine binding site of the NMDA receptors to blunt central sensitization.[100] This mechanism plays a major role in the treatment of postoperative pain. Rahmanian et al. found that 0.25 mg/kg IV ketamine following spinal anesthesia with intrathecal bupivacaine significantly decreased pain scores and delayed initiation of pain.[101] Menkiti et al. similarly found that 0.15 mg/kg IV ketamine prior to spinal anesthesia with intrathecal bupivacaine also decreased pain scores in the first 120 min, delayed initiation of pain, and decreased opioid consumption in the first 24 hours.[102] On the contrary, Bauchat et al. reported that pain scores and opioid consumption in the first 24 hours did not differ with respect to controls after a 10 mg IV ketamine bolus.[103] In this study, patients received spinal anesthesia with intrathecal bupivacaine and morphine. It is thought that intravenous ketamine may improve postoperative analgesia in patients who receive spinal anesthesia without intrathecal morphine.[83] In patients undergoing general anesthesia, preemptive IV ketamine 0.3 mg/kg has been shown to decrease opioid consumption and delay initiation of pain.[104] The main side effects of intravenous ketamine to consider are hallucinations and sedation and the subsequent effect on mother-baby bonding.

Magnesium Sulfate

Magnesium sulfate is used for the treatment of acute and chronic pain due to its role as a noncompetitive antagonist at the NMDA receptor.[105,106] Helmy et al. looked at preemptive 30 mg/kg IV magnesium sulfate infusion in patients undergoing cesarean section under general anesthesia and found no statistically significant difference on the postoperative pain score, on total opioid dose in the first 24 hours, or on time to initiation of pain when compared to the control. Paech et al. also reported no statistically significant difference in pain scores, time to initiation of pain, or opioid consumption in patients undergoing cesarean under neuraxial anesthesia treated with high-dose (50 mg/kg bolus then 2 g/h) or low-dose (25 mg/kg bolus followed by 1 g/h) magnesium sulfate.[107] However, Rezae et al. found that preemptive 50 mg/kg IV magnesium sulfate infusion, in patients undergoing cesarean section under general anesthesia, helped decrease postoperative pain scores for the first 24 hours.[108] Benefits also included decreased postoperative nausea, vomiting, and shivering.[108] The potential risks of magnesium sulfate for postoperative analgesia include hypermagnesemia, flushing, nausea, headaches, and dizziness.[106] Hutchins et al. recommend continuous hourly monitoring of deep-tendon reflexes, respiratory rate, oxygen saturation, and urine output to prevent toxic levels and effects.

Regional Techniques

Transversus Abdominis Plane Block

Regional techniques for managing postcesarean delivery pain are much less commonly utilized when compared to neuraxial opioids and other analgesic adjuvants. Transverse abdominis plane (TAP) block involves injecting local anesthetic into the fascial plane between the internal oblique and transversus abdominis muscles, which blocks T7–L1 nerves to the anterior abdominal wall to offer relief from somatic pain.[109] Kerai et al. examined three studies comparing TAP blocks to control for post cesarean section analgesia, and found that TAP blocks can reduce opioid consumption only in patients receiving general anesthesia or when intrathecal morphine is not used.[85,105] The authors also found two trials that supplemented intrathecal morphine with TAP block and concluded there was no advantage in doing so. However, larger studies with adequate power are needed to establish the possible benefit of adjuvant TAP block to intrathecal morphine.[85]

Iliohypogastric and Ilioinguinal Nerve Block

Iliohypogastric and ilioinguinal nerves originate from the L1 spinal root and run between the transverse abdominis and internal oblique muscles. Blocking these can provide anterior abdominal wall analgesia. Kerai et al. reviewed five studies on iliohypogastric and ilioinguinal nerve blocks for postcesarean analgesia and found that, in four of the five studies, the iliohypogastric and ilioinguinal nerve blocks were effective for postcesarean analgesia. One of these studies, conducted by Wolfson et al., showed that bilateral ilioinguinal and iliohypogastric nerve blocks led to lower pain scores and lower analgesic requirements in patients who received neuraxial anesthesia with intrathecal morphine.[110] Kiran et al. compared ultrasound-guided ilioinguinal iliohypogastric nerve blocks to TAP blocks following cesarean section under spinal anesthesia. The authors found that there were higher tramadol requirements in the ilioinguinal iliohypogastric block group than in the TAP block group.[111] However, the authors still considered the ilioinguinal iliohypogastric block effective because there was less tramadol use over a 24-hour period when compared to previous studies (63 mg[111] vs. 331 mg+/- 82mg[112]). However due to differences in local anesthetic dosing and block techniques, one can not make a recommendation of one block over the other.[109]

Quadratus Lumborum Block

The quadratus lumborum (QL) block is an interfascial plane block that involves a posterior approach to provide posterior abdominal wall analgesia.[109] The thoracolumbar fascia is a posterior extension of abdominal wall fascia that encloses the back muscles including the quadratus lumborum and facilitates spread to the paravertebral space and inhibition of sympathetic fibers and thus visceral pain analgesia. Literature on the QL block involves four different approaches depending on needle placement: QL1(lateral), QL2(posterior), transmuscular QL or QL3 (anterior), and intramuscular QL.[113] Blanco et al. recommended QL2 over QL1 because QL 2 had a more predictable spread into the paravertebral space on MRI imaging and was quicker and safer to perform.

The QL block was associated with significantly less opioid consumption at 6 and 12 hours and lower pain scores in postoperative cesarean patients under neuraxial anesthesia without intrathecal morphine.[114] If patients are unable to receive intrathecal morphine, Kang et al. recommends a combination QL 2 and 3 block.[115] Tamura et al. conducted a triple-blinded randomized trial comparing intrathecal morphine with QL block 2 after cesarean section. Posterior QL block in addition to intrathecal morphine was shown to have no additional benefit.[116] This is hypothesized to be due to minimal spread of local anesthetic into the paravertebral space. As there have only been a handful of studies looking at the QLB for post cesarean analgesia, we can not make a recommendation at this time.

Wound Infiltration

Subcutaneous wound infiltration with local anesthetic is an easy technique for obstetricians and it is recommended by the ACOG.[82] Wound infiltration can be either a single-shot technique or a catheter-based infusion. Wound infiltration with local anesthetic has been shown to decrease opioid consumption in the first 12 hours and lower pain scores for the first 6 hours.[117] A meta-analysis including catheters and single-shot local anesthetic infiltration showed that local anesthetic wound infiltration significantly decreased opioid consumption at 24 hours in patients who had not received intrathecal morphine.[118] The study did not find a difference between single-shot and catheter techniques. TAP blocks provide greater decrease in pain scores at 24 hours and more delayed pain initiation compared with wound infiltration with local anesthetics.[119] Adjuvants such as dexmedetomidine have also been shown to decrease pain scores, decrease the amount patients needing rescue analgesics, and delay initiation of pain.[120] Ketorolac, when added to a local anesthetic infusion, was shown to decrease pain scores at 24 hours and opioid consumption.[121] Prior to making a recommendation, more studies are needed to evaluate the efficacy of local wound infiltration, catheter placement, volume, and type of local anesthetic.

Box 21.1 Summary of Recommendations for Analgesia After Cesarean Delivery in the General Obstetric Population

---

Summary

- According to the SOAP and to the ASA Practice Guidelines for Obstetric Anesthesia[7] recommendations, low-dose neuraxial morphine is the preferred method for analgesia after cesarean delivery in healthy patients.
- Combination of morphine with multimodal analgesic regimens provides better analgesia and allows for reducing total neuraxial and systemic opioid use, thus reducing the risk of side effects such as nausea, vomiting, pruritus, and respiratory depression.
- Neuraxial opioids provide superior analgesia and do not increase the risk of respiratory depression compared to systemic opioids.
- Systemic opioids, nonopioid adjuvants, and peripheral nerve blocks have a very important role as part of a multimodal regimen for postcesarean delivery analgesia.

A summary of recommendations for analgesia after cesarean delivery in the general obstetric population is shown in Box 21.1.

References

1. Martin JA, Hamilton BE, Osterman MJK, Driscoll AK, Drake P. Births: Final data for 2017. *National vital statistics reports: from the Centers for Disease Control and Prevention, National Center for Health Statistics, National Vital Statistics System.* 2018;67(8):1–50.
2. Gamez H, B., Habib S, A. Predicting severity of acute pain after cesarean delivery: a narrative review. *Anesthesia & Analgesia.* 2018;126(5):1606–1614. doi:10.1213/ANE.0000000000002658.
3. Peahl AF, Smith R, Johnson TRB, Morgan DM, Pearlman MD. Better late than never: Why obstetricians must implement enhanced recovery after cesarean. *Obstet Gynecol.* 2019;221(2): 117.e–117.e7. doi:10.1016/j.ajog.2019.04.030.
4. King T, Choby B, El-Sayed Y. ACOG committee opinion no. 742 summary: Postpartum pain management. *Obstetrics & Gynecology.* 2018;132(1):252–253. doi:10.1097/AOG.0000000000002711.
5. Mcdonnell G, J., Curley H, G., Carney G, J., et al. The analgesic efficacy of transversus abdominis plane block after cesarean delivery: a randomized controlled trial. *Anesthesia & Analgesia.* 2008;106(1):186–191. doi:10.1213/01.ane.0000290294.64090.f3.
6. Stogicza A, Trescot AM, Racz E, Lollo L, Magyar L, Keller E. Inferior hypogastric plexus block affects sacral nerves and the superior hypogastric plexus. *ISRN Anesthesiology.* 2012;2012(2012). doi:10.5402/2012/686082.
7. Soc Obstet AP, Amer Soc Anesthesiologists, Task Fo. Practice guidelines for obstetric anesthesia: an updated report by the American Society of Anesthesiologists Task Force on Obstetric Anesthesia and the Society for Obstetric anesthesia And Perinatology. *Anesthesiology.* 2016;124(2):270–300. doi:10.1097/ALN.0000000000000935.
8. Bonnet M, Mignon A, Mazoit J, Ozier Y, Marret E. Analgesic efficacy and adverse effects of epidural morphine compared to parenteral opioids after elective caesarean section: a systematic review. *European Journal of Pain.* 2010;14(9):894.e–894.e9. doi:10.1016/j.ejpain.2010.03.003.

9. Sutton CD, Carvalho B. Optimal pain management after cesarean delivery. *Anesthesiology Clinics*. 2017;35(1):107–124. doi:10.1016/j.anclin.2016.09.010.

10. Guay J. The benefits of adding epidural analgesia to general anesthesia: a metaanalysis. *J Anesth*. 2006;20(4):335–340. doi:10.1007/s00540-006-0423-8.

11. Block BM, Liu SS, Rowlingson AJ, Cowan AR, Cowan JA, Wu CL. Efficacy of postoperative epidural analgesia: a meta-analysis. *JAMA*. 2003;290(18):2455–2463. doi:10.1001/jama.290.18.2455.

12. Kettner SC, Willschke H, Marhofer P. Does regional anaesthesia really improve outcome? *Br J Anaesth*. 2011;107:i90–i95. doi:10.1093/bja/aer340.

13. Yaksh TL, Rudy TA. Analgesia mediated by a direct spinal action of narcotics. *Science*. 1976;192(4246):1357. doi:10.1126/science.1273597.

14. Rahman A. Shnider and Levinson's anesthesia for obstetrics, 5th ed. *Anesthesiology*. 2015;122(1):182–184. doi:10.1097/ALN.0000000000000498.

15. Julius D, Basbaum AI. Molecular mechanisms of nociception. *Nature*. 2001;413(6852):203. doi:10.1038/35093019.

16. Bujedo BM. Recommendations for spinal opioids clinical practice in the management of postoperative pain. *J Anesthesiol Clin Sci*. 2013. doi:10.7243/2049-9752-2-28.

17. Bujedo BM. Spinal opioid bioavailability in postoperative pain. *Pain Practice*. 2014;14(4):350–364. doi:10.1111/papr.12099.

18. Nordberg G, Hedner T, Mellstrand T, Dahlström B. Pharmacokinetic aspects of intrathecal morphine analgesia. *Anesthesiology*. 1984;60(5):448–454. doi:10.1097/00000542-198405000-00010.

19. Palmer CM, Nogami WM, Van Maren G, Alves DM. Postcesarean epidural morphine: a dose-response study. *Anesthesia & Analgesia*. 2000;90(4):887–891. doi:10.1213/00000539-200004000-00021.

20. Singh SI, Rehou S., Marmai KL, Jones PM. The efficacy of 2 doses of epidural morphine for postcesarean delivery analgesia: A randomized noninferiority trial. *Anesthesia & Analgesia*. 2013;117(3):677–685. doi:10.1213/ANE.0b013e31829cfd21.

21. Dualé C, Frey C, Bolandard F, Barrière A, Schoeffler P. Epidural versus intrathecal morphine for postoperative analgesia after caesarean section. *Br J Anaesth*. 2003;91(5):690–694. doi:10.1093/bja/aeg249.

22. King MJ, Bowden MI, Cooper GM. Epidural fentanyl and 0.5% bupivacaine for elective caesarean section. *Anaesthesia*. 1990;45(4):285–288. doi:10.1111/j.1365-2044.1990.tb14733.x.

23. Cohen S, Lowenwirt I., Pantuck CB, Amar D, Pantuck EJ. Bupivacaine 0.01% and/or epinephrine 0.5 microg/ml improve epidural fentanyl analgesia after cesarean section. *Anesthesiology*. 1998;89(6):1354–1361. doi:10.1097/00000542-199812000-00012.

24. Ginosar Y, Riley ET, Angst MS. The site of action of epidural fentanyl in humans: The difference between infusion and bolus administration. *Anesthesia & Analgesia*. 2003;97(5):1428–1438. doi:10.1213/01.ANE.0000081793.60059.10.

25. D'Angelo R, Gerancher JC, Eisenach JC, Raphael BL. Epidural fentanyl produces labor analgesia by a spinal mechanism. *Anesthesiology*. 1998;88(6):1519–1523. doi:10.1097/00000542-199806000-00016.

26. Cohen S, Pantuck CB, Amar D, Burley E, Pantuck EJ. The primary action of epidural fentanyl after cesarean delivery is via a spinal mechanism. *Anesthesia & Analgesia*. 2002;94(3):674–679. doi:10.1097/00000539-200203000-00036.

27. Grass JA, Sakima NT, Schmidt R, Michitsch R, Zuckerman RL, Harris AP. A random-ized, double-blind, dose-response comparison of epidural fentanyl versus sufentanil an-algesia after cesarean section. *Anesthesia & Analgesia*. 1997;85(2):365–371. doi:10.1097/00000539-199708000-00022.

28. Rosen MA, Dailey PA, Hughes SC, et al. Epidural sufentanil for postoperative analgesia after ce-sarean section. *Anesthesiology*. 1988;68(3):448–453. doi:10.1097/00000542-198803000-00024.

29. Grass JA, Sakima NT, Schmidt R, Michitsch R, Zuckerman RL, Harris AP. A randomized, double-blind, dose-response comparison of epidural fentanyl versus sufentanil analgesia after cesarean section. *Anesth Analg*. 1997;85(2):365–371. Accessed Oct 14, 2019. doi:10.1097/00000539-199708000-00022.

30. De Leon-Casasola OA, Lema MJ. Postoperative epidural opioid analgesia: what are the choices? *Anesthesia & Analgesia*. 1996;83(4):867–875. doi:10.1213/00000539-199610000-00038.

31. Chestnut DH, Choi WW, Isbell TJ. Epidural hydromorphone for postcesarean analgesia. *Obstetrics & Gynecology*. 1986;68(1):65–69.

32. Dougherty TB, Baysinger CL, Henenberger JC, Gooding DJ. Epidural hydromorphone with and without epinephrine for post-operative analgesia after cesarean delivery. *Anesthesia & Analgesia*. 1989;68(3):318–322. doi:10.1213/00000539-198903000-00024.

33. Angst M, Drover D. Pharmacology of drugs formulated with DepoFoam™. *Clin Pharmacokinet*. 2006;45(12):1153–1176. doi:10.2165/00003088-200645120-00002.

34. Carvalho B, Roland LM, Chu LF, Campitelli VA, Riley ET. Single-dose, extended-release epidural morphine (DepoDur™) compared to conventional epidural morphine for post-cesarean pain. *Anesthesia & Analgesia*. 2007;105(1):176–183. doi:10.1213/01.ane.0000265533.13477.26.

35. Apfelbaum J, Horlocker T, Agarkar M, et al. Practice guidelines for the prevention, detec-tion, and management of respiratory depression associated with neuraxial opioid admin-istration: An updated report by the American Society of Anesthesiologists Task Force on Neuraxial Opioids and the American Society of Regional Anesthesia and Pain Medicine. *Anesthesiology*. 2016;124(3):535–552. doi:10.1097/ALN.0000000000000975.

36. Gerancher JC, Nagle PC. Management of accidental spinal administration of extended-release epidural morphine. *Anesthesiology*. 2008;108(6):1147–1149. doi:10.1097/ALN.0b013e31817307c7.

37. Nagle PC, Gerancher JC. DepoDur ® (extended-release epidural morphine): A review of an old drug in a new vehicle. *Techniques in Regional Anesthesia and Pain Management*. 2007;11(1):9–18. doi:10.1053/j.trap.2007.02.011.

38. Hallworth SP, Fernando R, Bell R, Parry MG, Lim GH. Comparison of intrathecal and ep-idural diamorphine for elective caesarean section using a combined spinal-epidural tech-nique. *Br J Anaesth*. 1999;82(2):228–232. doi:10.1093/bja/82.2.228.

39. Roulson CJ, Bennett J, Shaw M, Carli F. Effect of extradural diamorphine on analgesia after caesarean section under subarachnoid block. *Br J Anaesth*. 1993;71(6):810–813. doi:10.1093/bja/71.6.810.

40. Ngan Kee WD, Lam KK, Chen PP, Gin T. Comparison of patient-controlled epidural anal-gesia with patient-controlled intravenous analgesia using pethidine or fentanyl. *Anaesth Intensive Care*. 1997;25(2):126–132. doi:10.1177/0310057X9702500203.

41. Wu CL, Cohen SR, Richman JM, et al. Efficacy of postoperative patient-controlled and continuous infusion epidural analgesia versus intravenous patient-controlled

analgesia with opioids: A meta-analysis. *Anesthesiology*. 2005;103(5):1079–1088. doi:10.1097/ 00000542-200511000-00023.

42. Cooper DW, Ryall DM, Mchardy FE, Lindsay SL, Eldabe SS. Patient-controlled extradural analgesia with bupivacaine, fentanyl, or a mixture of both, after caesarean section. *Br J Anaesth*. 1996;76(5):611–615. doi:10.1093/bja/76.5.611.

43. Sakura S, Sumi M, Shinzawa M, Toyota K, Kosaka Y. The addition of epinephrine increases intensity of sensory block during epidural anesthesia with lidocaine. *Anesthesiology*. 1998;89:834A. doi:10.1097/00000542-199809150-00009.

44. Tagaloa LA, Butwick AJ, Carvalho B. A survey of perioperative and postoperative anesthetic practices for cesarean delivery. *Anesthesiology Research and Practice*. 2009;2009:510642.

45. Vercauteren M, Vereecken K, La Malfa M, Coppejans H, Adriaensen H. Cost-effectiveness of analgesia after caesarean section. A comparison of intrathecal morphine and epidural PCA. *Acta Anaesthesiol Scand*. 2002;46(1):85–89. doi:10.1034/j.1399-6576.2002.460115.x.

46. Sviggum P, H., Arendt W, K., Jacob K, A., et al. Intrathecal hydromorphone and morphine for postcesarean delivery analgesia: Determination of the ED90 using a sequential allocation biased-coin method. *Anesthesia & Analgesia*. 2016;123(3):690–697. doi:10.1213/ ANE.0000000000001229.

47. Palmer CM, Emerson S, Volgoropolous D, Alves D. Dose-response relationship of intrathecal morphine for postcesarean analgesia. *Anesthesiology*. 1999;90(2):437–444. doi:10.1097/ 00000542-199902000-00018.

48. Uchiyama A, Nakano S, Ueyama H, Nishimura M, Tashiro C. Low dose intrathecal morphine and pain relief following caesarean section. *International Journal of Obstetric Anesthesia*. 1994;3(2):87–91. doi:10.1016/0959-289X(94)90175-9.

49. Berger JS, Gonzalez A, Hopkins A, et al. Dose–response of intrathecal morphine when administered with intravenous ketorolac for post-cesarean analgesia: A two-center, prospective, randomized, blinded trial. *International Journal of Obstetric Anesthesia*. 2016;28:3–11. doi:10.1016/j.ijoa.2016.08.003.

50. Sultan P, Halpern SH, Pushpanathan E, Patel S, Carvalho B. The effect of intrathecal morphine dose on outcomes after elective cesarean delivery: A meta-analysis. *Anesthesia & Analgesia*. 2016;123(1):154–164. doi:10.1213/ANE.0000000000001255.

51. Belzarena SD. Clinical effects of intrathecally administered fentanyl in patients undergoing cesarean section. *Anesthesia & Analgesia*. 1992;74(5):653–657. doi:10.1213/ 00000539-199205000-00006.

52. Dahl JB, Jeppesen IS, Jørgensen H, Wetterslev J, Møiniche S. Intraoperative and postoperative analgesic efficacy and adverse effects of intrathecal opioids in patients undergoing cesarean section with spinal anesthesia: A qualitative and quantitative systematic review of randomized controlled trials. *Anesthesiology*. 1999;91(6):1919. doi:10.1097/00000542-199912000-00045.

53. Hunt CO, Naulty JS, Bader AM, et al. Perioperative analgesia with subarachnoid Fentanyl–Bupivacaine for cesarean delivery. *Anesthesiology*. 1989;71(4):535–540. doi:10.1097/ 00000542-198910000-00009.

54. Chu CC, Shu SS, Lin SM, et al. The effect of intrathecal bupivacaine with combined fentanyl in cesarean section. *Acta Anaesthesiol Sin*. 1995;33(3):149–154. Accessed Oct 14, 2019.

55. Chen X, Qian X, Fu F, Lu H, Bein B. Intrathecal sufentanil decreases the median effective dose (ED50) of intrathecal hyperbaric ropivacaine for caesarean delivery. *Acta Anaesthesiol Scand*. 2010;54(3):284–290. doi:10.1111/j.1399-6576.2009.02051.x.

56. Karaman S, Kocabas S, Uyar M, Hayzaran S, Firat V. The effects of sufentanil or morphine added to hyperbaric bupivacaine in spinal anaesthesia for caesarean section. *Eur J Anaesthesiol.* 2006;23(4):285–291. doi:10.1017/S0265021505001869.

57. Lee JH, Chung KH, Lee JY, et al. Comparison of fentanyl and sufentanil added to 0.5% hyperbaric bupivacaine for spinal anesthesia in patients undergoing cesarean section. *Korean journal of anesthesiology.* 2011;60(2):103–108. doi:10.4097/kjae.2011.60.2.103.

58. Wilwerth M, Majcher J-L, Van der Linden, P. Spinal fentanyl vs. sufentanil for post-operative analgesia after c-section: A double-blinded randomised trial. *Acta Anaesthesiol Scand.* 2016;60(9):1306–1313. doi:10.1111/aas.12738.

59. Braga, A. de F. de Assunção, Braga, F. S. da Silva, Potério GMB, Pereira RIC, Reis E, Cremonesi E. Sufentanil added to hyperbaric bupivacaine for subarachnoid block in caesarean section. *Eur J Anaesthesiol.* 2003;20(8):631–635. Accessed Oct 14, 2019. doi:10.1017/s0265021503001017.

60. Marroquin B, Feng C, Balofsky A, et al. Neuraxial opioids for post-cesarean delivery analgesia: Can hydromorphone replace morphine? A retrospective study. *International Journal of Obstetric Anesthesia.* 2017;30:16–22. doi:10.1016/j.ijoa.2016.12.008.

61. Yu SC, Ngan Kee WD, Kwan ASK. Addition of meperidine to bupivacaine for spinal anaesthesia for caesarean section. *BJA: International Journal of Anaesthesia.* 2002;88(3):379–383. doi:10.1093/bja/88.3.379.

62. Saravanan S, Robinson APC, Dar AQ, Columb MO, Lyons GR. Minimum dose of intrathecal diamorphine required to prevent intraoperative supplementation of spinal anaesthesia for caesarean section. *Br J Anaesth.* 2003;91(3):368–372. doi:10.1093/bja/aeg197.

63. Kelly MC, Carabine UA, Mirakhur RK. Intrathecal diamorphine for analgesia after caesarean section: A dose finding study and assessment of side-effects. *Anaesthesia.* 1998;53(3):231–237. doi:10.1046/j.1365-2044.1998.00307.x.

64. Allen TK, Mishriky BM, Klinger RY, Habib AS. The impact of neuraxial clonidine on postoperative analgesia and perioperative adverse effects in women having elective caesarean section–a systematic review and meta-analysis. *Br J Anaesth.* 2018;120(2):228–240. doi:10.1016/j.bja.2017.11.085.

65. Maheshwari N, Gautam S, Kapoor R, Prakash R, Jafa S, Gupta R. Comparative study of different doses of clonidine as an adjuvant with isobaric levobupivacaine for spinal anaesthesia in patients undergoing caesarean section. *Journal of Obstetric Anaesthesia and Critical Care.* 2019;9(1):9–13. doi:10.4103/joacc.JOACC_36_18.

66. Bajwa SJ, Bajwa SK, Kauer J. Comparison of epidural ropivacaine and ropivacaine clonidine combination for elective cesarean sections. *Saudi Journal of Anaesthesia.* 2010;4(2):47–54. doi:10.4103/1658-354X.65119.

67. Hughes SC, Rosen MA, Shnider SM, Abboud K, TK, Stefani SJ, Norton M. Maternal and neonatal effects of epidural morphine for labor and delivery. *Anesthesia & Analgesia.* 1984;63(3):319–324. doi:10.1213/00000539-198403000-00007.

68. Courtney MA, Bader AM, Hartwell B, Hauch M, Grennan MJ, Datta S. Perioperative analgesia with subarachnoid sufentanil administration. *Reg Anesth.* 1992;17(5):274.

69. Carvalho B., Cohen SE, Lipman SS, Fuller A, Mathusamy AD, Macario A. Patient preferences for anesthesia outcomes associated with cesarean delivery. *Anesthesia & Analgesia.* 2005;101(4):1182–1187. doi:10.1213/01.ane.0000167774.36833.99.

70. Yeh H, Chen L, Lin C, et al. Prophylactic intravenous ondansetron reduces the incidence of intrathecal morphine-induced pruritus in patients undergoing cesarean delivery. *Anesthesia & Analgesia*. 2000;91(1):172–175. doi:10.1213/00000539-200007000-00032.

71. Somrat C, Oranuch K, Ketchada U, Siriprapa S, Thipawan R. Optimal dose of nalbuphine for treatment of Intrathecal-Morphine induced pruritus after caesarean section. *J Obstet Gynaecol Res*. 1999;25(3):209–213. doi:10.1111/j.1447-0756.1999.tb01149.x.

72. Heffernan AM, Rowbotham DJ. Postoperative nausea and vomiting—time for balanced antiemesis? *Br J Anaesth*. 2000;85(5):675.

73. Kafer ER, Brown JT, Scott D, et al. Biphasic depression of ventilatory responses to CO_2 following epidural morphine. *Anesthesiology*. 1983;58(5):418–427. doi:10.1097/00000542-198305000-00005.

74. Halpern S, Arellano R, Preston R, et al. Epidural morphine vs hydromorphone in post-caesarean section patients. *Can J Anaesth*. 1996;43(6):595–598. doi:10.1007/BF03011773.

75. D'Angelo R, Smiley RM, Riley ET, Segal S. Serious complications related to obstetric anesthesia: The serious complication repository project of the society for obstetric anesthesia and perinatology. *Anesthesiology*. 2014;120(6):1505–1512. doi:10.1097/ALN.0000000000000253.

76. Bauchat JR, Weiniger CF, Sultan P, et al. Society for Obstetric Anesthesia and Perinatology consensus statement: monitoring recommendations for prevention and detection of respiratory depression associated with administration of neuraxial morphine for cesarean delivery analgesia. *Anesthesia & Analgesia*. 2019;129(2):458–474. doi:10.1213/ANE.0000000000004195.

77. Liang CC, Chang SD, Chang YL, Chen SH, Chueh HY, Cheng PJ. Postpartum urinary retention after cesarean delivery. *International Journal of Gynecology & Obstetrics*. 2007;99(3): 229–232. doi:10.1016/j.ijgo.2007.05.037.

78. Bateman BT, Franklin JM, Bykov K, et al. Persistent opioid use following cesarean delivery: patterns and predictors among opioid-naïve women. *Obstet Gynecol*. 2016;215(3):353.–353.e18. doi:10.1016/j.ajog.2016.03.016.

79. Hudcova J, McNicol E, Quah C, Lau J, Carr DB. Patient controlled opioid analgesia versus conventional opioid analgesia for postoperative pain. *Cochrane Database of Systematic Reviews*. 2006(4):CD003348. doi:10.1002/14651858.CD003348.pub2.

80. Chestnut DH, Wong CA, Tsen LC, et al. *Chestnut's obstetric anesthesia: Principles and practice*. 6th ed. Philadelphia, PA: Elsevier; 2019.

81. Baker C, Bird J, Cain K, et al. Post-operative pain management. https://www.mdanderson.org/documents/for-physicians/algorithms/clinical-management/clin-management-post-op-pain-web-algorithm.pdf. Updated 2018.

82. King T, Choby B, El-Sayed Y. ACOG committee opinion no. 742 summary: Postpartum pain management. *Obstetrics & Gynecology*. 2018;132(1):252–253. doi:10.1097/AOG.0000000000002711.

83. Carvalho B, Butwick AJ. Postcesarean delivery analgesia. *Best Practice & Research Clinical Anaesthesiology*. 2017;31(1):69–79. doi:10.1016/j.bpa.2017.01.003.

84. Sachs HC. The transfer of drugs and therapeutics into human breast milk: An update on selected topics. *Pediatrics*. 2013;132(3):e796. doi:10.1542/peds.2013-1985.

85. Kerai S, Saxena KN, Taneja B. Post-caesarean analgesia: What is new? *Indian J Anaesth*. 2017;61(3):200–214. doi:10.4103/ija.IJA_313_16.

86. Niklasson B, Arnelo C, Georgsson Öhman S, Segerdahl M, Blanck A. Oral oxycodone for pain after caesarean section: A randomized comparison with nurse-administered IV morphine in a pragmatic study. *Scandinavian Journal of Pain*. 2015;7(1):17–24. doi:10.1016/j.sjpain.2015.01.003.

87. Davis KM, Esposito MA, Meyer BA. Oral analgesia compared with intravenous patient-controlled analgesia for pain after cesarean delivery: A randomized controlled trial. *Obstet Gynecol.* 2006;194(4):967–971. doi:10.1016/j.ajog.2006.02.025.

88. McDonnell NJ, Paech MJ, Browning RM, Nathan EA. A randomised comparison of regular oral oxycodone and intrathecal morphine for post-caesarean analgesia. *International Journal of Obstetric Anesthesia.* 2010;19(1):16–23. doi:10.1016/j.ijoa.2009.03.004.

89. Oderda GM, Evans RS, Lloyd J, et al. Cost of opioid-related adverse drug events in surgical patients. *J Pain Symptom Manage.* 2003;25(3):276–283. doi:10.1016/S0885-3924(02)00691-7.

90. Chou R, Gordon DB, de Leon-Casasola OA., et al. Management of postoperative pain: A clinical practice guideline from the American Pain Society, the American Society of Regional Anesthesia and Pain Medicine, and the American Society of Anesthesiologists' committee on regional anesthesia, executive committee, and administrative council. *Journal of Pain.* 2016;17(2):131–157. doi:10.1016/j.jpain.2015.12.008.

91. Urman RD, Boing EA, Pham AT, et al. Improved outcomes associated with the use of intravenous acetaminophen for management of acute post-surgical pain in cesarean sections and hysterectomies. *Journal of Clinical Medicine Research.* 2018;10(6). doi:10.14740/jocmr3380w.

92. Altenau B, Crisp C, Devaiah G, Lambers D. Randomized control trial of IV acetaminophen for post cesarean delivery pain control. *Obstet Gynecol.* 2017;216(1):S24. doi:10.1016/j.ajog.2016.11.925.

93. Munishankar B, Fettes P, Moore C, Mcleod GA. A double-blind randomised controlled trial of paracetamol, diclofenac or the combination for pain relief after caesarean section. *International Journal of Obstetric Anesthesia.* 2008;17(1):9–14. doi:10.1016/j.ijoa.2007.06.006.

94. Rawlinson A, Kitchingham N, Hart C, McMahon G, Ong SL, Khanna A. Mechanisms of reducing postoperative pain, nausea and vomiting: A systematic review of current techniques. *Evid Based Med.* 2012;17(3):75. doi:10.1136/ebmed-2011-100265.

95. Ong CKS, Seymour RA, Lirk P, Merry AF. Combining paracetamol (acetaminophen) with nonsteroidal antiinflammatory drugs: A qualitative systematic review of analgesic efficacy for acute postoperative pain. *Anesthesia & Analgesia.* 2010;110(4):1170–1179. doi:10.1213/ANE.0b013e3181cf9281.

96. Kissin I. Preemptive analgesia. *Anesthesiology.* 2000;93(4):1138–1143. doi:10.1097/00000542-200010000-00040.

97. Wischnik A, Manth S, Lloyd J, Bullingham R, Thompson J. The excretion of ketorolac tromethamine into breast milk after multiple oral dosing. *Eur J Clin Pharmacol.* 1989;36(5):521–524. doi:10.1007/BF00558080.

98. Pavy TJG, Paech MJ, Evans SF. The effect of intravenous ketorolac on opioid requirement and pain after cesarean delivery. *Anesth Analg.* 2001;92(4):1010–1014.

99. Felder L, Saccone G, Scuotto S, et al. Perioperative gabapentin and post cesarean pain control: A systematic review and meta-analysis of randomized controlled trials. *European Journal of Obstetrics & Gynecology and Reproductive Biology.* 2019;233:98–106. doi:10.1016/j.ejogrb.2018.11.026.

100. Radvansky BM, Shah K, Parikh A, Sifonios AN, Le V, Eloy JD. Role of ketamine in acute postoperative pain management: A narrative review. *BioMed research international.* 2015;2015:749837. doi:10.1155/2015/749837.

101. Rahmanian M, Leysi M, Ali AH, Mirmohammadkhani M. The effect of low-dose intravenous ketamine on postoperative pain following cesarean section with spinal anesthesia: A randomized clinical trial. *Oman Medical Journal.* 2015;30(1):11–16. doi:.5001/omj.2015.03.

102. Menkiti ID, Desalu I, Kushimo OT. Low-dose intravenous ketamine improves post-operative analgesia after caesarean delivery with spinal bupivacaine in African parturients. *International Journal of Obstetric Anesthesia*. 2012;21(3):217–221. doi:10.1016/j.ijoa.2012.04.004.

103. Bauchat JR, Higgins N, Wojciechowski KG, McCarthy RJ, Toledo P, Wong CA. Low-dose ketamine with multimodal postcesarean delivery analgesia: A randomized controlled trial. *International Journal of Obstetric Anesthesia*. 2011;20(1):3–9. doi:10.1016/j.ijoa.2010.10.002.

104. Helmy N, Badawy AA, Hussein M, Reda H. Comparison of the preemptive analgesia of low dose ketamine versus magnesium sulfate on parturient undergoing cesarean section under general anesthesia. *Egyptian Journal of Anaesthesia*. 2015;31(1):53–58. doi:10.1016/j.egja.2014.12.006.

105. Vuckovic S, Srebro D, Savic Vujovic K, Prostran M. The antinociceptive effects of magnesium sulfate and MK-801 in visceral inflammatory pain model: The role of NO/cGMP/K+ATP pathway. *Pharm Biol*. 2015;53(11):1621–1627. doi:10.3109/13880209.2014.996821.

106. Hutchins D, Rockett M. The use of atypical analgesics by intravenous infusion for acute pain: Evidence base for lidocaine, ketamine and magnesium. *Anaesthesia & Intensive Care Medicine*. 2019;20(8):415–418. doi:10.1016/j.mpaic.2019.05.011.

107. Paech MJ, Magann EF, Doherty DA, Verity LJ, Newnham JP. Does magnesium sulfate reduce the short- and long-term requirements for pain relief after caesarean delivery? A double-blind placebo-controlled trial. *Obstet Gynecol*. 2006;194(6):1596–1602. doi:10.1016/j.ajog.2006.01.009.

108. Rezae M, Naghibi K, Taefnia A. Effect of pre-emptive magnesium sulfate infusion on the post-operative pain relief after elective cesarean section. *Advanced Biomedical Research*. 2014;3(1):164. doi:10.4103/2277-9175.139127.

109. Patel SD, Sharawi N, Sultan P. Local anaesthetic techniques for post-caesarean delivery analgesia. *International journal of obstetric anesthesia*. 2019;40:62. doi:10.1016/j.ijoa.2019.06.002.

110. Wolfson A, Lee AJ, Wong RP, Arheart KL, Penning DH. Bilateral multi-injection iliohypogastric-ilioinguinal nerve block in conjunction with neuraxial morphine is superior to neuraxial morphine alone for postcesarean analgesia. *J Clin Anesth*. 2012;24(4):298–303. doi:10.1016/j.jclinane.2011.09.007.

111. Kiran L, Sivashanmugam T, Kumar V, Krishnaveni N, Parthasarathy S. Relative efficacy of ultrasound-guided ilioinguinal-iliohypogastric nerve block versus transverse abdominis plane block for postoperative analgesia following lower segment cesarean section: a prospective, randomized observer-blinded trial. (original article). *Anesthesia: Essays and Researches*. 2017;11(3):713. doi:10.4103/0259-1162.206855.

112. Sakalli M, Ceyhan A, Uysal HY, Yazici I, Başar H. The efficacy of ilioinguinal and iliohypogastric nerve block for postoperative pain after caesarean section. *Journal of research in medical sciences: the official journal of Isfahan University of Medical Sciences*. 2010;15(1):6–13.

113. Ueshima H, Otake H, Lin J. Ultrasound-guided quadratus lumborum block: An updated review of anatomy and techniques. *BioMed Research International*. 2017;2017. doi:10.1155/2017/2752876.

114. Blanco R, Ansari T, Girgis E. Quadratus lumborum block for postoperative pain after caesarean section: A randomised controlled trial. *Eur J Anaesthesiol*. 2015;32(11):812–818. doi:10.1097/EJA.0000000000000299.

115. Kang W, Lu D, Yang X, et al. Postoperative analgesic effects of various quadratus lumborum block approaches following cesarean section: A randomized controlled trial. *Journal of Pain Research*. 2019;12:2305. doi:10.2147/JPR.S202772.

116. Tamura T, Yokota S, Ando M, Kubo Y, Nishiwaki K. A triple-blinded randomized trial comparing spinal morphine with posterior quadratus lumborum block after cesarean section. *International journal of obstetric anesthesia*. 2019;40:32–38. doi:10.1016/j.ijoa.2019.06.008.

117. Niklasson B, Börjesson A, Carmnes U, Segerdahl M, Öhman SG, Blanck A. Intraoperative injection of bupivacaine-adrenaline close to the fascia reduces morphine requirements after cesarean section: A randomized controlled trial. *Acta Obstet Gynecol Scand*. 2012;91(12):1433–1439. doi:10.1111/j.1600-0412.2012.01480.x.

118. Adesope O, Ituk U, Habib AS. Local anaesthetic wound infiltration for postcaesarean section analgesia: A systematic review and meta-analysis. *Eur J Anaesthesiol*. 2016;33(10):731–742. doi:10.1097/EJA.0000000000000462.

119. Aydogmus M, Sinikoglu S, Naki M, Ocak N, Sanlı N, Alagol A. Comparison of analgesic efficiency between wound site infiltration and ultra-sound-guided transversus abdominis plane block after cesarean delivery under spinal anaesthesia. *Hippokratia*. 2014;18(1):28–31.

120. Bhardwaj S, Devgan S, Sood D, Katyal S. Comparison of local wound infiltration with ropivacaine alone or ropivacaine plus dexmedetomidine for postoperative pain relief after lower segment cesarean section. *Anesthesia: Essays and Researches*. 2017;11(4):940. doi:10.4103/aer.AER_14_17.

121. Carvalho B, Lemmens HJ, Ting V, Angst MS. Postoperative subcutaneous instillation of low-dose ketorolac but not hydromorphone reduces wound exudate concentrations of interleukin-6 and interleukin-10 and improves analgesia following cesarean delivery. *Journal of Pain*. 2013;14(1):48–56. doi:10.1016/j.jpain.2012.10.002.

22

Neonatal Assessment and Resuscitation

Fatoumata Kromah, Darshna Bhatt, Nayef Chahin, Miheret Yitayew,
and Joseph Khoury

Neonatal Assessment

Risk Identification

During pregnancy and the perinatal period, maternal and fetal well-being is monitored to identify risk factors that may impact maternal or fetal/neonatal outcome. Pregnant women are assessed for pre-existing disorders and pregnancy-related conditions that may result in vascular endotheliopathy and inflammatory states, which may increase the risk of fetal growth restriction, fetal death, or a poor neonatal outcome. Common antenatal fetal surveillance tests include maternal fetal movement assessment, nonstress test, contraction stress test, biophysical profile, and the umbilical artery Doppler velocimetry (Table 22.1). Other antenatal fetal surveillance tests are performed for high-risk pregnancies complicated by conditions such as diabetes, hypertension, and fetal growth restriction (FGR).[2]

Fetal well-being is often an indication of maternal well-being. Fetal assessment allows for correction of maternal hemodynamics and factors that will optimize intrauterine fetal conditions. In the intrapartum period, fetal monitoring may lead to identification of fetal intolerance to the stress of labor and delivery and allow for management of intrauterine hypoxia and uteroplacental insufficiency. Fetal monitoring in the intrapartum period includes the use of the electronic fetal heart rate (FHR) monitor, fetal scalp electrodes, sampling of the umbilical cord gases, fetal pulse oximetry, electrocardiogram, and ultrasonography. Advancement in antenatal ultrasonography has allowed obstetricians and maternal-fetal medicine specialists to diagnose congenital fetal abnormalities earlier, which guides care for these high-risk pregnancies. Non-reassuring fetal assessments increase the probability of needing neonatal resuscitation and thus may dictate delivery mode and timing of delivery. A non-reassuring fetal assessment may also guide maternal intervention and anesthetic management. Other intrapartum risk factors such as preterm labor, abnormal fetal presentation, and meconium-stained amniotic fluid also increase the risk for neonatal resuscitation.[3] Understanding antepartum and intrapartum risk factors that may affect the fetus' ability to transition from intrauterine to extrauterine life allows for mobilization of resources and better preparation at birth. Studies of closed obstetric anesthesia malpractice claims indicate poor tracing and anesthesia delay due to poor communication as causes of newborn brain injury.[4] Early communication and dissemination of information between the multidisciplinary teams may facilitate anesthetic intervention and optimization of maternal hemodynamics, which may positively impact fetal and neonatal outcomes. When at-risk neonates are identified and the need for resuscitation is predicted, labor and delivery should take place at a facility with a neonatal intensive care unit (NICU). In institutions with a large volume of high-risk obstetric

Table 22.1 Antenatal Fetal Surveillance Tests

Antepartum Tests	Reassuring signs of fetal well-being
Maternal perception of fetal movement	10 distinct fetal movements in a period of up to 2 hours
Contraction stress test (CST)	Lack of decelerations with uterine contractions
Nonstress test (NST)	2 or more fetal heart rate accelerations of 15 beats per minute above baseline and for 15 seconds from the baseline in a 20- to 40-minute period
Biophysical profile (BPP)	A total biophysical score of 8 or 10
Umbilical artery Doppler velocimetry	High-velocity diastolic flow

In general, various antepartum fetal assessments are utilized to monitor pregnancies in which the risk of fetal demise is increased.

patients, labor and delivery of at-risk mothers and fetuses should be carefully planned and discussed in a multidisciplinary fashion. In the event of an unanticipated delivery of an at-risk fetus, the presence of skilled personnel and equipment for newborn life support may prevent long-term consequence of fetal hypoxemia and mortality.

Personnel and Equipment

One of the main causes of fetal death is fetal asphyxia. The American Academy of Pediatrics (AAP) and American College of Obstetricians and Gynecologists (ACOG) guidelines state that at least one person skilled in performing the initial steps of newborn resuscitation and positive pressure ventilation (PPV) should be present at every delivery.[5] This person's sole responsibility should be the care of the newborn.[5] It is recommended that hospitals with labor and delivery units have written policies identifying the personnel responsible for neonatal resuscitation. It is also recommended that all personnel, including obstetric anesthesiologists, working in the delivery area receive basic training in neonatal resuscitation and be Neonatal Resuscitation Program (NRP) certified. This is an important consideration because the obstetric anesthesiologist, who is skilled in airway management, may be required to help with unanticipated newborn resuscitation prior to the arrival of the NICU team or in cases of difficult airway management. However, according to the ACOG Committee Opinion on Optimal Goals for Anesthesia Care in Obstetrics, the surgeon and the obstetric anesthesiologist have primary responsibilities to maternal care.[6] A single anesthesiologist should not be responsible for both maternal and fetal resuscitative care except in an unforeseen emergency. Another individual or a second anesthesia provider must assume the role for neonatal resuscitation.[6] Resuscitation of a newborn is a team effort. Some facilities have multidisciplinary neonatal resuscitation teams composed of various team member from pediatrics, anesthesiology, obstetrics and gynecology, respiratory therapy, and nursing. Teamwork is pivotal in neonatal resuscitation and knowing the role of each team member is vital in ensuring that newborn standards of care are provided. A collaborative effort among all providers present is essential to a successful neonatal resuscitation. For the resuscitation team to remain efficient and cohesive, simulation practice should be done on a regular basis.

Initial newborn resuscitation measures utilize simple, easy-to-use equipment such as a radiant warmer, warm towel, pulse oximeter and probe, oropharyngeal airways, suction catheter, bulb syringe, oxygen source with flowmeter, and face masks. Not only is it important that all personnel working in the delivery area receive basic training in neonatal resuscitation, but it is equally important for personnel to maintain familiarity with the equipment available in the delivery area. This can be accomplished by maintaining standardized equipment and layout in each delivery area.

Initial Newborn Assessment

Routine newborn care involves rapid assessment and evaluation of the newborn's appearance, pulse, grimace, activity and respiratory effort, which identify the need for further resuscitative measures. Immediate newborn assessment follows the Apgar scoring system established in 1953 by Dr. Virginia Apgar, who was an anesthesiologist. The Apgar score provides a standardized approach to identify newborns who may require immediate attention and resuscitation. It evaluates five important parameters: breathing, heart rate, color, muscle tone, and reflex irritability. Each evaluated parameter is rated on a scale from 0 to 2 and is assessed at the first and fifth minute of life, and later if indicated. The two most important parameters are respiratory efforts and heart rate. Reassuring neonatal assessment indicators include adequate respiratory efforts, a heart rate greater than 100 beats per minute (bpm), a vigorously moving neonate with flexed extremities resistant to extension, irritability with stimulation such as rubbing of the back, and pink color. An Apgar score greater than 8 is a reassuring sign of neonatal well-being and the infant may remain with the mother. Scores less than 8 are concerning for neonatal distress, and the newborn may require further management. If resuscitation is required, the resuscitation team should be notified immediately and three guiding questions (term gestation, tone, and breathing/crying) need to be communicated and addressed as well as an accurate time of birth.

Neonatal Resuscitation

Overview and Principles of Resuscitation

The Neonatal Resuscitation Program (NRP) is a set of guidelines based on the American Academy of Pediatrics and the American Heart Association (AHA) guidelines for newborn cardiopulmonary resuscitation. The majority of newborns undergo normal physiologic transition at birth and adapt to extrauterine life with little to no intervention. At birth, approximately 10% of neonates require some intervention to regain regular breathing. Extensive resuscitation which includes chest compressions is required approximately 1% of the time.[7] Approximately 0.06% require intervention with drugs such as epinephrine.[8] In adults, most cases of cardiac arrest are secondary to a cardiac etiology or trauma, with resuscitation focused on recovery of cardiac function. However, in newborns, the primary etiology is respiratory, as the heart is usually healthy. Respiratory failure, leading to hypoxia, hypercarbia, and subsequent cardiac arrest, is the main reason resuscitation is required at this age. Respiratory failure in neonates can start prenatally or can occur postnatally. Prenatal failure occurs when there is a significant acute or chronic stress at the uteroplacental bed. Placental respiration failure may be initiated by an abruption, cord compression, or ruptured cord. In this case, the fetus will become hypoxic and hypercarbic, leading to acidosis. Fetal monitoring will reveal loss of heart rate variability, decreased fetal movement, and fetal bradycardia. At that point the fetus will attempt to breathe by gasping. If the fetus is delivered shortly after the onset of symptoms and in early respiratory failure, tactile stimulation may be enough to induce spontaneous respirations. This is referred to as primary apnea. If delivery is delayed and stimulation is not enough to restore breathing, the newborn may present in secondary apnea. At this stage, assisted ventilation, chest compressions, and medications may be necessary to initiate spontaneous respirations, oxygenation, and ventilation. Since respiratory failure is the main cause of cardiac arrest in the fetus and newborn, recovery of oxygenation and ventilation is the primary focus of neonatal resuscitation.

Initial Steps of Resuscitation

1. Temperature Control: The presence of a higher surface-to-volume ratio in newborns, especially those born prematurely, increases the risk of hypothermia after delivery. Hypothermia increases the risk for neonatal morbidity and mortality.[9,10] For neonates born close to or at term, moving the neonate to a warming table and drying, placing a hat on, and wrapping the newborn with a warm blanket should be sufficient enough to maintain euthermia. However, for newborns born prematurely, those thermoregulatory measures are not enough. Current guidelines recommend that any fetus born prior to 32 weeks' gestational age (GA) should be immediately placed in a polyethylene bag or wrap after birth, and then placed on top of a warming mattress and warming table. It is imperative to keep the newborn covered up to the neck while in the bag or wrap to prevent evaporative heat loss. The bag or wrap should not be removed during resuscitation, and auscultation should be done through the bag or wrap. To avoid extreme body heat, it is useful to place a temperature sensor under the bag or wrap, to monitor the neonate's temperature, and adjust as needed. The ideal neonatal body temperature is between 36.5 and 37.5°C. The room temperature also plays an important role in thermoregulation. It is recommended to keep the temperature in the delivery and NICU area between 23°C and 25°C.

2. Delayed Cord Clamping: Delayed cord clamping allows blood to continue to flow between the placenta and newborn for 30 to 60 seconds after delivery.[13] This is known as placental transfusion.[11] A criterion for delayed cord clamping is a gestational age of 23–34 weeks as determined by best dating and singleton pregnancy. Delayed cord clamping in premature infants has been associated with decreased mortality, lower risk of intraventricular hemorrhage, and decreased need for blood transfusions.[12] Continuous and open communication between the neonatal and obstetrics teams is critical during this period of time. To ensure that the procedure is done safely and there is no harm to the newborn, exclusion criteria for delayed cord clamping include multiple gestations, suspected major congenital anomalies, suspected or confirmed abruption, significant maternal bleeding, fetal/neonatal bradycardia, and lack of neonatal respiratory effort.

Positive Pressure Ventilation

Once a newborn is handed over to the neonatal team, it is imperative to assess the patient's heart rate and respirations. This assessment should be quick and not take more than 30 seconds. If the neonate's heart rate is over 100 bpm, and the neonate does not have adequate and spontaneous respirations, PPV should be initiated. Establishing adequate ventilation and oxygenation to the newborn is the most critical step for a successful resuscitation. As the newborn is assessed, a pulse oximeter probe should be connected to the neonate's right palm, to measure preductal saturations. Pulse oximetry is a vital assessment of resuscitative measures. Target saturation guidelines are standardized and present on the NRP algorithm to guide neonatal resuscitation. Supplemental oxygen should be provided to maintain saturation within these guidelines. For initial resuscitation, a newborn born at or past 35 weeks gestational age should be started on a FiO_2 of 21%. Newborns delivered at gestational age less than 35 weeks should be started on a FiO_2 between 21% and 30%. Once it is established that the neonate is in respiratory distress and has not improved after one minute of tactile stimulation, it is imperative that the team provides supportive measures to improve neonatal respirations.

Continuous Positive Pressure Ventilation (CPAP) is used to maintain lung patency in a neonate with spontaneous respiratory effort and a heart rate over 100 bpm. If the neonate has a poor respiratory effort, labored breathing, or a heart rate below 100 bpm, PPV should be initiated. As ventilation is the most crucial step in neonatal resuscitation, it is imperative that the provider knows how to deliver effective PPV. The most common techniques of PPV utilize either a self-inflating bag, a flow-inflating bag, or a T-piece resuscitator. We will not go into the details of each device in this chapter; however, it is important to note that there are major differences among the various modalities. The benefit of the T-piece resuscitator is that it reliably and consistently provides a preset pressure to the neonate. This is more difficult to accomplish with the bag ventilation technique. A comprehensive study showed that neonates ≥ 26 weeks GA were less likely to require intubation when resuscitated with a T-piece resuscitator compared to a self-inflating bag (17% vs 26%).[13] Despite the advantages and disadvantages of each method of providing PPV, the expertise of the provider plays a major role in the adequacy of ventilation. This puts a greater emphasis on the importance of training and exposure of the provider to these devices. During PPV, it is important to ensure that the neonate's airway is patent and free of obstruction. The airway should be cleared of secretions and the head should be appropriately positioned to ensure patency of the airway and deliver adequate PPV. The provider should ensure that the correct mask size is used during resuscitation to ensure a proper seal. The mask should be big enough to rest on the chin and nose but should not compress the neonate's eyes. Care should also be taken to not compress the neonate's soft neck tissues, as this may obstruct the neonate's airway or cause a vasovagal response (Figure 22.1). The rate of ventilation should be 40–60 times per minute. One easy way to remember that is by counting out loud "Breath, two, three, Breath…." The provider should say breath as they compress the bag or occlude the T-piece cap.[7] Starting peak inspiratory pressure (PIP) should be 20 to 25 cm H_2O. The initial peak end expiratory pressure (PEEP) should be 5 cm H_2O. If PPV does not lead to an improvement, the provider should ensure that ventilation is being delivered effectively. The most common causes for ineffective ventilation include a leak around the mask, airway obstruction, and inadequate pressures. In order to address these problems, the provider should adjust the Mask, Reposition

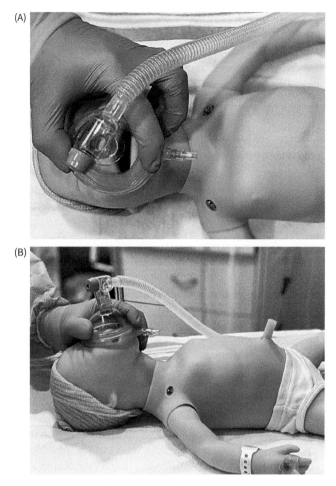

Figure 22.1 Proper placement and securement of mask during PPV.

the neonate's head and neck (reposition the airway), Suction the mouth and nose, Open the mouth, increase the Pressures provided, and consider an Alternate airway management. The acronym commonly used for the described steps is MR. SOPA.[7]

Alternate Airway Management

An alternate airway should be considered in any newborn who does not respond to PPV, or when chest compressions need to be initiated. Alternate airway devices include an endotracheal (ET) tube or a laryngeal mask. Laryngeal masks are used when an endotracheal intubation is unsuccessful or not possible due to anatomy. Its use in preterm infants is limited due to size. Neonatal ET tubes have a uniform diameter and are not cuffed. Selecting the correct size of the ET tube is critical to allow minimal leakage with adequate pressures to ensure proper ventilation. For preterm infants weighing below 1000 grams and/or below 28 weeks GA, a 2.5 mm ET tube should be used. For infants weighing 1000–2000 grams, or 28–34 weeks GA, a 3.0 mm ET tube should be used. Lastly, for infants greater than 2000 grams or greater than 34 weeks GA, a 3.5 mm ET tube is recommended. [7] Selecting the correct blade for intubation helps to optimize the successful rate for intubation. A No. 1 blade is usually used for term neonates, while a No. 0 blade is used for preterm neonates. Some providers prefer to use a No. 00 blade for extremely preterm infants. ET tubes have markers on them to guide the provider and indicate proper insertion depth. A formula for approximating insertion depth is: weight in kg + 6. For example, if the patient weighs 2 kg, the ET tube should be inserted to 8 cm at the level of the neonate's gums. After placement and securement, a chest x-ray should be obtained to confirm proper positioning of the ET tube. The ET tube is properly positioned when the tapered end is above the bifurcation of the carina, between the first and second thoracic vertebrae.

Chest Compressions

Poor ventilation in the newborn will eventually lead to cardiac compromise and cardiac arrest. Chest compressions should be initiated if the heart rate remains less than 60 bpm for at least 30 seconds after initiation of effective PPV. Effective PPV most commonly means ventilation through a properly positioned ET tube or laryngeal mask. Effective chest compressions require the provider to utilize both hands with the palms of the hands encircling the newborn's chest. The provider's fingers should be positioned behind the back of the neonate to provide a firm surface during chest compressions. The provider's thumbs should be placed side-by-side or on top of each other along an imaginary line connecting the nipples, and over the middle of the sternum, above the xiphoid[7] (see Figure 22.2).

Once compressions are initiated, the neonate's chest is compressed about a third of the diameter of the chest, and then released to allow for refilling of the heart. The provider should allow for full recoil of the neonate's chest wall, but the provider's thumbs should not lose contact with the neonate's chest. The compression rate should be 90 times per minute. While doing compressions there should be coordination between the team member providing ventilation and the team member performing chest compressions. Each cycle should be 3 compressions and 1 breath every 2 seconds.[7] The rhythm used is "one-and-two-and-three-and-breathe-one-and-two-and-three-and-breathe."[7] It is important for both team members to speak clearly and loud enough so that they can hear each other and be coordinated. The heart rate should be checked after 60 seconds (which is considered one cycle) of chest compressions and ventilation. Heart rate should be assessed by auscultation, or, if available, by electrocardiogram (ECG). ECG is the preferred method for monitoring heart rate during resuscitation. Chest compressions should be halted once the heart rate is maintained above 60 bpm.

Medications

During resuscitation, if proper PPV is provided to a newborn, the probability that the neonate will require chest compressions is low and the probability of needing medications is even lower (less than 0.1%).[7,14] The most commonly used mediation during resuscitation is epinephrine. Epinephrine is a catecholamine with inotropic (increases cardiac contractility), lusitropic (myocardial relaxation), chronotropic (increases heart rate), and vasoconstrictor

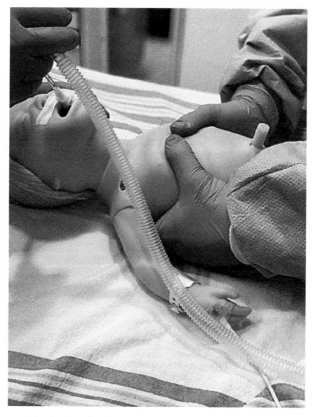

Figure 22.2 The provider's thumbs should be placed side-by-side or on top of each other along an imaginary line connecting the nipples, and over the middle of the sternum, above the xiphoid.

properties.[15] The vasoconstriction property caused by the α-adrenergic receptor plays a major role in resuscitation. Increased vasoconstriction leads to an increase in blood pressure and improved coronary blood flow during resuscitation.[15] Animal studies have shown that chest compressions alone are not enough to provide adequate cerebral perfusion, and resuscitation is more effective and has a more positive outcome when epinephrine is utilized.[16,17] Once chest compressions are initiated an intravenous line (IV) or preferably an umbilical venous catheter (UVC) should be placed to allow for venous access and administration of epinephrine. See Table 22.2 for recommendations for epinephrine use.

Volume Expanders

Volume expanders should be used if there is any history of blood loss perinatally or postnatally. Loss of blood leads to hypovolemic shock, which can only be corrected with adequate volume expansion. Volume expanders are crystalloid fluids (normal saline) or red blood cells. A peripheral IV is not recommended as a route to infuse volume expanders. Dosing is 10 ml/kg, given rapidly via UVC. If the first bolus dose not lead to improvement, a second bolus may be required.

Table 22.2 Recommendations for Epinephrine Use During Neonatal Resuscitation

Indication	60 seconds of adequate chest compressions and ventilation fails to increase neonate's heart rate over 60 bpm
Concentration	Only the 1:10,000 preparation should be used in neonatal resuscitation
Route of Administration	IV: Most effective and recommended Administer rapidly and follow with a flush
	ET: Less effective, utilize only if IV access cannot be established
Dose	IV dose: 0.1–0.3 ml/kg/dose (0.01–0.03 mg/kg/dose)
	ET dose: 0.5–1 ml/kg/dose (0.05–0.1 mg/kg/dose)
Frequency	If the heart rate remains below 60 bpm, repeat epinephrine dose every 3–5 minutes

Special Circumstances

Resuscitation of the Preterm Newborn

The preterm neonate poses a different challenge to the provider, as special considerations arise due to a more difficult transition to extrauterine life. Due to the preterm neonate's unique anatomy and physiology, special care should focus on temperature control, oxygen exposure, assisted ventilation, energy homeostasis, and intraventricular hemorrhage prevention. To help maintain euthermia NRP recommends, for all neonates born less than 32 weeks GA, to adjust room temperature to approximately 23°C to 25°C (74°F to 77°F) and use a thermal mattress and polyethylene bag or wrap[7] (see Figure 22.3). It is also important to turn on a servo-control radiant warmer and place a hat. Cardiovascular monitoring is recommended for rapid, reliable, and continuous assessment. When providing PPV, an initial inflating pressure of 20 to 25 cm H_2O and a PEEP of 5 cm H_2O is recommended.[7] Care should be taken to maintain saturations within the NRP guidelines.[7]

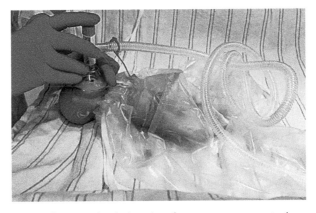

Figure 22.3 Premature infant in polyethylene bag for temperature control.

Meconium-Stained Amniotic Fluid

Meconium is a mix composite of fetal intestinal and skin cells, vernix caseosa, enzymes, bile acids, and amniotic fluid. Meconium is frequently passed from the fetal intestine into the amniotic fluid before 20 weeks of gestation and then again at term. The presence of meconium-stained amniotic fluid (MSAF) is reported to be unusual in preterm births and present in 38% of term deliveries. The presence of meconium may be indicative of fetal distress. Babies born with MSAF are at a higher risk of needing resuscitation. In such cases it is recommended that at least two qualified personnel be present at the delivery. The current NRP recommendation for management of nonvigorous neonates born with MSAF is to avoid delay in resuscitation. Intubation for tracheal suctioning of MSAF is only recommended for airway obstruction preventing effective ventilation.[7,18]

Pneumothorax and Airway Obstruction

Pneumothoraces early in the neonatal period are more common than any other time in life. Pneumothoraces can be spontaneous, but most commonly are associated with the use of PPV in the setting of prematurity and lung pathology such as meconium aspiration syndrome (MAS), lung hypoplasia, and respiratory distress syndrome (RDS). The accumulation of small amounts of air in the pleural space can be asymptomatic or cause minimal respiratory distress. Larger accumulations may manifest with sudden cardio-respiratory collapse leading to increased oxygen requirement, severe respiratory distress, and bradycardia, making this a life-threatening emergency. Transillumination of the chest is a noninvasive, quick, and simple bedside screening tool that can easily diagnose a pneumothorax. In a dark room with light shining on the neonate's chest, there will be a greater and brighter halo noted on the affected (pneumothorax) side versus the nonaffected side. Most small pneumothoraces will resolve on their own, but larger ones resulting in cardiorespiratory compromise require emergent evacuation of the air via needle and chest tube decompression. Needle decompression requires entry of the needle into the pleural space at the 2nd intercostal space along the mid-clavicular line and/or placement of a chest tube at the 4th intercostal space along the mid-axillary line to release the tension created by the air[7,19,20] (see Figure 22.4).

Airway obstruction is another life-threatening neonatal emergency requiring prompt recognition and management. Obstruction can be due to the presence of thick meconium secretions, blood, mucus, or vernix. These secretions may be suctioned out with a suction catheter or a direct tracheal suction using a meconium aspirator. Anatomical malformations, as seen in neonates with Pierre-Robin sequence (PRS) or choanal atresia, can also lead to airway obstruction.

Congenital Malformations

Congenital diaphragmatic hernia (CDH) results from interruptions in development of the diaphragm, creating a communication between the chest and abdominal cavity which allows abdominal content (mainly stomach, liver, and intestines) to move up into the chest cavity and interfere with normal lung development. At birth, newborns with CDH present with respiratory distress, hypoxemia, and sometimes a scaphoid abdomen. If suspected at birth, prompt intubation and placement of an oro/nasogastric tube is essential to prevent overdistention of abdominal contents in the chest cavity.

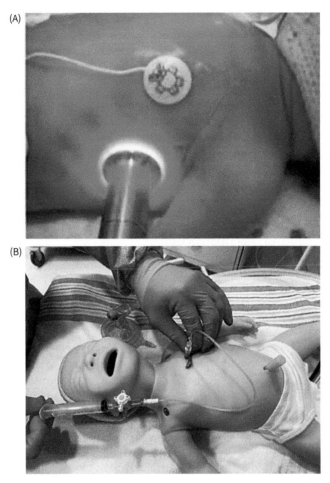

Figure 22.4 Transillumination of the chest and demonstration of adequate needle decompression.

Gastroschisis and omphaloceles are abdominal wall defects. Management of these cases requires placing an oro/nasogastric tube for decompression and covering the defect (ideally with either a polyethylene bag or wrap) to prevent evaporative losses. The neonate should be immediately transferred to a NICU.

Defects in closure of the neural tube can occur as well and lead to the formation of myelo-meningoceles, exposing the spinal cord to extrauterine trauma. If encountered in the delivery room, it is recommended to place the neonate in a prone position and cover the defect with a polyethylene bag/wrap to prevent further damage, as well as to prevent evaporative and heat loss. Neonates with neural tube defects are at a higher risk of developing latex allergies, thus it is strongly recommended to use latex free gloves in their care.[7,18,21]

Maternal Narcotic or Anesthetic Exposure

Narcotics used for pain relief during labor have the potential of crossing the placenta into the fetal circulation, increasing the risk of neonatal respiratory depression. If encountered, the focus should be on maintaining adequate ventilation either via PPV or if needed ET intubation. Not enough evidence exists to support the routine use of narcotic antagonists during neonatal resuscitation.

Ethical Implications

Discontinuing Resuscitation

Neonatal intensive care is an area of medicine that is prone to ethical dilemmas, as this area of medicine often deals with life-or-death situations. Providers are often faced with the question of when to stop resuscitation and, given the complexity of this topic, differences of opinions often arise.[22] Multiple stakeholders are included in the ethics of neonatal resuscitation, with the parents and the neonate being the most central and vulnerable. At the center of these conversations are questions related to the quality of life associated with severe physical and/or cognitive impairments.[22]

According to the NRP,

> If the responsible physicians believe that there is no chance for survival, initiation of resuscitation is not an ethical treatment option and should not be offered. In conditions associated with a high risk of mortality or significant burden of morbidity for the baby, caregivers should discuss the risks and benefits of life-sustaining treatment and allow the parents to participate in the decision whether attempting resuscitation is in their baby's best interest. If there is agreement between the parents and the caregivers that intensive medical care will not improve the chances for the newborn's survival or will pose an unacceptable burden on the child, it is ethical to provide compassionate palliative care and not initiate resuscitation."[7]

Withholding Resuscitation and Decision Making

Beliefs and biases, whether subconscious or conscious, sometimes cloud physician perspectives. This becomes particularly challenging when parental opinion is in stark contrast to the physician providing care. In this situation, employment of a shared decision-making model can be helpful. It is important for any provider who may need to have this difficult conversation with parents of a critically ill neonate to have a framework within which to have these challenging conversations. Walter and Ross discuss the idea of relational autonomy, where the relationship between the provider(s) and the patients' families is both dynamic and fluid.[23] With each patient and their family, there will be different conceptions of autonomy, which then have different implications for the role of providers.[22,24] Building on this idea of relational autonomy, Lantos offers a model that is driven by open-ended questions that can help elucidate parental values, fears, goals, and hope, which can provide key elements essential to the decision-making process.[22] Malone and Sisk propose a model of parental hope and optimism, where both of these elements are appreciated as discrete concepts. In their model, maintaining specific hopes that parents have for their child is central and should be acknowledged. Delineating the difference between the concepts of hope and optimism may help parents reach a specific decision or accept a certain inevitable outcome.[23] In these complex situations, utilizing components of different shared decision-making models helps to facilitate conversation. Open communication with parents allows them the opportunity to appreciate the choices they face and how those choices align with their own values, such that together the best decision for the neonate can be made.

Post-resuscitation Care

Neonates who require resuscitation at birth are at a higher risk for having difficulty in transitioning to extrauterine life. This may lead to multiple organ-system dysfunctions. Anticipation of the development of multiple organ-system dysfunction and/or the need for respiratory support beyond the initial resuscitation warrants close cardiorespiratory monitoring. The newborn's condition, progress towards normal transition, and presence of identifiable risk factors will dictate the amount of time needed for post-resuscitation care.[17,25,26]

Neonatal Neurologic Assessment

The neurologic examination of a newborn is affected by several factors including but not limited to gestational age, maternal anesthesia or narcotic administration, and neonatal congenital disorders. Initial neurologic assessment of the newborn begins by observing the newborn in the delivery room. The newborn should be grossly examined for spinal deformities. [27-29]

Hypoxic ischemic encephalopathy (HIE) remains a significant cause of neonatal mortality and long-term morbidity.[30] Hypoxic-ischemic insult occur due to acute peripartum or intrapartum events that lead to systemic hypoxemia and/or interruption in blood flow. Such events include placental abruption, cord prolapse, uterine rupture, feto-maternal hemorrhage, maternal trauma, or cardio-respiratory arrest.[31] Timely recognition of these peripartum risk factors is essential, as affected newborns may require immediate extensive resuscitation postdelivery. Management of HIE includes therapeutic hypothermia, which is done via whole body cooling or selective head cooling. [32,33] All newborns who may potentially meet criteria for therapeutic hypothermia should be started on passive cooling (avoid radiant warmer, clothing) and referred to a center with such capability within the first 6 hours of life.[32-34]

Conclusion

Earlier recognition of signs of maternal and fetal distress have resulted in improved maternal and fetal outcomes. Time of birth and transition to extrauterine life can pose a challenge for some neonates and, as such, it is important to understand newborn physiology. Being familiar and competent with those skills taught by NRP will aid the provider in properly stabilizing a newborn who requires further assistance. In order to successfully resuscitate a neonate, the effort must be multidisciplinary and collaborative. Maintenance of skills necessitates frequent simulation and practice, which allows providers to practice skills and be familiar with their designated roles during resuscitation. The obstetric anesthesiologist should be cognizant of the standard equipment and layout and should maintain NRP proficiency. In conclusion, the role of the providers, including obstetric anesthesiologists, is pivotal in ensuring that the best care is provided to this vulnerable patient population.

References

1. National Center for Health Statistics, United States. Health, United States, 2009 with special features on medical technology. Hyatsville, MD: National Center for Health Statistics; 2010. Retrieved October 11, 2019, from https://www.cdc.gov/nchs/data/hus/hus09.pdf#019.

2. American College of Obstetricians and Gynecologists. ACOG practice bulletin number 145: antepartum fetal surveillance. *Obstet Gynecol.* 2014;124:182–92.

3. Aziz K, Chadwick M, Baker M, Andrews W. Ante- and intra-partum factors that predict increased need for neonatal resuscitation. *Resuscitation.* 2008;79:444–452. doi:10.1016/j.resuscitation.2008.08.0.

4. Davies JM, Posner KL Lee LA, Cheney FW, Domino KB. Liability associated with obstetric anesthesia: a closed claims analysis. *Anesthesiology.* 2009;110:131–139. doi:10.1097/ALN.0b013e318190e16a.

5. American Academy of Pediatrics, American College of Obstetricians and Gynecologists. Guidelines for perinatal care. 8th ed. Elk Grove Village, IL: AAP- American College of Obstetricians and Gynecologists;2017:22

6. American College of Obstetricians and Gynecologists Committee on Obstetric Practice and American Society of Anesthesiologists Committee on Obstetric Anesthesia. ACOG committee opinion no. 433. Optimal goals for anesthesia care in obstetrics. *Obstet Gynecol.* 2009;113:1197–1199.

7. Textbook of Neonatal Resuscitation (NRP), 7th Ed By American Academy of Pediatrics and American Heart Association Edited by Gary M. Weiner and Jeanette Zaichkin Book | Published in 2016 ISBN (paper): 978 1 61002-024-4 ISBN (electronic): 978-1-61002-025-1.

8. Wyllie J, Perlman JM, Kattwinkel J, Atkins DL, Chameides L, Goldsmith JP, Guinsburg R, Hazinski MF, Morley C, Richmond S, Simon WM, Singhal N, Szyld E, Tamura M, Velaphi S, Neonatal Resuscitation Chapter Collaborators Part 11: neonatal resuscitation: 2010 international consensus on cardiopulmonary resuscitation and emergency cardiovascular care science with treatment recommendations. *Resuscitation.* 2010;81(Suppl 1):e260–e287. doi:10.1016/j.resuscitation.2010.08.029.

9. Miller SS, Lee HC, Gould JB. Hypothermia in very low birth weight infants: distribution, risk factors and outcomes. *J Perinatol.* 2011;31(Suppl 1):S49–S56. doi:10.1038/jp.2010.177.

10. Chitty H, Wyllie J. Importance of maintaining the newly born temperature in the normal range from delivery to admission. *Semin Fetal Neonatal Med.* 2013;18(6):362–368. doi:10.1016/j.siny.2013.08.002.

11. Rabe H, Diaz-Rossello JL, Duley L, Dowswell T. Effect of timing of umbilical cord clamping and other strategies to influence placental transfusion at preterm birth on maternal and infant outcomes. *Cochrane Database Syst Rev.* 2012;(8):CD003248.

12. Backes CH, Rivera BK, Haque U, et al. Placental transfusion strategies in very preterm neonates: a systematic review and meta-analysis. *Obstet Gynecol.* 2014;124(1):47–56.

13. Szyld E, Aguilar A, Musante GA, Vain N, Prudent L, Fabres J, Carlo WA, Delivery Room Ventilation Devices Trial Group. Comparison of devices for newborn ventilation in the delivery room. *J Pediatr.* 2014, 165(2):234–239. e233.

14. Kapadia VS, Wyckoff MH. Drugs during delivery room resuscitation–what, when and why? *Semin Fetal Neonatal Med.* 2013;18(6):357–361.

15. Vali P, Mathew B, Lakshminrusimha S. Neonatal resuscitation: evolving strategies. *Matern Health, Neonatol and Perinatol.* 2015;1:4. https://doi.org/10.1186/s40748-014-0003-0

16. Solevåg AL, Dannevig I, Wyckoff M, Saugstad OD, Nakstad B. Return of spontaneous circulation with a compression:ventilation ratio of 15:2 versus 3:1 in newborn pigs with cardiac arrest due to asphyxia. *Arch Dis Child Fetal Neonatal Ed.* 2011;96(6):F417–F421.

17. Sobotka K, Polglase G, Schmölzer G, et al. Effects of chest compressions on cardiovascular and cerebral hemodynamics in asphyxiated near-term lambs. *Pediatr Res.* 2015;78:395–400. https://doi.org/10.1038/pr.2015.117.

18. Martin RJ, Fanaroff AA, Walsh MC. Fanaroff and Martin's neonatal-perinatal medicine: diseases of the fetus and infant. Amsterdam: Elsevier; 2019.

19. Bruschettini M, Romantsik O, Ramenghi L, Zappettini S, O'Donnell C, Calevo M. Needle aspiration versus intercostal tube drainage for pneumothorax in the newborn. *Cochrane Database of Syst Rev.* 2016(1):CD011724.

20. Smithhart W, Wyckoff MH, Kapadia V, Jaleel M, Kakkilaya V, Brown LS, Nelson DB, Brion LP. Delivery Room Continuous Positive Airway Pressure and Pneumothorax. *Pediatrics.* 2019 Sep;144(3):e20190756. doi:10.1542/peds.2019-0756. Epub 2019 Aug 9. PMID: 31399490.

21. Adaikalam SA, Higano NS, Tkach JA, et al. Neonatal lung growth in congenital diaphragmatic hernia: evaluation of lung density and mass by pulmonary MRI. *Pediatric Research.* 2019 Nov;86(5):635–640. doi:10.1038/s41390-019-0480-y.

22. Lantos, JD. Ethical problems in decision making in the neonatal ICU. *N Engl J Med.* 2018;379(19):1851–1860. doi:10.1056/NEJMra1801063.

23. Walter JK, Ross LF. Relational autonomy: moving beyond the limits of isolated individualism. *Pediatrics.* 2014;133(Suppl 1):S16–S23.

24. Mackenzie C, Stoljar N, eds. *Relational autonomy: feminist perspective on autonomy, agency, and the social self.* New York: Oxford University Press, 2000:12.

25. Akinloye O, O'Connell C, Allen A, El-Naggar W. Post-resuscitation care for neonates receiving positive pressure ventilation at birth. *Pediatrics.* 2014;134(4); E1057–62.

26. Wyckoff M et al. Part 13: neonatal resuscitation: 2015 American Heart Association guidelines update for cardiopulmonary resuscitation and emergency cardiovascular care (reprint). *Pediatrics.* 2015;136(Suppl 2):S196–S218.

27. Yang M. Newborn neurologic examination. *Neurology.* 2004;62(7):E15–E7.

28. Volpe JJ. Chapter 9—Neurological Examination: Normal and Abnormal Features. In *Volpe's Neurology of the Newborn* (6th ed.). 2018:191–221.e8. Elsevier.

29. Weprin BE, Oakes WJ. Coccygeal pits. *Pediatrics.* 2000;105(5):e69–e.

30. Glass HC. Hypoxic-ischemic encephalopathy and other neonatal encephalopathies. *CONTINUUM: Lifelong Learning in Neurology.* 2018;24(1):57–71.

31. Nelson KB, Bingham P, Edwards EM, Horbar JD, Kenny MJ, Inder T, Pfister RH, Raju T, Soll RF. Antecedents of neonatal encephalopathy in the Vermont Oxford Network Encephalopathy Registry. *Pediatrics.* 2012;130(5):878–886. doi:10.1542/peds.2012-0714. Epub 2012 Oct 15.

32. Shankaran S. Neonatal encephalopathy: treatment with hypothermia. *NeoReviews.* 2010;11(2):e85–e92.

33. Long M, Brandon DH. Induced hypothermia for neonates with hypoxic-ischemic encephalopathy. *Journal of Obstetric, Gynecologic & Neonatal Nursing.* 2007;36(3):293–298.

34. Gomella TL, ed. *Neonatology: management, procedures, on-call problems, diseases and drugs.* 7th ed. New York; McGraw-Hill Education; 2013.

23

Postpartum Complications in Obstetric Anesthesia

Lucy Li, Jingping Wang, Alan D. Kaye, and Henry Liu

Introduction

The typical patient encountered in obstetric anesthesia is a healthy woman of childbearing age who in usual circumstances would have minimal anesthetic or surgical risk. However, the obstetric anesthesiologist must be prepared to manage a wide variety of urgent and emergent postpartum complications, which can arise from both obstetric and anesthetic-related causes.

Pregnancy and the postpartum period are characterized by major physiological changes, and patient factors and the progression of labor and delivery can place the parturient at increased risk for a range of obstetric complications (Table 23.1).[1,2] Labor analgesia is most commonly delivered with neuraxial methods: epidurals and spinals are reliable and effective at providing pain control during labor and delivery, and studies have shown neuraxial is associated with less morbidity and mortality than general anesthesia.[1,2] However, complications after neuraxial anesthesia do exist and vary widely in their severity and incidence. The majority of postpartum complications are relatively common and transient, like postpartum back soreness and headache, while some complications are extremely rare and initially present similarly to benign complications but eventually lead to devastating outcomes. It is imperative for the anesthesiologists to be vigilant of all these potential postpartum complications in the obstetric practice and to recognize and manage them expediently. This chapter will discuss some of the most common postpartum complications that the anesthesia practitioner will encounter and their best management.

Common Complications after Obstetric Anesthesia

Hemorrhage

Incidence

Postpartum hemorrhage is one of the top five causes of maternal mortality around the world and one of the most common severe morbidities encountered in obstetric anesthesia.[3,4] Incidence varies depending upon the definition used and is estimated to occur in 1–5% of deliveries worldwide.[1] In 2010, hemorrhage was the third-leading cause of maternal mortality in the United States at 12%, after cardiovascular diseases and cardiomyopathy.[1] In developing countries, postpartum hemorrhage is the leading cause of maternal mortality (Table 23.2).[1,4]

Table 23.1 Postpartum Complications in Obstetric Anesthesia

	Incidence	Causes and Etiologies	Diagnosis	Management
Postpartum Hemorrhage	1–5%	Uterine atony, retained placenta and products of conception, obstetric lacerations, uterine inversion, use of tocolytics prior to delivery	Obstetric exam	Large-bore intravenous access, rapid resuscitation with fluids and blood products, uterotonic agents, bimanual uterine massage, dilation and evacuation, laceration repair, uterine replacement/reversion, surgical or interventional radiology procedures
Postdural Puncture Headache	0.7% (1% of epidurals, < 1% of spinals)	Unintentional dural puncture leading to CSF loss faster than CSF production	Physical exam	Minimize CSF leakage by covering epidural needle hole or reinserting stylet, bed rest, supine position, fluid hydration, caffeine, analgesics and anti-emetics, epidural blood patch
Neurological Complications	1% (permanent injury in 0.2 to 1.2 in 100,000)	Peripheral neuropathies secondary to direct trauma or obstetric compression, transient neurological symptoms, epidural or spinal hematoma, cauda equina syndrome, transverse myelitis, anterior spinal syndrome, paraplegia	Physical exam, imaging (MRI, CT)	Supportive treatment (analgesics, warm compresses, physical therapy), surgical decompression, corticosteroids
Infection	1 in 60,000	Meningitis and arachnoiditis, epidural abscess	Lumbar puncture, imaging (MRI, CT, myelogram), cultures	Removal of epidural catheter, anti-*Staphylococcal* antibiotics, surgical decompression or percutaneous drainage
Amniotic Fluid Embolism	2 to 6 in 100,000	Anaphylactoid-like maternal response to fetal elements in amniotic fluid	Clinical diagnosis of exclusion	Cardiopulmonary resuscitation, delivery of fetus via cesarean delivery, supportive care, circulatory support, intubation and mechanical ventilation, blood products, uterotonic agents

Pathophysiology and Diagnosis

Postpartum hemorrhage has various definitions worldwide. Classically, it is defined as an estimated blood loss of greater than 500 mL after vaginal birth or greater than 1000 mL after cesarean delivery. In 2017, the American College of Obstetrician and Gynecologists redefined postpartum hemorrhage as an estimated blood loss of greater than 1000 mL or bleeding associated with signs or symptoms of hypovolemia in the first 24 hours postpartum, regardless of delivery route.

Table 23.2 Causes of Postpartum Hemorrhage and Their Risk Factors

Cause	Risk Factors
Uterine atony	High parity, use of tocolytics (e.g., oxytocin, terbutaline, or magnesium sulfate) during labor, chorioamnionitis
Retained placenta and products of conception	Maternal age ≥ 30, delivery at 24 to 27 weeks, stillbirth, delivery in a teaching hospital
Obstetric lacerations	Primiparity, occiput posterior position, labor induction, labor augmentation, epidural anesthesia, midline episiotomy, forceps delivery, vacuum-assisted delivery
Uterine inversion	Placenta accreta, placental implantation at the fundus of the uterus, excessive traction on the umbilical cord prior to placental separation from the uterus
All causes of postpartum hemorrhage	Preeclampsia, maternal bleeding or clotting disorders, overdistention of the uterus (e.g., secondary to fetal macrosomia, multiple gestations, polyhydramnios), forceps delivery, prolonged labor

The most common causes of postpartum hemorrhage are uterine atony, retained placenta and products of conception, obstetric lacerations, uterine inversion, and use of tocolytics prior to delivery.[5]

Postpartum uterine atony refers to when a uterus does not adequately contract after delivery, and it is responsible for 75 to 90% of cases of postpartum hemorrhage.[1,4–7] It is the leading cause of maternal mortality worldwide.[8,9] Risk factors include high parity, fetal macrosomia, multiple gestations, prolonged labor, use of tocolytics like terbutaline or magnesium sulfate during labor, and chorioamnionitis. Other complications like retained placenta and products of conception occur in 3.3% of vaginal deliveries.[10] Obstetric lacerations of the vagina, cervix, and perineum are very common after vaginal delivery, and significant bleeding from lacerations is often difficult to estimate.

Uterine inversion is very rare, occurring in 1 in 3000 to 5000 all deliveries and is an obstetric emergency.[5,10] In addition to significant hemorrhage, patients can have severe pain. Risk factors include placenta accreta, placental implantation at the fundus of the uterus, and excessive traction on the umbilical cord prior to placental separation from the uterus.

There are many factors associated with overall increased risk of hemorrhage postpartum including preeclampsia, maternal bleeding or clotting disorders, overdistention of the uterus secondary to multiple gestations or polyhydramnios, assisted delivery with forceps, and prolonged third stage of labor (Table 23.2).

Differential Diagnosis

Given the many causes of postpartum hemorrhage, it is important to discern the primary insulting factor. If a postpartum patient is hypotensive, other causes of shock must be considered, include severe sepsis, pulmonary embolism, venous air embolism, amniotic fluid embolism, and severe complications of preeclampsia.

Treatment

For all cases of postpartum hemorrhage, the first steps to management require obtaining large-bore intravenous access and rapid resuscitation with fluids and blood products.

The obstetrician often needs to examine the patient to determine the cause of hemorrhage, so supplementation to residual neuraxial or additional anesthesia beyond the residual neuraxial may be necessary with opioids and/or analgesia and sedatives. Care should be taken if neuraxial supplementation is undertaken in a hypovolemic bleeding patient, and the anesthesiologist should be prepared to induce general anesthesia for further management of hemorrhage in the operating room.

In cases of uterine atony, bimanual uterine massage should be performed by the obstetrician and uterotonic agents should be administered. Pharmacologic agents include oxytocin (Pitocin), ergot alkaloids like methylergonovine (Methergine), prostaglandins like prostaglandin $F_{2\alpha}$ (Hemabate), and prostaglandin E_1 (misoprostol). Oxytocin is routinely administered to all patients after delivery as prophylaxis against uterine atony and is also its first-line treatment. It increases uterine smooth muscle tone and is available as 30 IU diluted in 500 mL to 1000 mL of fluids for intravenous delivery. Care should be taken not to deliver oxytocin as a rapid bolus, as this can cause hypotension, tachycardia, headache, antidiuretic effects leading to pulmonary edema, and even cardiovascular collapse and death. Methylergonovine is administered intramuscularly in doses of 0.2 mg, repeated every 2 to 4 hours as needed for a maximum dose of 1 mg; the medication is contraindicated in hypertension. Prostaglandin $F_{2\alpha}$ is also given intramuscularly in doses of 0.25 mg repeated every 15 to 90 minutes as needed for a maximum dose of 2 mg; it is contraindicated in patients with asthma. It can also be given directly into the myometrium by the obstetrician. Prostaglandin E_1 increases myometrial intracellular free calcium concentration to improve uterine tone and can be given to patients with both hypertension and asthma, at a dose of 1000 mcg which can be given orally or sublingually, vaginally, or rectally (Table 23.3).

If hemorrhage is secondary to retained placenta or products of conception, major obstetric laceration, or uterine inversion, additional anesthesia is often required for manual extraction or dilation and evacuation, laceration repair, or uterine replacement, respectively. If a patient is hemodynamically stable, an existing epidural or induction of a spinal anesthetic can be utilized to provide anesthesia for the procedure. If the patient is hemodynamically unstable, general anesthesia is required via rapid-sequence induction.

With a retained placenta, additional uterine relaxation is sometimes necessary via pharmacological means to assist the obstetrician in extraction. Nitroglycerin 40 to 80 mcg can be administered intravenously with caution, watching for hypotension in the already hypovolemic patient. Nitroglycerin can also be given sublingually as tablets: the usual dose is 1 to 2 tablets, with each tablet containing 300 to 400 mcg of nitroglycerin. If the patient is intubated under general endotracheal anesthesia, inhalational gases at 2 MAC can also help achieve uterine relaxation. Uterine relaxation is typically not necessary for extraction of retained products of conception.

In cases of major laceration, patients usually require augmentation of anesthesia to facilitate repair by the obstetrician. This is often achieved by dosing additional local anesthetic through an existing epidural catheter.

Uterine inversion often requires uterine relaxation, as with a retained placenta, so the obstetrician can perform uterine replacement. On rare occasions, uterine replacement is not successful with vaginal maneuvers alone and laparotomy is required. After uterine reversion, the uterus is examined for any defects necessitating repair or retained products of conception. In any instance where patients are given uterine relaxants, uterine atony can follow and the patient may require uterotonics.

Table 23.3 Pharmacologic Treatment of Postpartum Hemorrhage

Drug	Dosing	Contraindications and Adverse Reactions	Considerations
Uterotonics for uterine atony			
Oxytocin (Pitocin)	30 IU diluted in 500 to 1000 mL NS delivered IV	Rapid bolus can lead to hypotension, tachycardia, headache, antidiuretic effects leading to pulmonary edema, cardiovascular collapse, death	Prophylaxis and first-line treatment
Methylergonovine (Methergine)	0.2 mg IM, repeated every 2 to 4 hours as needed (maximum dose 1 mg)	Hypertension	
Prostaglandin F$_{2a}$ (Hemabate)	0.25 mg IM or into myometrium, repeated every 15 to 90 minutes as needed (maximum dose 2 mg)	Asthma	
Prostaglandin E$_1$ (misoprostol)	1000 mcg orally, sublingually, vaginally, or rectally		
Uterine relaxants for retained placenta and products of conception or uterine inversion			
Nitroglycerin	40 to 80 mcg IV or 600 to 800 mcg sublingually	Can cause hypotension in already hypovolemic patient	
Inhaled anesthetic gases	2 to 3 MAC	Can cause hypotension in already hypovolemic patient	Utilized if patient is intubated under general anesthesia

If hemorrhage is not controlled with pharmacological therapy or the obstetric interventions already discussed, more invasive methods need to be undertaken.[11] The obstetrician can place compression sutures, perform internal iliac (hypogastric) or uterine artery ligation, or place a balloon catheter filled with warm saline in the uterine cavity to tamponade intrauterine bleeding.[12] If the patient is stable for transport, interventional radiology can perform balloon occlusion or embolization of the internal iliac or uterine arteries to prevent or treat hemorrhage.[12] These methods have success rates of 85 to 90%.[11] In rare cases, a patient may ultimately require laparotomy and hysterectomy for control of bleeding (Box 23.1).

Headache

Incidence
Headache is common in pregnancy, particularly in the postpartum period after patients have undergone hormonal and physiological changes and received neuraxial anesthesia and vasoactive medications. During this period, patients are often subject to irregular sleep schedules and food intake and psychosocial stressors, further increasing the risk of developing headaches. Estimates of the frequency of etiologies of postpartum headache have ranged widely, with studies showing the most common causes to be primary headache disorder (2-50%), preeclampsia (12-24%), and postdural puncture headache (16-21%).[8,13–15]

Box 23.1 Invasive Management Options for Postpartum Hemorrhage

Surgical interventions
  Obstetric laceration repair
  Manual uterine replacement/reversion
  Compression sutures
  Internal iliac (hypogastric) or uterine artery ligation
  Uterine tamponade with intrauterine balloon catheter filled with warm saline
  Laparotomy and hysterectomy

Interventional radiology procedures
  Balloon occlusion of internal iliac or uterine artery
  Embolization of internal iliac or uterine artery

If a normotensive postpartum patient who received neuraxial anesthesia develops headache, postdural puncture headache (PDPH) must be evaluated for. The chance of PDPH with epidural catheter placement after dural puncture is higher than after spinal placement, as epidurals are generally placed with a 18-gauge needle while spinals are placed with much smaller 25- to 29-gauge needles.[7] Unintentional dural puncture occurs in 1.5% of labor epidurals, and the resulting chance of PDPH is greater than 75%.[7,11] The incidence of PDPH with spinals is less than 1%.[16]

Pathophysiology and Diagnosis

Unintentional dural puncture, or a "wet tap," during lumbar epidural placement occurs when the epidural needle passes through the epidural space, punctures the dura, and enters the subarachnoid space. A wet tap can also occur if the epidural catheter punctures the dura during placement or at any time thereafter. Cases are usually immediately recognized by pouring of cerebrospinal fluid (CSF) from the epidural needle or aspiration from the epidural catheter, although PDPH can also occur without overt signs of dural puncture if only the tip of the epidural needle scratches through the dura. PDPH can also occur with intentional dural puncture for spinal anesthesia or myelography.

It is believed that CSF leakage from the defect leads to a rate of CSF loss faster than its production. The loss of CSF is thought to create traction on the structures supporting the brain, blood vessels, and cranial nerves, all of which contain very pain-sensitive fibers that lead to the pain of PDPH. CSF loss is also thought to decrease intracranial pressure, leading to a compensatory cerebral vasodilation that can also be painful.

PDPH usually occurs within 12 to 72 hours following dural puncture. The typical spinal headache is bilateral, located in the frontal, retroorbital, or occipital regions, and extends to the neck. Pain quality is usually throbbing and constant. Classically, the severity of the pain is associated with body position: pain is aggravated when the patient is upright—sitting or standing—and alleviated by lying supine, but it can be the opposite.[17] Pain can be associated with photophobia, nausea and vomiting, neck pain, dizziness; occasionally, patients have diplopia, tinnitus, and hearing loss due to traction on the cranial nerves, although this is rare. Seizures can also occur but are uncommon.

The risk of dural puncture increases with increased depth to a patient's epidural space and more attempts at epidural placement. The risk of PDPH increases with larger needle size, usage of cutting-point needles (compared to non-cutting pencil-point needles), needle bevel oriented in the short axis of the spine (as the needle will cut longitudinal dural fibers rather than separate them), and patient factors like young age, low BMI, history of prior PDPH, and vaginal delivery. Factors that protect against unintentional dural puncture include higher practitioner skill level and loss of resistance to saline.

Differential Diagnosis

In any patient with a headache and elevated blood pressure, preeclampsia must be ruled out. The disease can present postpartum, usually within the first 48 hours after delivery but at times up to more than a week postpartum.

Parturient may have headache even without dural puncture after lumbar epidural placement. This can occur due to injection of significant amounts of air into the epidural space when using loss-of-resistance technique with air or saline mixed with air. These headaches are usually self-limited.

If patients do not have findings consistent with PDPH or preeclampsia and have no focal neurological signs, a primary headache disorder is most likely. Tension-type headaches and musculoskeletal and cervicogenic headaches are common given the sleep deprivation and fatigue, irregular food intake, and stress that often characterizes the postpartum period. Migraines are common postpartum as well, particularly in women with a history of migraines.

Differential diagnosis should also include other serious causes of headache secondary to intracranial processes like infection and subarachnoid hemorrhage particularly if a patient has focal neurologic deficits. Other rarer causes of headache in the postpartum period include pituitary mass and hemorrhage, cerebral venous sinus thrombosis, and vertebral artery dissection.

Diagnostic approach to determine the etiology of a postpartum headache is similar to those in a nonpregnant patient.[13] Patients with a suspected secondary headache or danger signs like systemic signs and symptoms and focal neurological deficits should receive imaging, and those with concern for infection or subarachnoid hemorrhage should receive lumbar puncture.

Treatment

If dural puncture occurs during epidural placement, CSF leakage should first be minimized by covering the epidural needle hole or reinserting the stylet. If an epidural anesthetic is desired, a repeat attempt can be made at a different interspace; vigilance is necessary given the possibility that a spinal anesthetic can occur with injection of medication through the epidural catheter despite correct placement at another level. There is also the option to convert to continuous spinal anesthesia by placing an intrathecal catheter, with care taken in regard to appropriate neuraxial local anesthetic and opioid dosing for a spinal anesthetic. Placement of an intrathecal catheter can still provide excellent labor analgesia and avoids multiple attempts at epidural placement and the possibility of another unintentional dural puncture.

If PDPH occurs after dural puncture, conservative treatment for mild cases includes bed rest and keeping the patient supine; intravenous or oral fluid hydration; caffeine sodium benzoate; oral analgesics including acetaminophen, NSAIDs, opioids; and anti-emetics. Laying the patient flat decreases the hydrostatic pressure that drives CSF leakage out of the dural hole and minimizes pain. Hydration and caffeine both stimulate production of CSF, and caffeine also vasoconstricts and minimizes compensatory cerebral vasodilation. Caffeine in the amount of 300 to 500 mg is recommended either orally or intravenously (added to 1000 mL of intravenous fluids and administered at 200 mL per hour). Valsalva straining can worsen pain, so patients should avoid heavy lifting and can be given soft diets and bowel regimens to help minimize bearing down [Figure 23.1].

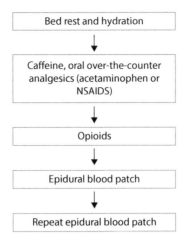

Figure 23.1 Management Algorithm of Postdural Puncture Headache.

Patients with moderate or severe PDPH that interferes with sitting or standing and activities of daily living or those who have failed conservative therapy after 24 hours should be offered an epidural blood patch. About 20 to 30 mL of autologous blood is sterilely drawn from the patient and then sterilely and slowly injected via epidural needle into the epidural space. This is performed at the level or one interspace below the level of the dural puncture, as studies have shown that the blood will spread preferentially cephalad to the level of injection.[18] About 15 mL of blood spreads over a mean distance of nine spinal segments.[18] Patients may feel pressure during injection; if the patient feels paresthesia or severe back pain, injection should stop immediately.

The blood patch stops further leakage of CSF by either mass effect or coagulation. Like neuraxial anesthesia, blood patch is contraindicated in patients on anticoagulation or with coagulopathy or infection at the site of injection or systemically. Patients often feel immediate relief, although it may take hours to achieve full effect as CSF production begins to match CSF loss and intracranial pressure normalizes. Roughly 90% of patients experience relief from one blood patch. Of the nonresponders, another 90% will have relief after a second blood patch, which is usually placed 24 to 48 hours after the first.[6,10] Patients can experience a mild residual headache or back discomfort afterwards. Some studies have utilized prophylactic epidural blood patches to reduce the development of PDPH in parturient prior to onset of headache, but this is not part of current treatment recommendations.[19]

If left untreated, 70% of PDPH spontaneously resolve in 7 days and 90% in 6 months as the dural defect heals on its own.[6] There have been rare occasions requiring surgical repair of the puncture site.

Neurologic Complications

Incidence

Analyses of the American Society of Anesthesiologists Closed Claims database reveals that the most common claims in obstetric anesthesia involve nerve injury following neuraxial anesthesia.[1] A 1969 review found that transient and permanent nerve injury likely occurs in 0.02% to 1% of epidural anesthetics, and more recent studies have found that this incidence

Table 23.4 Rare Neurological Complications of Neuraxial Anesthesia

	Incidence	Pathophysiology	Onset	Diagnosis	Treatment
Epidural or spinal hematoma	1 in 150,000 epidurals, 1 in 220,000 spinals	Mass effect leading to direct compression, pressure injury, and ischemia to spinal cord and nerves	Within 48 hours	MRI or CT	Emergent neurosurgical decompression within 6 to 12 hours of diagnosis
Cauda equina syndrome	0.1 in 10,000	Ischemic compression via mass effect (from hematoma or infection), direct neurotoxicity, prolonged exposure of nerves to high concentrations and high dose of local anesthetics	Variable depending on insult	MRI	Corticosteroids (limited data)
Transverse myelitis	Unknown	Unknown, with neuraxial techniques suggested as possible cause	Acute (within hours to days) or subacute (1 to 2 weeks)	MRI or myelogram	Physical therapy, exercise, corticosteroids
Anterior spinal syndrome	Unknown	Ischemia from profound hypotension, vasoconstrictors	Following insult	MRI or arteriogram	Correction of hypotension or vasoconstriction
Paraplegia	0.1 in 10,000	Direct trauma to spinal cord, ischemia from profound hypotension	Following insult	Physical exam, MRI	Correction of hypotension

has likely not changed in the time since this review.[20–23] These more recent studies have found that epidural anesthesia is more likely to be associated with peripheral neuropathy than spinal anesthesia.[21] Serious neurologic complications are extremely rare and their exact incidence after neuraxial anesthesia remains unknown (Table 23.4).[24,25]

Pathophysiology and Diagnosis

Peripheral neuropathies after labor neuraxial anesthesia can be due to direct trauma from the needle or catheter to nerve roots. Development of a persistent neurological deficit after neuraxial anesthesia has been associated with pain during placement of needle or catheter, pain on injection, and multiple attempts during a difficult placement.[26,27] Thus, pain on placement requires redirection of the needle or catheter.

Differential Diagnosis

Nerve injury in the postpartum period may be related to neuraxial anesthesia or it may be secondary to obstetric causes.[1,28,29] It is important to discern whether injury is related to obstetrical cause, and if necessary to obtain neurological consultation to help identify the source of injury.

Lateral femoral cutaneous neuropathy, or meralgia paresthetica, can ensue due to entrapment of the nerve as it courses under the inguinal ligament.[29] During pregnancy, expansion of the abdominal wall and increased lumbar lordosis can cause entrapment. During labor, as the patient flexes the hip during labor and delivery, the nerve may also be injured. During cesarean delivery, the nerve may be injured by surgical retraction or cutting. Since the nerve does not contain motor fibers, symptoms of meralgia paresthetica are restricted to pain and/

or sensory changes as numbness and tingling, and diminished sensation over the upper lateral thigh. Sensory changes are unilateral in 80% of cases.[29] The disease is benign and self-limited in most patients. Persistent symptoms can be treated with low-dose amitriptyline or injection of local anesthetic at the level of the inguinal ligament.

Foot drop can occur postpartum from compression injury at the level of the lumbar root, lumbosacral plexus, sciatic nerve, or common peroneal nerve.[30] Lumbosacral plexus injuries can occur from direct compression by the fetal head during labor or from assisted delivery. Sciatic nerve lesions have been theorized to be secondary to compression while the patient is in the left uterine displacement position during labor or cesarean delivery. The common peroneal nerve can be injured during labor from pressure to the lateral leg either with poor positioning in stirrups or during pushing when the patient hyperflexes their knee and holds the lateral leg with their hands. Risk of these compression injuries is increased after epidural placement as the patient is less likely to notice prolonged pressure to the lateral leg. Recovery depends on the kind of compressive injury sustained, taking 3 to 6 months for pure demyelinating injury and longer for axonal injury. Supportive management includes physical therapy and orthotics for the ankle and foot.

Some postpartum back soreness may occur after epidural or spinal placement. Placement of an epidural or spinal needle can lead to tissue trauma as it passes through skin, subcutaneous tissue, and ligaments, leading to localized inflammation and reflexive muscle spasms. Symptoms can also be secondary to relaxation of ligaments in the back that occur with neuraxial anesthesia. Soreness is usually over the placement site and mild and self-limited. Studies have shown that persistent new-onset back pain has no association with neuraxial placement, as postpartum back pain rates were found to be the same in patients who received epidurals and patients who received systemic analgesia during labor.[6,31] Supportive treatment includes over-the-counter analgesics like acetaminophen, NSAIDs, warm and cold compresses.

Transient neurological symptoms (TNS) are thought to be due to concentration-dependent neurotoxicity of local anesthetics, and they are most commonly associated with hyperbaric lidocaine, although they have also been seen with other local anesthetics like bupivacaine, mepivacaine, and tetracaine. Other risk factors include obesity and lithotomy position. Symptoms begin after resolution of a spinal, usually 12 to 24 hours after uneventful spinal placement, with patients experiencing unilateral or bilateral radicular pain that begins in the buttocks and radiates down the legs without associated sensory or motor deficits. Pain is usually described by patients to be aching or burning in quality and ranges from mild to severe. Full spontaneous recovery is usually within 7 days and symptoms can be managed conservatively with NSAIDs, muscle relaxants, opioids, and warm compresses.

With any neurological deficits or back pain, there are some very rare neurological complications of neuraxial anesthesia that must be ruled out as they can lead to permanent neurologic sequelae if not expediently treated. These include epidural and spinal hematoma, cauda equina syndrome, transverse myelitis, anterior spinal artery syndrome, and paraplegia.

Bleeding in the vertebral canal can occur with epidural or spinal placement or epidural catheter removal. Minor bleeding is common secondary to trauma to epidural veins from the needle or catheter, but usually has no clinical ramifications. The largest study on incidence from the United Kingdom National Health Service audit reports that clinically significant hematoma occurs in 1 in 150,000 of epidurals and 1 in 220,000 of spinals.[1,10,21] Risk increases in patients with abnormal coagulation from bleeding disorders, significant thrombocytopenia, platelet dysfunction, anticoagulant therapy, and difficult neuraxial placement. Thus, anticoagulation status should be checked at time of placement and time of catheter removal.

Trauma to epidural or spinal veins can lead to hematoma formation. Formation of a hematoma leads to a mass effect that causes direct compression of neural tissue and pressure injury and ischemia to the spinal cord and nerves. Signs and symptoms usually present within 48 hours of the inciting event and include sharp radicular back pain or pressure along with progressive development of neurological deficits like motor weakness, sensory loss, and bladder and bowel dysfunction. Persistent neuraxial blockade that lasts longer than expected should also raise suspicion of a hematoma. If there is concern regarding an epidural or spinal hematoma, close monitoring of signs and symptoms is necessary, with urgent MRI or CT imaging performed for definitive diagnosis. An epidural or spinal hematoma is a surgical emergency and requires immediate treatment to avoid permanent neurological damage. Good neurological recovery is obtainable in patients who receive neurosurgical decompression within 6 to 12 hours of diagnosis.

Cauda equina syndrome is caused by ischemic compression via mass effect (as from an abscess or hematoma), direct neurotoxicity, or prolonged exposure of nerves to high concentrations and high doses of local anesthetics.[6] Incidence is 0.1 in 10,000 neuraxial anesthetics.[6,30,32] Signs and symptoms include radicular lower back pain, motor deficits, patchy sensory deficits, and bladder and bowel dysfunction. Diagnosis is with MRI, and treatment includes corticosteroids, although data is limited on their effectiveness. Neurologic recovery is variable, and permanent neurologic deficits often ensue.

Transverse myelitis is another rare complication of neuraxial anesthesia that leads to lower back pain, motor deficits, sensory changes like allodynia, and bladder and bowel dysfunction.[7] Symptoms can either begin acutely within hours to days or over 1 to 2 weeks. Diagnosis is with MRI or myelogram. Treatment includes physical therapy and exercise as well as corticosteroids, and recovery is variable: some patients achieve recovery within 2 to 12 weeks of symptom onset, but if there is no improvement within 3 to 6 months, future significant recovery is usually unlikely.

Paraplegia after neuraxial anesthesia is reported to occur in 0.1 in 10,000 neuraxial anesthetics.[7,22,30,32] Causes include direct trauma to the spinal cord from the needle and ischemia of the spinal cord due to profound hypotension. In cases of severe hypotension, anterior spinal artery syndrome is a possible complication due to the anterior cord's single arterial blood supply from the artery of Adamkiewicz. Patients experience painless motor and sensory loss with preservation of proprioception (as that is carried by the posterior spinal column). Diagnosis is with MRI and arteriogram, and treatment is with correction of hypotension or other insults like vasospasm. Like cauda equina syndrome and transverse myelitis, recovery is variable.

Treatment

Transient paresthesia during placement usually resolves immediately and does not lead to persistent nerve injury. Most neuropathies resolve spontaneously within 6 weeks to 2 months. Supportive treatment includes analgesics like acetaminophen and NSAIDs and warm and cold compresses.

Infection

Incidence

Infection and sepsis caused 11% of pregnancy-related death in 2010 in the United States.[1] The majority of these cases are related to chorioamnionitis, which occurs in 1–2% of pregnancies.[1] Serious infections related to neuraxial placement are incredibly rare, estimated at 0.6 per 10,000 epidural anesthetics and less than 0.3 per 10,000 spinal anesthetics.[6,20,21,32] Estimates of the incidence of epidural abscess in the obstetric population varies widely from 1 in 500,000 to 1 in 6500 epidurals.[1,21,33] Risk of infection increases in compromised immune states like pregnancy and diabetes and in patients who are immunocompromised or already have systemic infection.[7]

Pathophysiology and Diagnosis

Meningitis and arachnoiditis, infections of the subarachnoid space, can occur due to contamination from the equipment, the patient's skin flora, or the anesthesiologist placing the neuraxial anesthesia. The most common infectious causes are *Staphylococcus* species tracked from the patient's skin during placement and oral flora like *Streptococcus viridans* from the proceduralist.[34,35]

Meningitis symptoms include fever, headache, neck stiffness, and confusion. Diagnosis is made with lumbar puncture and cerebrospinal fluid studies, and initial empiric antibiotic regimens should cover both gram-positive and gram-negative bacteria, with further tailoring of antibiotic therapy based on cultures and susceptibilities.[34]

Patients with arachnoiditis experience symptoms of lower back pain that worsens with activity and sometimes motor and sensory deficits, and onset can occur up to years after the initial insult. Diagnosis is made with MRI or myelogram. Symptoms are managed with analgesics, physical therapy, and exercise; in some cases, steroid injections and electrical stimulation may help alleviate symptoms. Unfortunately, treatment usually does not yield significant improvement, with most patients developing a chronic pain disorder from arachnoiditis.

Both meningitis and arachnoiditis can be noninfectious, with cases of chemical irritation in the early twentieth century caused by disinfectant detergent solutions that are no longer in use in modern preparations.[1,7]

Epidural abscesses are most commonly caused by *Staphylococcus aureus* and *Staphylococcus epidermis* in the postpartum population.[33,36] Similar to meningitis and arachnoiditis, the source of infection can be from contamination of equipment, patient, or proceduralist during neuraxial placement, as well as from hematogenous spread from an area of infection into the epidural space. The exact mechanisms of spinal cord damage are unclear, as neurological damage is often out of proportion to the degree of spinal cord compression by the abscess. It is thought that direct compression and ischemia via compression or infarction of vessels both play important roles in the evolution of neurological injury.

Symptom progression has four classic stages: fever and localized lower back tenderness, nerve root and radicular pain, neurological deficits including motor and sensory deficits and bladder and bowel dysfunction, and paraplegia or paralysis. Onset of symptoms of an epidural abscess was found in one series to occur in 5 days on average, although presentation can range from 2 days to weeks after epidural catheter insertion.

Laboratory tests can help establish diagnosis, including leukocytosis and elevated erythrocyte sedimentation rate. Lumbar puncture can reveal studies suggesting infection. Cultures can be sent from the epidural catheter tip, the catheter placement site, and from the blood. Confirmation of the diagnosis is made with neurological imaging with MRI or CT scan.

Differential Diagnosis

Differential diagnosis includes postpartum peripheral neuropathies, backache, and epidural or spinal hematoma. A high index of suspicion is necessary given the devastating consequences of unrecognized and untreated epidural abscess.

Treatment

Prevention is key for infections related to neuraxial placement. Strict aseptic technique is essential. If a family member is present during placement, they must also wear a mask and be instructed to not contaminate the neuraxial equipment tray. With regards to epidural abscess prevention, general methods include daily evaluation of epidural catheter dressings, minimizing manipulation and opening of the closed catheter system, utilizing a micropore filter to guard against bacterial migration into the system, and removing catheters or changing the catheter within a defined time, usually after 4 days of initial placement [Box 23.2].

Prognosis and recovery correlates to the degree of neurological dysfunction at the time of diagnosis and initiation of treatment, so rapid diagnosis and treatment are crucial to attaining neurological recovery. Associated fever and back pain which are common in obstetric patients can lead to delayed diagnoses and worse outcome in postpartum epidural abscesses. If so, the epidural catheter should be removed and cultured, and anti-*Staphylococcal* antibiosis should be initiated with consultation with infectious diseases specialists. Antibiotic therapy is necessary for prolonged periods of 6 to 12 weeks, with transition from intravenous to oral antibiotics at 3 to 4 weeks. Treatment may sometimes involve early surgical decompression with posterior laminotomy or laminectomy and washout, so neurosurgical consultation should be made early. The goal is to remove pus, debride infected tissue, and drain any affected areas. Percutaneous drainage is possible if the abscess is well defined by imaging, and it is often chosen over open surgery if the abscess is multicompartmental. In some patients—generally those with no or minor neurological signs—antibiotics alone may be sufficient, although if a patient is managed medically, there are specific criteria for antibiotic selection.[37]

Box 23.2 Strategies to Prevent Infection in Neuraxial Anesthesia

During neuraxial placement
Strict aseptic technique
Facemasks for all individuals in room where neuraxial anesthesia is being placed
Instruction of any family member present during placement regarding sterile technique

After neuraxial placement
Daily evaluation of epidural catheter dressing
Minimize manipulation and opening of closed catheter system
Micropore filter to guard against bacterial migration into system
Remove or change catheter within defined time interval (usually 4 days after initial placement)

Embolism

Incidence
Amniotic fluid embolism (AFE) is a rare and often fatal condition, estimated in various reports to range from 2 in 100,000 to 6 in 100,000 live births.[6,8,10] The true incidence is unknown as it is a diagnosis of exclusion that is frequently made postmortem. The mortality rate is high, with some series citing an 86% overall mortality rate and a mortality exceeding 50% in the first hour of diagnosis.[1,8] In the United States, 12% of pregnancy-related deaths were due to amniotic fluid or thrombotic pulmonary embolism in 2010.[1]

Pathophysiology and Diagnosis
AFE occurs due to amniotic fluid entry into the maternal circulation, with entry occurring at any break in the uteroplacental membranes at any stage of labor or delivery—whether a spontaneous vaginal delivery or cesarean delivery, following pathologies like placental abruption or uterine rupture, or in the postpartum period. Amniotic fluid contains fetal elements and chemical mediators like prostaglandins and leukotrienes that when introduced to the mother's circulation, leads to an anaphylactoid-like maternal systemic response with activation of proinflammatory mediators.

AFE consists of three major disease processes: acute pulmonary embolism, disseminated intravascular coagulation (DIC), and uterine atony. Patients present with sudden hemodynamic collapse that consists of two stages of shock. Right heart failure occurs first secondary to a transient pulmonary hypertension due to maternal release of vasoactive substances, and then left heart failure occurs due to direct myocardial depression and ischemic injury to the left ventricle. Hypoxia and respiratory distress arise from pulmonary hypertension and both cardiogenic and noncardiogenic pulmonary edema. Patients have generalized bleeding and can have neurological manifestations like altered mental status and seizures.

Previously, definitive diagnosis was made by testing for fetal elements in the maternal circulation via aspiration from a central line or at autopsy, but fetal squamous cells have been found in the circulation of otherwise healthy pregnant women during labor and delivery. Therefore, AFE remains a clinical diagnosis of exclusion with no definitive diagnostic test.

Differential Diagnosis
Presentation of acute shock and respiratory distress in the parturient should always raise suspicion of amniotic fluid embolism. However, the differential diagnoses should always include other potential causes of sudden cardiovascular collapse like acute thrombotic pulmonary embolism, venous air embolism, massive hemorrhage, sepsis, or severe complications of preeclampsia like intracranial hemorrhage, pulmonary edema, heart failure, hepatic rupture, and DIC (Box 23.3).

Treatment
Management of AFE requires cardiopulmonary resuscitation, immediate delivery of the fetus via cesarean delivery (which improves both maternal and fetal outcomes), and supportive care. ACLS guidelines for the pregnant patient in cardiac arrest include left uterine displacement and performing compressions 2 to 3 cm higher on the sternum for those in the third trimester.[10] Delivery of the fetus within 5 minutes of cardiac arrest improves neonatal

---

Box 23.3 Differential Diagnosis for Amniotic Fluid Embolism

Acute thrombotic pulmonary embolism
Venous air embolism
Massive hemorrhage
Sepsis
Complications of preeclampsia
Intracranial hemorrhage
Pulmonary edema
Heart failure
Hepatic rupture
DIC

---

survival and assists maternal resuscitation. After resuscitation and delivery, patients generally require intubation, mechanical ventilation, circulatory support with fluids and vasopressors, and further care in the intensive care unit. Some patients require cardiopulmonary bypass and extracorporeal membrane oxygenation for treatment of refractory AFE. DIC is managed with platelets and coagulation factors guided by laboratory tests and uterine atony is treated with uterotonic agents. Mortality rates remain high, and 75% of survivors have permanent neurologic sequelae after AFE [Figure 23.2].[11]

Other

There are several other postpartum complications after obstetric anesthesia that bear mention.

Horner Syndrome

Horner syndrome occurs in 1 to 4% of epidural anesthetics.[10] Upper thoracic sympathetic blockade leads to the triad of ptosis, miosis, and anhidrosis, as well as enophthalmos. Symptoms typically resolve on their own.

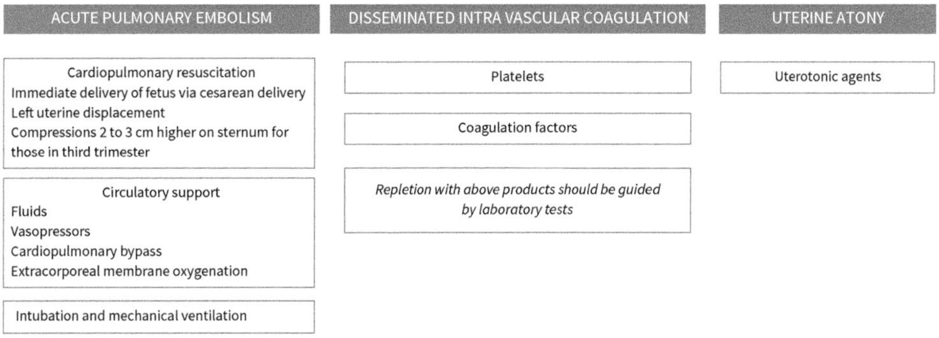

ACUTE PULMONARY EMBOLISM	DISSEMINATED INTRA VASCULAR COAGULATION	UTERINE ATONY
Cardiopulmonary resuscitation Immediate delivery of fetus via cesarean delivery Left uterine displacement Compressions 2 to 3 cm higher on sternum for those in third trimester	Platelets	Uterotonic agents
Circulatory support Fluids Vasopressors Cardiopulmonary bypass Extracorporeal membrane oxygenation	Coagulation factors	
Intubation and mechanical ventilation	*Repletion with above products should be guided by laboratory tests*	

Figure 23.2 Management of Amniotic Fluid Embolism.

Urinary Retention

Blockade of the S2, S3, and S4 nerve roots by local anesthetic can lead to urinary retention in up to a third of patients who receive epidurals and spinals, although symptoms are less pronounced in women compared to men who receive neuraxial anesthestics.[1,6] Local anesthetic blockade of these sacral nerve roots weakens the detrusor muscle which usually contracts during urination, thus interfering with normal voiding reflex. Opioids used in neuraxial mixes can further inhibit the detrusor muscle and reduce the urge to urinate. Patients can receive intermittent straight catheterizations or a urinary catheter, and bladder function will spontaneously return once the sensory level resolves. If bladder dysfunction continues, it is a possible sign of serious neurological complications like those discussed earlier in this chapter.

Epidural Catheter Breakage

Epidural catheter remnants can be left inside of tissue if a catheter is removed through the needle. If a catheter must be removed while the epidural needle is still in place, the two should be removed together. If a portion of a catheter breaks off, management depends on the location of the breakage. If the piece is within the superficial tissues, it should be removed surgically. If an asymptomatic catheter piece is within the epidural space, it can be safely left there and the patient observed, as the catheter is not reactive in absence of infection, and surgical removal will lead to more complications than conservative management.

Cardiovascular Disease

Due to the major cardiovascular changes that occur in the postpartum period, 2% of pregnant patients with existing heart disease will decompensate during this period.[1] Historically, the majority of these patients are those with rheumatic heart disease, but as more patients with congenital heart disease have survived infancy with surgical correction, an increasing number of pregnant patients present with corrected congenital disease. In the United States in 2010, cardiovascular disease was the leading cause of maternal mortality at 27%.[1]

When considering anesthetic options for these patients, the primary goal is to minimize the physiologic stress of labor. Pregnant patients with cardiac disease are divided into two primary groups: those who benefit from early neuraxial anesthesia and the sympathectomy's reduction in systemic vascular resistance, and those who do not.[1] Cardiac lesions that improve with neuraxial include aortic and mitral insufficiency, chronic heart failure, and congenital lesions with left-to-right shunting, as the sympathectomy reduces preload, afterload, and pulmonary congestion, and it can create an increase in cardiac output. Cardiac lesions that worsen with neuraxial include aortic stenosis, primary pulmonary hypertension, and congenital lesions with right-to-left or bidirectional shunting, as these disease states do not tolerate the reductions in preload or afterload seen in sympathectomy. For the patients in this second group, labor analgesia includes neuraxial opioids, systemic analgesics, regional nerve blocks, and general anesthesia.

Summary

The postpartum period is the denouement of a long journey for the parturient, but it requires the same level of provider vigilance as those periods preceding it. A wide range of obstetric and anesthesia-related postpartum complications fall under the purview of an obstetric anesthesiologist, and it is extremely important for the practitioner to be intimately familiar with their diagnoses, differentiation, and management.

References

1. Aromaa U, Lahdensuu M, Cozanitis DA. Severe complications associated with epidural and spinal anaesthesias in Finland 1987–1993 A study base on patient insurance claims. *Acta Anaesthesiol Scand.* 1997;41(4):445–452.

2. Auroy Y, Benhamou D, Bargues L, Ecoffey C, Falissard B, Mercier FJ, Bouaziz H, Samii K. Major complications of regional anesthesia in France: The SOS Regional Anesthesia Hotline Service. *Anesthesiology.* 2002;97(5):1274–1280.

3. Auroy Y, Narchi P, Messiah A, Litt L, Rouvier B, Samii K. Serious complications related to regional anesthesia: results of a prospective survey in France. *Anesthesiology.* 1997;87(3):479–486.

4. Baer ET. Postdural puncture bacterial meningitis. *Anesthesiology.* 2006;105(2):381–393.

5. Brull R, McCartney CJ, Chan VW, El-Beheiry H. Neurological complications after regional anesthesia: contemporary estimates of risk. *Anesth Analg.* 2007;104(4):965–974.

6. Burke D, Wildsmith JAW. Meningitis after spinal anaesthesia. *Br J Anaesth.* 1997;78(6):635–636.

7. Butterworth JF, Mackey DC, Wasnick JD, eds. *Morgan & Mikhail's clinical anesthesiology.* 5th ed. New York, NY: McGraw-Hill Education; 2013.

8. Chestnut DH, Wong CA, Tsen LC, Ngan Kee WD, Beilin Y, Mhyre J, eds. Obstetric *Anesthesia: Principles and Practice.* 6th ed. Philadelphia, PA: Elsevier; 2019.

9. Cook TM, Counsell D, Wildsmith JAW. Major complications of central neuraxial block: report on the Third National Audit Project of the Royal College of Anaesthetists. *Br J Anaesth.* 2009; (2):179–190.

10. Dahlgren N, Tornebrandt K: Neurological complications after anaesthesia. A follow-up of 18,000 spinal and epidural anaesthetics performed over three years. *Acta Anaesthesiol Scand.* 1995;39(7):872–880.

11. Dawkins CJM. An analysis of the complications of extradural and caudal block. *Anaesthesia.* 1969;24(4):554–563.

12. Doumouchtsis SK, Papgeorghiou AT, Arulkumaran S. Systematic review of conservative management of postpartum hemorrhage: what to do when medical treatment fails. *Obstet Gynecol Surv.* 2007;62(8):540–547.

13. Georgiou C. Balloon tamponade in the management of postpartum hemorrhage: a review. *Br J Obstet Gynaecol.* 2009;116:748–757.

14. Goldszmidt E, Kern R, Chaput A, Macarthur A. The incidence and etiology of postpartum headaches: a prospective cohort study. *Can J Anaesth.* 2005;52(9):971–977.

15. Grewal S, Hocking G, Wildsmith JAW. Epidural abscesses. *Br J Anaesth.* 2006; 96(3):292–302.

16. Knight M, Berg C, Brocklehurst P, Kramer M, Lewis G, Oats J, Roberts CL, Spong C, Sullivan E, van Roosmalen J, Zwart J. Amniotic fluid embolism incidence, risk factors and outcomes: a review and recommendations. *BMC Pregnancy Childbirth.* 2012;10:12–17.

17. Liu H, Kaye AD, Comarda N, Li MM. Paradoxical postural CSF leak-induced headache: report of two cases. *J Clin Anesth.* 2008;20(5):383–385

18. Lee LA, Posner KL, Domino KB, Caplan RA, Cheney FW. Injuries associated with regional anesthesia in the 1980s and 1990s: a closed claims analysis. *Anesthesiology.* 2004; 101(1): 143–152.

19. Leys D, Lesoin F, Viaud C, Pasquier F, Rousseaux M, et al. Decreased morbidity from acute bacterial spinal epidural abscess using computed tomography and nonsurgical treatment in selected patients. *Ann Neurol.* 1985;17(4):350–355.

20. Longnecker DE, Newman MF, Zapol WM, Mackey SC, Sandberg WS, eds. *Anesthesiology.* 3rd ed. New York, NY: McGraw-Hill Education; 2017.

21. MacKay AP, Berg CJ, Liu X, Duran C, Hoyert DL. Changes in pregnancy mortality ascertainment: United States, 1999–2005. *Obstet Gynecol.* 2011;118(1):104–110.

22. Miller RD, Cohen NH, Eriksson LI, Fleisher LA, Wiener-Kronish JP, Young WL, eds. *Miller's anesthesia.* 8th ed. Philadelphia, PA: Elsevier; 2015.

23. Moen V, Dahlgren N, Irestedt L. Severe neurological complications after central neuraxial blockades in Sweden 1990–1999. *Anesthesiology.* 2004;101:950–959.

24. Munnur U, Suresh MS. Backache, headache, and neurologic deficit after regional anesthesia. *Anesthesiol Clin North Am.* 2003;21(1):71–86.

25. Pian-Smith MCM, Leffert L, eds. *Obstetric anesthesia.* New York: PocketMedicine.com, Inc.; 2005.

26. Pino RM, ed. *Clinical anesthesia procedures of the Massachusetts General Hospital.* 9th ed. Boston, MA: Wolters Kluwer; 2016.

27. Reynolds F. Neurological infections after neuraxial anesthesia. *Anesthesiol Clin.* 2008;26(1): 23–52.

28. Rodgers A, Walker N, Schug S, McKee A, Kehlet H, van Zundert A, Sage D, Futter M, Saville G, Clark T, MacMahon S. Reduction of postoperative mortality and morbidity with epidural or spinal anaesthesia: results from overview of randomized trials. *BMJ.* 2000;321(7275):1493.

29. Sax TW, Rosenbaum RB. Neuromuscular disorders in pregnancy. *Muscle Nerve.* 2006;34: 559–571.

30. Sheldon WR, Blum J, Vogel JP, Souza JP, Gülmezoglu AM, Winikoff B, WHO Multicountry Survey on Maternal and Newborn Health Research Network. Postpartum haemorrhage management, risks, and maternal outcomes: findings from the World Health Organization Multicountry Survey on Maternal and Newborn Health. *Br J Obstet Gynaecol.* 2014;121, Suppl: 1–5.

31. Stein MH, Cohen S, Mohiuddin MA, Dombrovskiy V, Lowenwirt I. Prophylactic vs therapeutic blood patch for obstetric patients with accidental dural puncture-a randomized controlled trial. *Anaesthesia.* 2014;69:320–326.

32. Stella CL, Jodicke CD, How HY, Harkness UF, Sibai BM. Postpartum headache: is your workup complete? *Am J of Obstet Gynecol.* 2007;196:318.e1–318.e7.

33. Szeinfeld M, Ihmeidan IH, Moser MM, Machado R, Klose KJ, Serafini AN. Epidural blood patch: evaluation of the volume and spread of the blood injected into the epidural space. *Anesthesiology.* 1986;64:820–822.

34. Van de Velde M, Scherpers R, Berends N, Vandermeersch E, De Buck F. Ten years of experience with accidental dural puncture and post-dural puncture headache in a tertiary obstetric anaesthesia department. *Int J Obstet Anesth.* 2008;17(4):329–335.

35. Vgontzas A, Robbins MS. A hospital based retrospective study of acute postpartum headache. *Headache.* 2018;58:845–851.

36. Watson P. Postparum hemorrhage and shock. *Clin Obstet Gynecol.* 1980;23(4):985–1001.

37. Wong CA. Nerve injuries after neuraxial anaesthesia and their medicolegal implications. *Best Pract Res Clin Obstet Gynaecol.* 2010;24(3):367–381.

24

Trauma and Critical Care During Pregnancy

Gavin T. Best, Melissa A. Nikolaidis, and Yi Deng

Trauma

Epidemiology

Trauma occurs in approximately 6–9% of parturients in the developed world and is the leading nonobstetric cause of both maternal and fetal demise.[1,2] Blunt trauma, including motor vehicle accidents (MVAs), falls, assaults, and burns, accounts for 69% of all traumas, while penetrating trauma varies from 1.5% to 35% depending on the report.[1] Assault, specifically domestic violence, is underreported and may represent greater incidence than currently acknowledged. Fetal demise mirrors the maternal pattern, with the majority occurring through motor vehicle accidents (MVAs), followed by penetrating trauma (specifically gunshot wounds). Studies have shown that 70% of abdominal gunshot wounds lead to fetal injury, with mortality as high as 65%. Fetal loss during trauma is most commonly attributed to prolonged hypotension or hypoxemia of the mother, while other causes include direct uterine trauma/rupture, placental abruption, or maternal death.

Prehospital Care

During the prehospital phase, providers should inquire about pregnancy status for all women of child-bearing age. Advanced gestational age should prompt lateral decubitus positioning of the patient. Left "tilt" using a ramp or sheets (Figure 24.1) can mobilize the uterus off the inferior vena cava (IVC) and potentially improve cardiac output by as much as 30%.[3] A ramp with additional precautions (i.e., cervical collar) is preferred when spinal fracture is suspected.

Initial Hospital Assessment

Upon arrival to the trauma center, the patient should undergo standard trauma evaluation including primary and secondary surveys as well as laboratory/imaging studies. Mendez-Figueroa et al. proposed an algorithm for workup of these patients in 2013 (Figure 24.2).[4] A multidisciplinary approach is paramount, with obstetrician and neonatologist being consulted early to ensure the best possible outcomes.

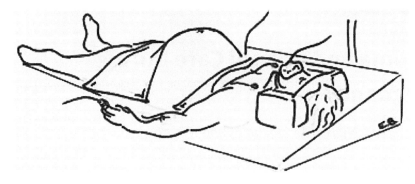

Figure 24.1 A ramp or other object can be used to tilt the patient to the left. This moves the gravid uterus off the IVC for improved venous return. Some ramps include neck stabilizers for suspected cervical trauma.[2]

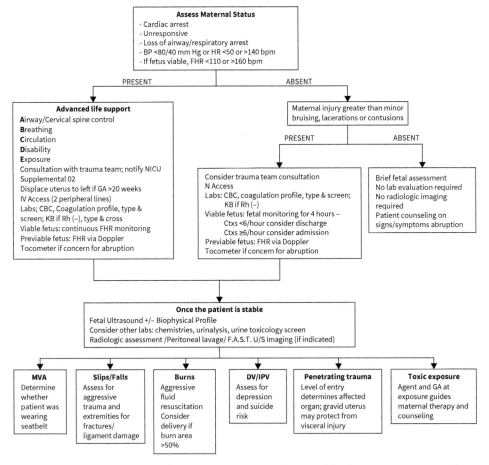

Assess Maternal Status
- Cardiac arrest
- Unresponsive
- Loss of airway/respiratory arrest
- BP <80/40 mm Hg or HR <50 or >140 bpm
- If fetus viable, FHR <110 or >160 bpm

PRESENT — ABSENT

Advanced life support
Airway/Cervical spine control
Breathing
Circulation
Disability
Exposure
Consultation with trauma team; notify NICU
Supplemental 02
Displace uterus to left if GA >20 weeks
IV Access (2 peripheral lines)
Labs; CBC, Coagulation profile, type & screen; KB if Rh (–), type & cross
Viable fetus: continuous FHR monitoring
Previable fetus: FHR via Doppler
Tocometer if concern for abruption

Maternal injury greater than minor bruising, lacerations or contusions

PRESENT — ABSENT

Consider trauma team consultation
N Access
Labs: CBC, coagulation profile, type & screen; KB if Rh (–)
Viable fetus: fetal monitoring for 4 hours –
    Ctxs <6/hour consider discharge
    Ctxs ≥6/hour consider admission
Previable fetus: FHR via Doppler
Tocometer if concern for abruption

Brief fetal assessment
No lab evaluation required
No radiologic imaging required
Patient counseling on signs/symptoms abruption

Once the patient is stable
Fetal Ultrasound +/– Biophysical Profile
Consider other labs: chemistries, urinalysis, urine toxicology screen
Radiologic assessment /Peritoneal lavage/ F.A.S.T. U/S Imaging (if indicated)

MVA	**Slips/Falls**	**Burns**	**DV/IPV**	**Penetrating trauma**	**Toxic exposure**
Determine whether patient was wearing seatbelt	Assess for aggressive trauma and extremities for fractures/ligament damage	Aggressive fluid resuscitation Consider delivery if burn area >50%	Assess for depression and suicide risk	Level of entry determines affected organ; gravid uterus may protect from visceral injury	Agent and GA at exposure guides maternal therapy and counseling

Figure 24.2 Proposed algorithm for obstetric trauma workup. BP = blood pressure, CBC = complete blood count, Ctxs = contractions, DV = domestic violence, FAST = focused assessment with sonography for trauma, FHR = fetal heart rate, GA = gestational age, HR = heart rate, IPV = intimate partner violence, ISS = injury severity score, IV = intravenous, KB = Kleihauer-Betke, MVA = motor vehicle accident, NICU = neonatal intensive care unit, O2 = oxygen, U/S = ultrasound.
Adapted from Mendez-Figueroa, Trauma in pregnancy.[4]

Primary Survey

The American College of Surgeons' Committee on Trauma recommends an "ABCDE" approach to the primary survey of trauma patient: Airway, Breathing, Circulation, Disability, and Exposure/Environmental control. This is the same regardless of pregnancy status. Frequent vital signs and intravenous access should be obtained. Once the patient is stabilized, then a secondary survey can be performed which includes obstetric and nonobstetric injuries as well as fetal well-being.

Secondary Survey

The secondary survey begins with a thorough history and physical examination including pregnancy course and gestational age. Gestational age can be estimated by fundal height if otherwise unavailable (Figure 24.3). The clinician should focus on key elements in a parturient exam including uterine tenderness, tone/contractions, and vaginal bleeding/discharge. Pelvic stability should be assessed, as pelvic fracture is the most common traumatic cause of fetal demise. A vaginal examination should be performed to inspect for blood or amniotic fluid. Blood in the vaginal vault could indicate placenta previa, abruption, or uterine rupture and, if detected, ultrasonography should be performed prior to manual cervical manipulation. In addition to traditional transvaginal ultrasonography, point-of-care ultrasound in trauma has gained widespread adoption, particularly the Focused Assessment

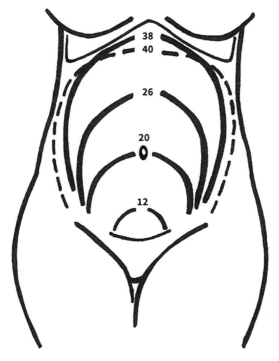

Figure 24.3 This image shows approximate uterine fundus location during pregnancy for purposes of gestational age estimation. Note at 40 weeks the fundus drops due to rotation of the infant and migration of the skull into the pelvis.

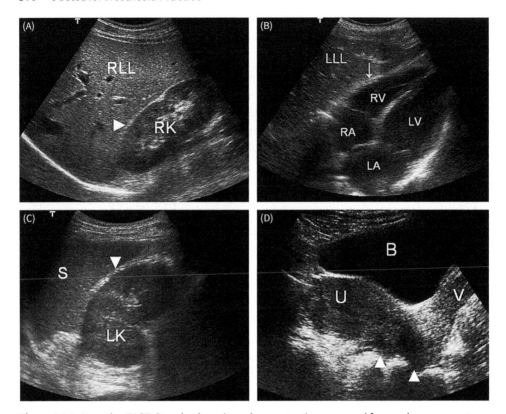

Figure 24.4 Negative FAST. Standard sections demonstrating a normal focused assessment with sonography in trauma (FAST) scan. (a) Subhepatic view. The probe is placed in a parasagittal plane demonstrating a longitudinal section of the right lobe of liver (RLL), right kidney (RK) and hepatorenal space (arrowhead) which contains no fluid. (b) Sub-xyphoid view. The probe is placed in a transverse plane just to the left of the xiphisternum and angled cranially under the costal margin. The left lobe of liver (LLL) acts as a "window" to the heart. The normal pericardium (arrow) demonstrates no fluid. LA left atrium; LV, left ventricle, RA, right atrium; RV, right ventricle. (c) Left upper quadrant view showing a normal spleen (S), left kidney (LK) and normal spleno-renal space (arrowhead). (d) Longitudinal section of the pelvic region in a female patient, showing the uterus (U) and vagina (V) posterior to a full bladder (B). The retro-uterine space, or pouch of Douglas (arrowhead), is fluid-free.

Used with permission from Smith J. Focused assessment with sonography in trauma (FAST): should its role be reconsidered? *Postgrad Med J.* 2010;*86*(1015):285–291.

with Sonography in Trauma (FAST; Figures 24.4 and 24.5) and Focused Assessment of Transthoracic Echocardiography (FATE) examinations (Figure 24.6) FAST exams, for example, have an 83% sensitivity for detecting intraperitoneal fluid in trauma cases for both the pregnant and nonpregnant patients.[5]

Laboratory and Imaging Studies

Standard trauma laboratory workups such as blood counts, serum chemistry, and coagulation profile—especially fibrinogen—should be obtained. It is important to remember,

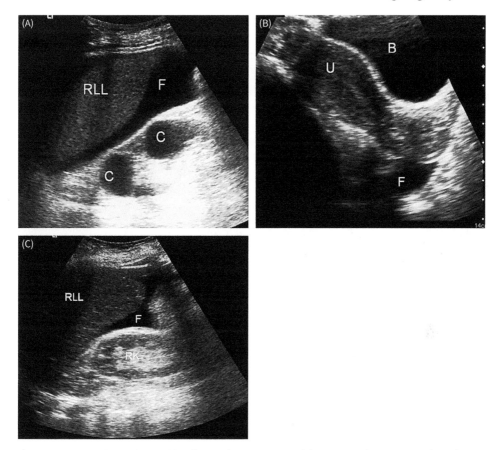

Figure 24.5 Positive FAST. Positive focused assessment with sonography in trauma (FAST) scans. (a) Longitudinal section through the right upper quadrant demonstrating free fluid (F) between the right lobe of liver (RLL) and right kidney following blunt abdominal trauma (BAT). The kidney contains two cysts (C). (b) Longitudinal section of a female pelvis, demonstrating fluid (F) in the pouch of Douglas behind the uterus (U) and bladder (B). (c) An example of a false-positive FAST scan. Following BAT, the fluid (F) is pre-existing ascites due to chronic liver disease, and not hemoperitoneum.

Used with permission from Smith J. Focused assessment with sonography in trauma (FAST): should its role be reconsidered? *Postgrad Med J.* 2010;*86*(1015):285–291.

however, that lab values during pregnancy often differ from "normal" nonpregnant values. (Table 24.1) For example, white cell count and fibrinogen levels tend to be elevated, while serum creatinine and platelet values will decrease. Patients may trend toward higher arterial pH due to respiratory alkalosis of pregnancy, which is partially compensated by lower serum bicarbonate levels.

The Kleihauer-Betke test should be performed in all Rh-negative pregnant women who sustained major trauma. While these patients are given anti-D immunoglobulin at the outset, this test can help quantify fetal blood in maternal circulation and guide further immunoglobulin administration (i.e., additional 300 mcg for every 30 mL of fetomaternal hemorrhage). The test should be repeated every 24 to 48 hours to monitor potential ongoing hemorrhage. Of note, it has not been proven useful in Rh-positive patients.[6,7]

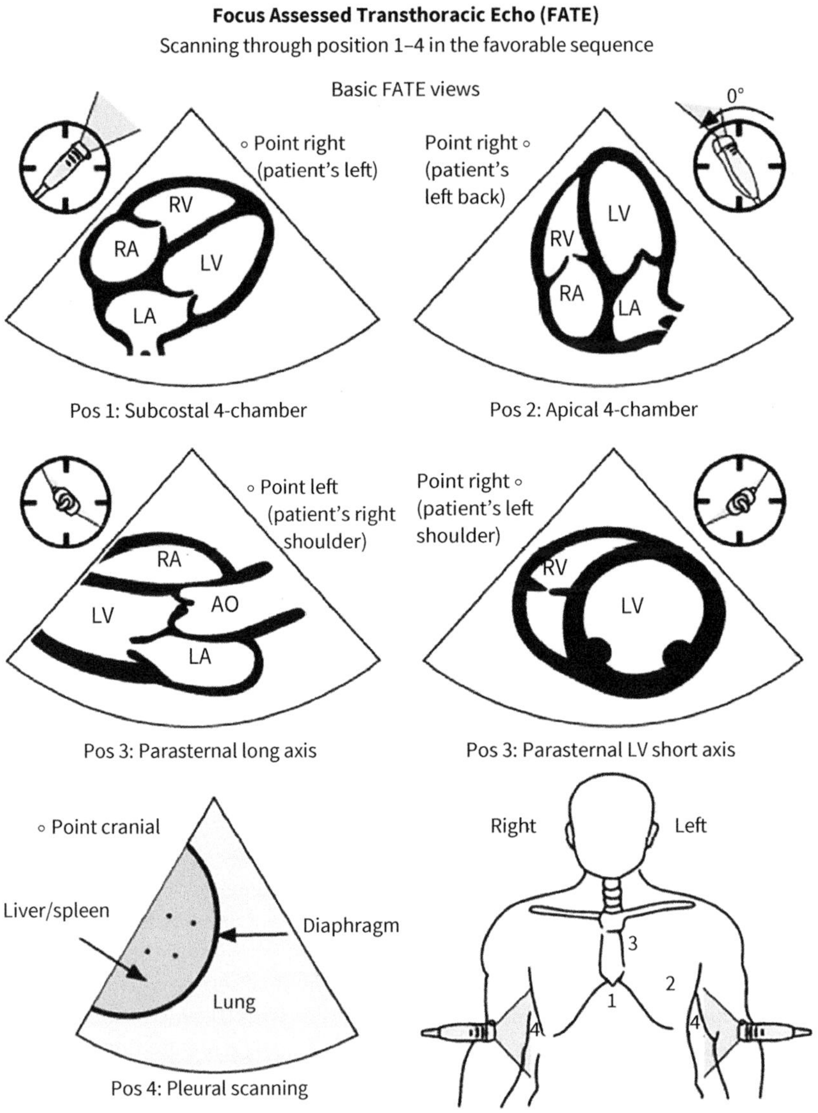

Focus Assessed Transthoracic Echo (FATE)
Scanning through position 1–4 in the favorable sequence

Basic FATE views

Point right
(patient's left)

RV
RA
LV
LA

Pos 1: Subcostal 4-chamber

0°

Point right
(patient's left back)

LV
RV
RA
LA

Pos 2: Apical 4-chamber

Point left
(patient's right shoulder)

RA
LV
AO
LA

Pos 3: Parasternal long axis

Point right
(patient's left shoulder)

RV
LV

Pos 3: Parasternal LV short axis

Point cranial

Liver/spleen
Diaphragm
Lung

Pos 4: Pleural scanning

Right   Left
3
2
1
4   4

Figure 24.6   FATE. The basic 4 views of focused assessment of transthoracic echocardiography (FATE) protocol. RA, right atrium; RV, right ventricle; LA, left atrium; LV, left ventricle.

Reprinted from Oveland N, Bogale N, Waldron B, Bech K, Sloth E. Focus assessed transthoracic echocardiography (FATE) to diagnose pleural effusions causing haemodynamic compromise. *Case Reports in Clin Med.* 2013;2(3):189–193.

Practitioners are often hesitant to obtain diagnostic imaging in pregnant patients due to concerns of radiation and contrast. Nevertheless, necessary imaging in the trauma setting should not be delayed because of this. The American College of Obstetricians and Gynecologists (ACOG) guideline suggests that radiation doses less than 5 rads/5 mSv (5× the dose from an abdomen/pelvis computed tomograph or 500× that of a chest rotengraph) will not increase the risk of fetal defects or loss.[2,6,8] In general, the clinician should minimize radiation exposure whenever possible (i.e. shield the abdomen), but not withhold critical diagnostic imaging if the situation warrants it.

Table 24.1 Normal Pregnancy Lab Values

	Normal Lab Values	
	Pregnant (3rd trimester)	Nonpregnant
Hematocrit	32–42%	37–48%
White Blood Cell Count	5,000–12,000/μL	4,000–11,000/μL
Fibrinogen	> 400 mg/dL	150–400 mg/dL
Serum HCO₃	17–20 mEq/L	23 mEq/L
Arterial pH	7.43 (7.40–7.45)	7.40
PaO_2	101–106 mm Hg	93 mm Hg
$PaCO_2$	26–30 mm Hg	37 mm Hg

HCOAcute Physiology And Chronic Health Evaluation

= serum bicarbonate

Monitoring After Trauma

Assuming no immediate critical or surgical intervention is required, monitoring of the parturient after a trauma work-up will depend on gestational age of the fetus. Any parturient with greater than 24 weeks of gestational age should receive immediate noninvasive fetal and uterine monitoring. Critical patients should be monitored in the intensive care unit regardless of gestational age. Patients with vaginal bleeding, frequent contractions, rupture of membranes, uterine tenderness, significant abdominal pain, atypical fetal heart tones, high-risk injury mechanism, or low serum fibrinogen should be monitored for at least 24 hours.[7]

Blunt Trauma

Direct injury to the fetus from blunt trauma is exceedingly rare, occurring in less than 1% of cases. Uterine musculature, amniotic fluid, and other maternal soft tissue act to disperse and absorb forces from the impact. Pelvic fractures, however, are associated with a high mortality rate, both through brisk hemorrhage into the retroperitoneal space and/or direct fetal injury.[1,6]

After the first trimester, the placenta retains its rigidity while myometrium becomes more elastic. This results in shearing forces along the interface during blunt trauma which can lead to placental abruption. The clinician must retain a high index of suspicion, as ultrasonography has poor sensitivity as a screening tool for abruption.[6]

Penetrating Thoracoabdominal Trauma

Gunshot and stab wounds make up the majority of penetrating trauma. In a parturient the growing uterus displaces other organs cranially and posteriorly, which helps shield them from many anterior penetrations. Additionally, the muscular uterine wall impedes bullets from through-and-through penetration into retroperitoneal space. Upper abdominal penetrations inversely tend to have poorer outcomes because of the high concentration of organs in that space. Finally, if a tetanus vaccine is being considered in a trauma patient, it is safe in pregnancy and should be administered according to protocol.[6]

Burn Injury

Burns in pregnant patients are treated similarly to nonpregnant patients. Primary management depends on total body surface area (TBSA) burned and medical comorbidities. Cesarean section should be considered in patients with burns greater than 50% TBSA and viable fetuses.[9] Clinicians must carefully titrate fluid administration due to high capillary leak and third-spacing, while managing electrolyte replacement, inhalation injury, carbon monoxide and cyanide poisoning, and high metabolic and pain profiles.

Critical Care

Pregnant patients make up less than 0.5–1.5% of intensive care unit (ICU) admissions in the United States.[3,10] The most common causes for admission are hypertensive disorders like preeclampsia/eclampsia; postpartum hemorrhage; sepsis, hemolysis, elevated liver enzymes, and low platelets (HELLP) syndrome; and acute respiratory distress syndrome (ARDS). Even then, these are more commonly seen in the immediate postpartum period than during the pregnancy.

Most mortality predictors, such as the Acute Physiology And Chronic Health Evaluation (APACHE) scores, overestimate mortality in the pregnant population.[3] This is because the normal physiologic changes that occur during pregnancy, such as respiratory alkalosis, tachycardia, tachypnea, and low hematocrit, contribute to higher illness severity scores in those matrices. While general ICU guidelines may apply to obstetric patients, most evidence-based ICU studies actually exclude them from their selection pool.

The following sections discuss general principles for management of the parturient in the ICU as well as considerations for critical conditions specific to these patients.

Airway Management and Mechanical Ventilation

Airway management in the pregnant patient is notably more difficult than in the nonpregnant patient. Hormonal changes lead to increased friability, bleeding, and edema in laryngeal mucus membranes. This, combined with difficult positioning due to increased breast size and body mass index, leads to eight times the number of failed intubations when compared to the nonpregnant population.[3] This is especially concerning given that pregnant patients have decreased functional residual capacity and increased minute ventilation due to an increased tidal volume. In parturients, desaturation occurs twice as fast and CO_2 has been shown to rise almost 2.5 times faster than in nonpregnant patients.[11]

When intubating a pregnant patient, it is important to have back-up methods of airway management whenever possible. The Difficult Airway Algorithm set forth by the American Society of Anesthesiologists should be strictly observed, and clinicians should have a low threshold to advance down the algorithm pathways.

Once the trachea has been intubated and mechanical ventilation initiated, it is important to use the patient's nonpregnant ideal body weight to calculate tidal volume.[3] While there is no clear evidence that alkalosis of pregnancy should be maintained during ventilation, severe respiratory alkalosis should be avoided due to its effects on uterine blood flow as discussed later in this chapter.[3,12]

Cardiovascular Support

Placental and fetal perfusion is heavily dependent upon maternal mean arterial pressure due to lack of autoregulation of uterine blood flow. Thus, maintenance of arterial pressure is paramount, and parturients in critical condition often require pharmacologic support to accomplish this. Ephedrine is often labeled the drug of choice in pregnant patients, but this is based on limited animal data.[3] Neither phenylephrine, norepinephrine, epinephrine, nor dopamine has been rigorously studied in humans, and all pose potential risk of causing uterine artery constriction. Nevertheless, all these medications have been successfully used in pregnant women.[3] Specific agents should be chosen based on clinician comfort and institutional protocol with careful titration to effect.

Obstetric Complications Requiring Critical Care

Hypertensive Emergencies/Preeclampsia

Hypertensive emergencies are one of the most common causes for ICU admissions among parturients and present on a spectrum from uncomplicated gestational hypertension to preeclampsia and eclampsia.[10,13,14] Preeclampsia/eclampsia complicates 10% of all pregnancies and eclampsia can occur before, during, or even after labor. Diagnostic criteria of preeclampsia include systolic blood pressure ≥ 140 or diastolic blood pressure ≥ 90 after 20 weeks' gestation *in a previously normotensive patient* with the new onset of one or more of the following: proteinuria, thrombocytopenia, serum creatinine > 1.1 mg/dL (or doubling from baseline), liver enzymes twice the upper limit of normal, pulmonary edema, and/or cerebral/visual symptoms.[15] In patients with essential hypertension, hyperuricemia indicates superimposed preeclampsia.[16] Severe preeclampsia with organ dysfunction is an indication for immediate delivery, and *delivery is the only cure for pregnancy-induced hypertensive disorders.*[17] Antihypertensive medications commonly used in pregnancy are listed in Table 24.2. Severely preeclamptic patients not yet in organ failure should be given intravenous (IV) magnesium sulfate (standard therapeutic range 4–7 mEq/L) for seizure prophylaxis if before 32 weeks gestation and corticosteroids to enhance fetal lung maturity if between 24 and 34 weeks. For seizing patients, magnesium sulfate is loaded for 4–6 g over 15 minutes followed by 1–2 g/h infusion.[18] Patients refractory to this treatment should receive standard seizure abortive medications (benzodiazepines, phenytoin, levetiracetam, etc.) and pursue delivery immediately.[10,19]

Table 24.2 Antihypertensives to be Used in Pregnant Patients

Antihypertensives Used for Urgent BP Control in Pregnancy		
Drug	Dose	Comments
Labetalol	10–20 mg IV, then 20–80 mg every 20–30 min. Max dose 300 mg	Considered first line in pregnancy
	Can infuse at 1–2 mg/min IV	Contraindicated in asthma, heart disease, or congestive heart failure
		FDA pregnancy category C
Hydralazine	5 mg IV or IM then 5–10 mg IV every 20–40 min	Hypotension, headaches, and fetal distress at high doses
	Can infuse at 0.5–10 mg/hr	FDA pregnancy category C
Nifedipine	10–20 mg PO; repeat in 30 min if needed; then 10–20 mg every 3–6 h	Tachycardia and headaches, potential peripheral edema
		FDA pregnancy category C
Nicardipine	Continuous infusion 3 mg/h. Increase by 0.5 mg every 20 min. Max dose 15 mg/h	Embryotoxicity seen in rabbits at high doses. Crosses the placenta. Fetal heart rate changes, hypotension, and fetal acidosis possible
	Once BP control achieved, titrate down	FDA pregnancy category C
Nitroglycerine	5 µg/min; double every 5 min	Venodilator, requires arterial pressure monitoring
		Potential for methemoglobinemia with prolonged use
		FDA pregnancy category C
Nitroprusside	0.25 µg/kg/min infusion increase by 0.25 µg/kg/min every 5 min	Requires continuous BP monitoring with arterial line Potential for cyanide toxicity with prolonged use
		FDA pregnancy category C

IV = intravenous, IM = intramuscular, hr = hour, PO = per os, min = minute, BP = blood pressure

HELLP Syndrome

Hemolysis, elevated liver enzymes, and low platelets (< 100,000/µL) make up the HELLP syndrome. It is commonly associated with preeclampsia and is also an indication for delivery followed by 48 hours of monitoring.[10,20] Neuraxial anesthesia can be used for delivery if placed early before platelet levels become prohibitive. HELLP must be differentiated from thrombotic thrombocytopenic purpura (TTP) among other conditions. TTP will usually have a lower platelet count, normal coagulation profile and fibrinogen, and higher lactic acid dehydrogenase.[10]

Obstetric Hemorrhage

Massive obstetric (OB) hemorrhage, commonly secondary to uterine atony or abnormal uterine placentation, will often necessitate transfusion of 10 or more units of packed red blood cells (pRBC) intraoperatively. The accepted transfusion ratio in obstetric literature is

2:1:1 pRBC:plasma:platelets, rather than the more widely used 1:1:1 ratio in traumatic hemorrhage. In the ICU, these patients should be monitored closely for transfusion-associated circulatory overload (TACO), transfusion-related acute lung injury (TRALI), electrolyte derangements, citrate toxicity, and continued bleeding.[10,21]

Amniotic Fluid Embolism

Amniotic fluid embolism (AFE) has an incidence < 1% but mortality of 60–90%. It is postulated to be caused by an anaphylactoid inflammatory reaction to fetal tissues in the maternal circulation, resulting in respiratory failure, cardiogenic collapse, and coagulopathy. Decline is rapid, and management is supportive with restrictive fluid management, replacement of coagulation factors, and mechanical ventilation as needed.[10,22]

Tocolytic Pulmonary Edema

Medications like magnesium sulfate, terbutaline, nifedipine, and indomethacin are used by obstetricians to prolong pregnancy. These tocolytics can induce pulmonary edema in a parturient partially aided by decreased oncotic pressure and increased hydrostatic pressure present in a normal parturient.[10,23] The incidence increases with prolonged exposure. Management of tocolytic-induced pulmonary edema includes discontinuing the offending agent, fluid restriction, gentle diuresis, and supportive respiratory care. Echocardiography can be helpful in ruling out cardiac-induced etiology.[10]

Pathologies Affected by Pregnancy

Cardiac Disease

Normal physiologic changes in pregnancy such as increased blood volume/cardiac output can worsen existing cardiac disease. The World Health Organization (WHO) classification can be salient in guiding treatment decisions (Table 24.3). Some conditions, like peripartum cardiomyopathy, are relatively common, and in most cases will resolve within a year of delivery (although those that do not are associated with > 85% mortality).[24,25] Others, such as pulmonary hypertension, introduce prohibitive risk and contraindicate pregnancy. Pulmonary hypertension can result in death in one third of pregnancies, although the risk can be mitigated by close monitoring, phosphodiesterase inhibitors, prostacyclins, and anticoagulation.[25–27] Patients with severe left-sided valvular stenosis can undergo balloon valvotomy after 20 weeks of gestation.[25] Those with chronic atrial fibrillation should be rate-controlled with β_1-blockers or calcium channel blockers and anticoagulated to prevent thromboembolic events.[25,27] Finally, patients with ascending aortic aneurysms should also be treated with beta blockers to reduce risk of dissection but should be delivered immediately if the aneurysm increases in size in the third trimester.[25,27]

Sepsis

Genital tract infections are implicated in 50% of cases involving sepsis during pregnancy and are more common postpartum. Pneumonia and acute pyelonephritis are also common culprits.[25,28] Clindamycin and aminoglycosides are the drug combination of choice for sepsis in pregnancy with third-generation cephalosporins, piperacillin-tazobactam, or amoxicillin-clavulanic acid acting as second-line agents.[25,28,29]

Table 24.3 World Health Organization Cardiac Disease in Pregnancy Classification

Class I	Class II	Class III	Class IV
Very low risk	Low to moderate risk	High risk	Extremely high risk: **pregnancy is contraindicated**
• uncomplicated mild pulmonary stenosis, patent ductus arteriosus and mitral valve prolapse • successfully repaired simple lesions (atrial or ventricular septal defect, patent ductus arteriosus, anomalous pulmonary venous drainage) • isolated atrial or ventricular ectopic beats	• unoperated atrial or ventricular septal defect • repaired tetralogy of Fallot • most arrhythmias • mild left ventricular impairment • hypertrophic cardiomyopathy • native or tissue valvular heart disease not considered WHO I or IV • Marfan syndrome without aortic dilatation • aorta < 45 mm in aortic disease associated with bicuspid aortic valve • repaired coarctation	• mechanical valve • systemic right ventricle • Fontan circulation • cyanotic heart disease (unrepaired) • other complex congenital heart disease • aortic dilatation 40–45 mm in Marfan syndrome • aortic dilatation 45–50 mm in aortic disease associated with bicuspid aortic valve.	• pulmonary arterial hypertension of any cause • severe systemic ventricular dysfunction (left ventricular ejection fraction < 30% • previous peripartum cardiomyopathy with residual impairment of left ventricular function • severe mitral stenosis and severe symptomatic aortic stenosis • Marfan syndrome with aorta dilated > 45 mm • aortic dilatation > 50 mm associated with bicuspid aortic valve • severe coarctation

Thromboembolism

Pregnancy is a hypercoagulable state with a ten-fold increase in risk of deep venous thrombosis and pulmonary embolus.[30] Fibrinogen is greatly increased, as are von Willebrand Factor, Factors VII, VIII, and IX. Anticoagulants like Protein S are decreased, further contributing to risk of thrombotic events.[8] Pregnant patients should be treated similarly to "high-risk" nonpregnant patients. Mechanical prophylaxis should be placed consistently on all patients, while heparin (low molecular weight preferred over unfractionated) is ideal for pharmacologic prophylaxis, as it does not cross the placenta.[3,25,31,32]

Acute Respiratory Distress Syndrome

ARDS has increased prevalence in pregnancy. If a parturient is intubated, the clinician should follow the ARDS Network's lung protective strategy (tidal volumes at 6 mL/kg with plateau pressures <30 cmH$_2$O).[23,25] Maintaining this plateau pressure can be difficult in the third trimester when intraabdominal pressures rise to around 14 mm Hg.[33]

Ensuring fetal health during maternal ARDS is complicated. Fetal oxygen levels most closely resemble maternal PaO$_2$ (not SaO$_2$). Overventilation causing maternal hypocapnia decreases uterine blood flow and ultimately results in fetal hypoxia. PaCO$_2$ of 30–45 mm Hg increases uterine blood flow, but PaCO$_2$ > 60 mm Hg decreases it and leads to elevated fetal intracranial pressure. Thus, permissive hypercapnia is not advised in pregnant patients.[12,23,25,34,35]

Emergency and Perimortem Cesarean Delivery

For potentially viable fetuses at or over 24 weeks gestation, emergency cesarean section should be considered when maternal death is imminent. Emergency section of an infant for specific indications like shock and acute maternal decompensation has been associated with a 45% fetal and 72% maternal survival.[36] Outlook is particularly good for the fetus with ongoing fetal heart tones during maternal resuscitation, emphasizing the importance of the fetal heart tone monitor. Conventional teaching states perimortem cesarean section should wait no longer than four minutes after cardiopulmonary resuscitation (CPR) is initiated to aid in resuscitation and improve chances of a positive outcome for both mother and baby. However, while chances of a normal infant drop precipitously after the 4–5-minute mark, the ACOG notes that chances of injury-free survival for both can still be as high as 50% even 25 minutes after CPR is initiated. Therefore, it is currently recommended that resuscitative hysterotomy be performed as soon as possible even if the 4-minute mark has passed.[37]

Summary

Trauma and critical illness are not uncommon in the pregnant population. Parturients will require different knowledge base and skillsets in these settings due to their altered physiology, but initial resuscitation is focused primarily on the health and survival of the mother. They require a careful understanding of conditions and treatments specific to these patients as well as care from an interdisciplinary team consisting of the trauma, obstetric, pediatric, anesthesiology, and intensive care physicians in order to ensure the highest chance of survival for both the mother and baby.

References

1. Petrone P, Jiménez-Morillas P, Axelrad A, Marini CP. Traumatic injuries to the pregnant patient: a critical literature review. *Eur J Trauma Emerg Surg.* 2019;45(3):383–392. doi:10.1007/s00068-017-0839-x.
2. Battaloglu E, Battaloglu E, Chu J, Porter K. Obstetrics in trauma. *Trauma.* 2015;17(1):17–23. doi:10.1177/1460408614530944.
3. Honiden S, Abdel-Razeq SS, Siegel MD. The Management of the critically ill obstetric patient. *J Intensive Care Med.* 2013;28(2):93–106. doi:10.1177/0885066611411408.
4. Mendez-Figueroa H, Dahlke JD, Vrees RA, Rouse DJ. Trauma in pregnancy: an updated systematic review. *Am J Obstet Gynecol.* 2013;209(1):1–10. doi:10.1016/j.ajog.2013.01.021.
5. Goodwin H, Holmes JF, Wisner DH. Abdominal ultrasound examination in pregnant blunt trauma patients. *J Trauma.* 2001;50(4):689–693; discussion 694. doi:10.1097/00005373-200104000-00016.
6. Mattox KL, Goetzl L. Trauma in pregnancy. *Crit Care Med.* 2005;33(10 Suppl):S385–9. doi:10.1097/01.ccm.0000182808.99433.55.

7. Jain V, Chari R, Maslovitz S, et al. Guidelines for the management of a pregnant trauma patient. *J Obstet Gynaecol Can.* 2015;37(6):553–574. http://www.ncbi.nlm.nih.gov/pubmed/26334607.

8. Rossignol M. Trauma and pregnancy: what anesthesiologist should know. *Anaesthesia, Crit care pain Med.* 2016;35 Suppl 1:S27–S34. doi:10.1016/j.accpm.2016.06.006.

9. Agarwal P. Thermal injury in pregnancy: predicting maternal and fetal outcome. *Indian J Plast Surg.* 2005;38(2):95–99. doi:10.4103/0970-0358.19774.

10. Guntupalli KK, Hall N, Karnad DR, Bandi V, Belfort M. Critical illness in pregnancy: part I: An approach to a pregnant patient in the ICU and common obstetric disorders. *Chest.* 2015;148(4):1093–1104. doi:10.1378/chest.14-1998.

11. Cheun JK, Choi KT. Arterial oxygen desaturation rate following obstructive apnea in parturients. *J Korean Med Sci.* 1992;7(1):6–10. doi:10.3346/jkms.1992.7.1.6.

12. Levinson G, Shnider SM, DeLorimier AA, Steffenson JL. Effects of maternal hyperventilation on uterine blood flow and fetal oxygenation and acid-base status. *Anesthesiology.* 1974;40(4):340–347. doi:10.1097/00000542-197404000-00007.

13. Soubra SH, Guntupalli KK. Critical illness in pregnancy: an overview. *Crit Care Med.* 2005;33(10 Suppl):S248–55. doi:10.1097/01.ccm.0000183159.31378.6a.

14. Pollock W, Rose L, Dennis C-L. Pregnant and postpartum admissions to the intensive care unit: a systematic review. *Intensive Care Med.* 2010;36(9):1465–1474. doi:10.1007/s00134-010-1951-0.

15. ACOG. ACOG practice bulletin no. 202: gestational hypertension and preeclampsia. *Obstet Gynecol.* 2019;133(1):e1–e25. doi:10.1097/AOG.0000000000003018.

16. American College of Obstetricians and Gynecologists, Task Force on Hypertension in Pregnancy. Hypertension in pregnancy. Report of the American College of Obstetricians and Gynecologists' Task Force on Hypertension in Pregnancy. *Obstet Gynecol.* 2013;122(5):1122–1131. doi:10.1097/01.AOG.0000437382.03963.88.

17. Powe CE, Levine RJ, Karumanchi SA. Preeclampsia, a disease of the maternal endothelium: the role of antiangiogenic factors and implications for later cardiovascular disease. *Circulation.* 2011;123(24):2856–2869. doi:10.1161/CIRCULATIONAHA.109.853127.

18. Sibai BM. Magnesium sulfate prophylaxis in preeclampsia: lessons learned from recent trials. *Am J Obstet Gynecol.* 2004;190(6):1520–1526. doi:10.1016/j.ajog.2003.12.057.

19. Dildy G, Belfort M. Complications of pre-eclampsia. In: Belfort M, Saade G, Foley M, Phelan J, Dildy G, eds. *Critical care obstetrics.* 5th ed. Oxford, England: Wiley-Blackwell; 2010:438–635.

20. Sibai BM. Diagnosis, controversies, and management of the syndrome of hemolysis, elevated liver enzymes, and low platelet count. *Obstet Gynecol.* 2004;103(5 Pt 1):981–991. doi:10.1097/01.AOG.0000126245.35811.2a.

21. Sihler KC, Napolitano LM. Complications of massive transfusion. *Chest.* 2010;137(1):209–220. doi:10.1378/chest.09-0252.

22. Kramer MS, Rouleau J, Liu S, Bartholomew S, Joseph KS, Maternal Health Study Group of the Canadian Perinatal Surveillance System. Amniotic fluid embolism: incidence, risk factors, and impact on perinatal outcome. *BJOG.* 2012;119(7):874–879. doi:10.1111/j.1471-0528.2012.03323.x.

23. Cole DE, Taylor TL, McCullough DM, Shoff CT, Derdak S. Acute respiratory distress syndrome in pregnancy. *Crit Care Med.* 2005;33(10 Suppl):S269–78. doi:10.1097/01.ccm.0000182478.14181.da.

24. Pearson GD, Veille JC, Rahimtoola S, et al. Peripartum cardiomyopathy: National Heart, Lung, and Blood Institute and Office of Rare Diseases (National Institutes of Health) workshop recommendations and review. *JAMA*. 2000;283(9):1183–1188. doi:10.1001/jama.283.9.1183.

25. Guntupalli KK, Karnad DR, Bandi V, Hall N, Belfort M. Critical illness in pregnancy part II: Common medical conditions complicating pregnancy and puerperium. *Chest*. 2015;148(5):1333–1345. doi:10.1378/chest.14-2365.

26. Duarte AG, Thomas S, Safdar Z, et al. Management of pulmonary arterial hypertension during pregnancy: a retrospective, multicenter experience. *Chest*. 2013;143(5):1330–1336. doi:10.1378/chest.12-0528.

27. European Society of Gynecology (ESG), Association for European Paediatric Cardiology (AEPC), German Society for Gender Medicine (DGesGM), et al. ESC Guidelines on the management of cardiovascular diseases during pregnancy: the Task Force on the Management of Cardiovascular Diseases during Pregnancy of the European Society of Cardiology (ESC). *Eur Heart J*. 2011;32(24):3147–3197. doi:10.1093/eurheartj/ehr218.

28. Sriskandan S. Severe peripartum sepsis. *J R Coll Physicians Edinb*. 2011;41(4):339–346. doi:10.4997/JRCPE.2011.411.

29. Barton JR, Sibai BM. Severe sepsis and septic shock in pregnancy. *Obstet Gynecol*. 2012;120(3):689–706. doi:10.1097/AOG.0b013e318263a52d.

30. Bourjeily G, Paidas M, Khalil H, Rosene-Montella K, Rodger M. Pulmonary embolism in pregnancy. *Lancet*. 2010;375(9713):500–512. doi:10.1016/S0140-6736(09)60996-X.

31. Chan W-S, Rey E, Kent NE, et al. Venous thromboembolism and antithrombotic therapy in pregnancy. *J Obstet Gynaecol Can*. 2014;36(6):527–553. http://www.ncbi.nlm.nih.gov/pubmed/24927193.

32. Bates SM, Greer IA, Middeldorp S, Veenstra DL, Prabulos A-M, Vandvik PO. VTE, thrombophilia, antithrombotic therapy, and pregnancy: Antithrombotic Therapy and Prevention of Thrombosis, 9th ed.: American College of Chest Physicians Evidence-Based Clinical Practice Guidelines. *Chest*. 2012;141(2 Suppl):e691S–e736S. doi:10.1378/chest.11–2300.

33. Fuchs F, Bruyere M, Senat M-V, Purenne E, Benhamou D, Fernandez H. Are standard intra-abdominal pressure values different during pregnancy? *PLoS One*. 2013;8(10):e77324. doi:10.1371/journal.pone.0077324.

34. Ivankovic AD, Elam JO, Huffman J. Effect of maternal hypercarbia on the newborn infant. *Am J Obstet Gynecol*. 1970;107(6):939–946. doi:10.1016/s0002-9378(16)34052-2.

35. Walker AM, Oakes GK, Ehrenkranz R, McLaughlin M, Chez RA. Effects of hypercapnia on uterine and umbilical circulations in conscious pregnant sheep. *J Appl Physiol*. 1976;41(5 Pt. 1):727–733. doi:10.1152/jappl.1976.41.5.727.

36. Morris JA, Rosenbower TJ, Jurkovich GJ, et al. Infant survival after cesarean section for trauma. *Ann Surg*. 1996;223(5):481–491. doi:10.1097/00000658-199605000-00004.

37. ACOG. Critical care in pregnancy. *Obstet Gynecol*. 2019;130(76):168–186.

25
Non-obstetric Surgery During Pregnancy

Arunthevaraja Karuppiah, Jessica Galey, and Shobana Bharadwaj

Introduction

Knowledge of the physiologic changes of pregnancy as well as fetoplacental physiology is imperative, as it impacts decision making during the entire anesthetic process. Rates of non-obstetric surgery performed during pregnancy have been estimated to be between 0.3% to 2.2% or approximately 100,000 cases annually in both the United States and Europe.[1,2,3] It is generally felt that only procedures of urgent or emergent nature are performed during pregnancy and women may present at all stages of pregnancy for both pregnancy-related and unrelated procedures.[1] Procedures that are not of urgent/emergent nature are generally delayed until the second trimester when the natural rate of spontaneous abortion and preterm labor falls the lowest.[4] Commonly encountered procedures that are pregnancy-related include cervical cerclage for cervical incompetence, ovarian cystectomy or torsion, and fetal conditions that may be amenable to surgical intervention. Other nonpregnancy-related procedures include acute intraabdominal disease (most commonly being appendicitis or cholecystitis) or procedures related to malignancy. In addition, maternal trauma is responsible for a large portion of patients with significant maternal morbidity and mortality.[5,6] Decisions for the timing of the procedure as well as intraoperative fetal monitoring must be multidisciplinary (Figure 25.1). Anesthetic management of these patients require modifications to accommodate the physiologic changes of pregnancy (Table 25.1), avoidance of teratogens, prevention of decreased uteroplacental perfusion and fetal oxygenation, and monitoring for preterm labor in the postoperative period.[3]

Fetal Considerations

Fetal Effects of Anesthetics

A wide variety of drugs are currently utilized during a standard anesthetic. Inhalational anesthetics as well as opioids and intravenous induction agents are lipid-soluble drugs, which can cross the placenta. These lead to fetal central nervous system (CNS) depression which is seen as a decrease in fetal heart-rate variability. In the absence of decelerations, the decreased variability is presumed to be due to an anesthetized fetus; however, if decelerations are present, other causes should be identified and appropriately treated. Administration of muscle relaxants is safe to the fetus because of minimal placental transfer.

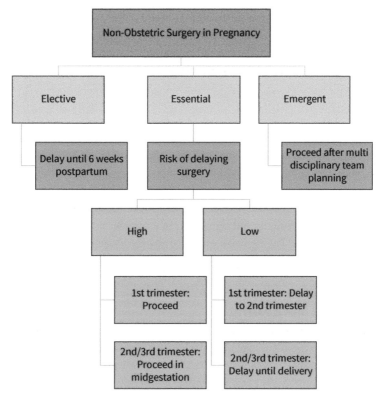

Figure 25.1 Timing of non-obstetric surgery in pregnancy.

Reversal agents are recommended to be given with caution as there are some studies indicating possible effects on the fetal heart rate. To date there is limited data on sugammadex administration in pregnancy.[3]

Teratogenicity and Fetal Safety

Clinical data indicate that surgery and anesthesia during pregnancy does not increase the risk of congenital anomalies and pregnancy loss.[1] There are however other risks, including the effects of the disease process itself, uteroplacental perfusion and fetal oxygenation, risk of preterm labor, and possible teratogenic effects of drugs administered during the perioperative period. Prospective clinical trials regarding the teratogenic effects of anesthetic agents are not possible, therefore data regarding teratogenicity is largely based on animal trials, retrospective studies, or data from exposed operating room personnel during pregnancy. Teratogenicity must also be considered in the context of the naturally high spontaneous abortion rate, estimated as 11–22% of pregnancies from 5–20 weeks' gestation.[7] The largest study available which investigated anesthetic type and pregnancy outcomes has indicated no higher incidence of congenital anomalies, and no specific anesthetic technique had a higher rate of adverse outcome.[1]

Maintenance of uteroplacental perfusion and fetal oxygenation are of utmost importance to ensure fetal safety during non-obstetric surgery. Blood flow to the fetus is directly dependent upon maternal oxygenation and circulation; therefore, the best way to ensure fetal well-being is maintenance of normal maternal physiology and rapid correction of derangements that may occur during the perioperative period. Mild reductions in maternal blood pressure or oxygenation can generally be tolerated by the fetus, but if severe alterations occur, fetal acidemia and possibly intrapartum fetal asphyxia may result. Situations such as maternal respiratory failure, or intraoperative problems such as difficult intubation or pulmonary aspiration, are important to consider. As with maternal hypoxemia, similarly, to maternal hypoxemia, significant maternal hypotension can lead to reduction in uteroplacental blood flow. This may arise during the perioperative period due to hemorrhage, aortocaval compression, deep level of general anesthesia, or sympathectomy due to a high neuraxial blockade. In addition, maintenance of normal maternal acid base status and $PaCO_2$ is necessary to ensure adequate gas exchange across the placenta.[3]

Fetal Heart Rate Monitoring

According to the American College of Obstetricians and Gynecologists (ACOG) and the American Society of Anesthesiologists (ASA) joint publication regarding intraoperative fetal heart rate monitoring, the previable fetus should have a doppler check of fetal heart rate pre- and postprocedure. The viable fetus should at least have electronic fetal heart rate monitoring and contraction monitoring pre- and postprocedure. Intraoperative fetal heart rate monitoring should be utilized on a case-by-case basis and should involve a multidisciplinary discussion between surgical, obstetric, anesthesiology, and neonatology teams (Figure 25.2). Considerations for intraoperative monitoring include: a viable fetus; the availability of equipment and personnel capable of monitoring and interpreting the tracing; physical feasibility, based on the site and type of surgery; the availability of

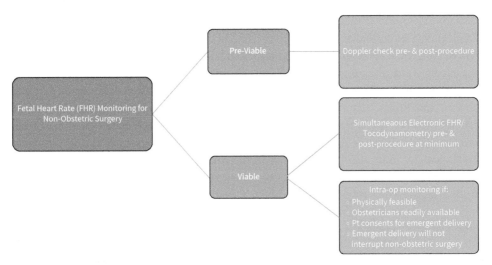

Figure 25.2 Fetal heart rate (FHR) monitoring during non-obstetric surgeries.

an obstetrician to perform an emergent cesarean section when required for fetal indications; and the nature of the surgery that would allow safe interruption, if required.[4] Interpretation of the fetal heart rate tracing during an anesthetic impacts anesthetic decision making as well as planning for possible intervention on behalf of the fetus. It is expected that the variability will decrease due to anesthetic agents; however, decelerations or bradycardia would indicate compromised uteroplacental perfusion and fetal hypoxia. Primary maneuvers during that event would involve maternal resuscitation including correction of hypotension, hypoxia, or any acid base disturbance, and if continued then emergent cesarean delivery may be warranted.

Maternal Physiology

Table 25.1 Physiological Changes During Pregnancy

Cardiovascular	Decreased BP, SVR, PVR Lack of autoregulation of uterine vasculature Aortocaval compression after 18–20 weeks of gestation Gallop rhythm, left axis deviation, systolic murmur, minor ST-T changes Increased blood volume, heart rate and cardiac output (50%)
Respiratory	Reduced FRC (20%), increased oxygen demand (20%) Mild chronic respiratory alkalosis ($PaCO_2$ = 28–32 mm Hg) Increased alveolar ventilation (30%) PaO_2 increases slightly or within normal range Vital capacity and dead space unchanged during pregnancy
Airway	Increased soft tissue in the neck, weight gain, and breast engorgement Increase in Mallampati score as pregnancy progresses Increased edema of the airway and vocal cord Increased vascularity of mucous membranes
Gastrointestinal	Incompetent lower esophageal sphincter tone Distorted gastric and pyloric anatomy Normal gastric emptying time until labor Increased gastric volume and acidity
Renal	Lower plasma creatinine due to increased glomerular filtration rate
Central nervous system	Engorged epidural venous plexus (Figure 25.3) Reduced epidural space volume Increased CSF pressure Increased sensitivity to opioids Decreased (40%) MAC requirements
Blood and coagulation	Relatively smaller increase in RBC (20%) than plasma volume (40%); leading to hemodilution Benign leukocytosis Hypercoagulable state with an increase in Fibrinogen, factors VII, VIII, X, XII and FDP Protein S (anticoagulant) is decreased and acquired resistance to protein C. Low platelet count

BP = blood pressure, SVR = systemic vascular resistance, PVR = pulmonary vascular resistance, FRC = functional residual capacity, PaO_2 = partial pressure of oxygen in blood, $PaCO_2$ = partial pressure of carbon dioxide in blood, CSF = cerebrospinal fluid, MAC = minimum alveolar concentration, RBC = red blood cells, FDP = fibrin degradation products

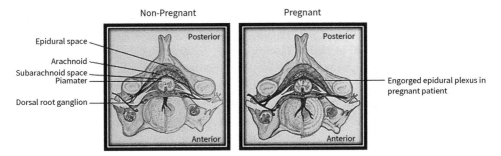

Figure 25.3 Epidural venous plexus.

Anesthetic Management

Maternal Monitoring

All pregnant patients should routinely be monitored using standard ASA monitoring throughout the intraoperative period. The use of invasive monitoring modalities should be guided by the predisposing medical or surgical condition. There is a good correlation between end-tidal CO_2 ($EtCO_2$) and $PaCO_2$ and the former gradient can be safely used to guide intraoperative ventilation in pregnant patients.[8] Uterine contractions can be monitored intraoperatively using external tocodynamometer when feasible. Tocodynamometry during the postoperative period is imperative as analgesics can mask awareness of early uterine contractions.

Preoperative Considerations

A multidisciplinary team-based approach is necessary to educate the patient and family about miscarriage, preterm labor, and the prospects of neonatal intensive care for the fetus. Adequate time should be spent during the preoperative period to reassure the mother concerning the safety of anesthetics and postoperative pain management. Preoperative assessment of a pregnant patient who require surgical interventions is similar to a nonpregnant patient with much emphasis on the following:

Aspiration prophylaxis: ASA adult fasting guidelines should be strictly followed for elective surgery. The gastric emptying has recently been shown to be normal during pregnancy until the onset of labor.[9,10] However, the risk of aspiration is still higher due to reduced gastric barrier pressure and lower esophageal sphincter tone. Pharmacological prophylaxis should be administered for patients over 18 weeks of gestation, or earlier, if at high risk for aspiration, with a combination of H_2-receptor blockers, metoclopramide, and nonparticulate antacids.[3]

Antibiotic prophylaxis: Depending on the specific procedure, antibiotic prophylaxis should be administered with careful attention to the fetal safety profile.[11]

Steroids for fetal lung maturity: Administration of a course of antenatal glucocorticoids 24–48 hours before surgery between 24 and 34 weeks of gestation can reduce perinatal morbidity/mortality if preterm birth occurs. Despite the potential benefits to the fetus, at times glucocorticoids are best avoided in the setting of systemic infection or inflammatory response.[11]

Thromboprophylaxis: Pregnancy as itself is a hypercoagulable state. Mechanical compression devices are recommended in all pregnant patients, and pharmacologic thromboprophylaxis is recommended for patients with additional risk factors.[12]

Premedication: Reassurance of the mother is the preferred method rather than resorting to medications for sedation prior to surgery. If necessary, benzodiazepines and opioids can be used.

Intraoperative Management

Core principles in the anesthetic management of a pregnant patient are avoidance of hypoxia, hypercarbia, hypocarbia, acidosis, hypothermia, hypoperfusion, hypotension, as well as mitigation of aortocaval compression. Pregnant patients beyond 18–20 weeks of gestation should be positioned with a 15° left uterine displacement when lying supine under any type of anesthesia (Figure 25.4).

Regional anesthesia is favored when possible owing to its minimal exposure of the mother and fetus to drugs.[13] Regional anesthesia also circumvents airway manipulation. Routine use of oxygen is recommended as well as $EtCO_2$ monitoring if sedation is given.

Appropriate maternal positioning during a general anesthetic must include patient positioning for airway control (Figure 25.5). A head-up tilt will aid in improving maternal functional residual capacity (FRC) and will also assist in securing the airway unhindered by enlarged breasts. It may also help prevent passive reflux at the induction of anesthesia. Denitrogenation (i.e., preoxygenation) should precede induction of anesthesia. Although there is no consensus, it is safer to use an endotracheal tube for longer or more extensive procedures. Although rapid-sequence induction with application of cricoid pressure has been a long-standing practice, some experts suggest that, in a fasting patient, it makes tracheal intubation more challenging.[14]

Anesthesia can be safely maintained using oxygen, nitrous oxide, and either propofol or halogenated agents. Both depolarizing or nondepolarizing muscle relaxing agents have a good safety record during pregnancy. The prolongation of the action of

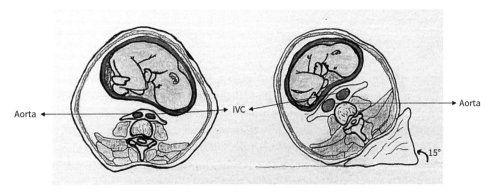

Figure 25.4 Left uterine displacement to avoid aortocaval compression.

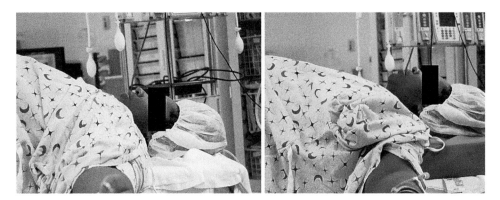

Figure 25.5 Ramped position for intubation in obese patients.

succinylcholine may not occur even though plasma choline esterase levels fall in pregnancy. Hyperventilation should be avoided; rather end-tidal CO_2 should be maintained in a normal range of 28 to 32 mm Hg in pregnant patients.[3] Hyperventilation decreases uteroplacental perfusion and shifts the maternal hemoglobin dissociation curve to the left. Minimum alveolar concentration (MAC) requirements for volatile agents are reduced in pregnancy. They relax the uterus proportionally to the MAC exposure and increase uterine blood flow. Simultaneously, significant hypotension associated with higher MAC levels compromises uterine perfusion.

Sympathetic stimulation due to pain may decrease uterine blood flow and should be addressed aptly. Recovery from anesthesia requires special attention in a pregnant patient, particularly of the airway and respiratory system, because most airway complications occur during emergence, extubation, or recovery. Neostigmine is preferred over sugammadex as a reversal agent. There is very limited evidence regarding the safety of sugammadex with regards to placental transfer, effects on maternal plasma progesterone, and fetal development during pregnancy.[15]

Fetal monitoring: Fetal heart rate monitoring may assist in maternal positioning and cardiorespiratory management and may influence a decision to deliver the fetus.[16] Consider sterile ultrasound as an option for intermittent FHR monitoring. Anesthetic agents reduce both the baseline fetal heart rate and variability, so readings must be interpreted in the context of administered drugs.

Postoperative Management

The provision of adequate postoperative analgesia is essential since pain has been shown to increase the risk of premature labor. Multimodal analgesia may include opioids, acetaminophen and nonsteroidal anti-inflammatory drugs (NSAIDs). Regional or neuraxial anesthesia can decrease the opioid consumption. Short-term exposure to opioids is considered safe even though they cross the placental barrier with the continuation of pregnancy after surgery. Long-term intrauterine exposure to opioids is well known to cause significant withdrawal symptoms in the newborn. Prolonged use of NSAIDs (> 48 hours), especially ibuprofen, should be avoided in the first trimester[3] and after 32 weeks of gestation.[11] Early ambulation,

---

Box 25.1 Summary of Anesthetic Management

Preoperative considerations
- Aspiration prophylaxis
- Reassurance and anxiolysis
- FHR monitoring—Doppler/electronic
- Initiation of DVT prophylaxis

Intraoperative considerations
- Regional Anesthesia preferred over general anesthesia when appropriate
- MAC and MLAC decreased
- Left uterine displacement prior to induction
- Be prepared for difficult airway
- Adequate preoxygenation prior to rapid-sequence Induction
- Maintain $PaCO_2$ at normal pregnancy levels (28–32 mmHg)
- Continuous FHR only if feasible, fetus is viable, emergency c-section anticipated; otherwise pre- and post procedure FHR/contraction monitoring

Postoperative considerations
- Ensure adequate reversal of muscle relaxants and ability to maintain airway
- Tocodynamometry to monitor uterine contraction
- Adequate postoperative pain control
- Continue DVT prophylaxis/early ambulation

---

when appropriate, in the postoperative period helps reduce the risk for developing venous thrombosis. In summary, the anesthetic management goals are to ensure maternal safety, fetal well-being, and maintain pregnancy (Box 25.1).

Special Considerations

Laparoscopy

Laparoscopy has been safely performed in pregnant patients for gynecologic and nongynecologic problems during any trimester.[17,18] However, concerns of risks exist for uterine or fetal injury, hypotension and placental hypoperfusion from abdominal insufflation, fetal acidosis from carbon dioxide absorption, and technical challenges. Initial abdominal access can be safely accomplished with an open (Hasson), Veress needle, or optical trocar technique, by surgeons experienced with these techniques, if the location is adjusted according to fundal height, via ultrasound guided subcostal approach. CO_2 insufflation of 10–15 mm Hg can be safely used for laparoscopy in the pregnant patient. The level of insufflation pressure should be adjusted to the patient's physiology. Intraoperative CO_2 monitoring by capnography should be used during laparoscopy in the pregnant patient to help avoid fetal acidosis.[19] The end-tidal carbon dioxide ($EtCO_2$) monitoring adequately reflects maternal acid-base status and is safe and efficacious. $EtCO_2$ should be maintained at maternal physiologic levels[8]

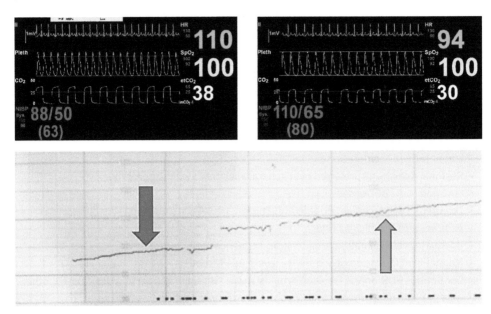

Figure 25.6 FHR change in the setting of maternal hypotension and hypercarbia. Arrow (red): Intraoperative decrease in fetal heart in the setting of maternal hypotension and hypercarbia. Arrow (green): FHR to baseline after correction of hypotension and hypercarbia.

(Figure 25.6). Vasopressors may be needed to treat hypotension from pneumoperitoneum, aortocaval compression, or the use of the reverse Trendelenburg position.

Preterm Labor

Pregnant patients undergoing non-obstetric surgery are at risk for preterm delivery due to the surgery, manipulation of the uterus, or the disease process itself. Prophylactic tocolytics are not routinely used. Monitoring of uterine contractions using external tocodynamometer postoperatively aids in the timely institution of tocolytic therapy. Inhalation agents used for maintenance of anesthesia have a theoretical advantage of suppressing myometrial irritability by smooth muscle relaxation.[3] Symptoms of uterine contractions may be masked if patients are on high dose narcotics for postoperative analgesia. Intravenous magnesium sulfate used for tocolysis or fetal cerebral neuroprotection in the immediate postoperative period has the potential to re-establish neuromuscular blockade.[20]

Maternal Cardiac Arrest

Maternal cardiac arrest is rare, and the reversible causes of cardiac arrest are similar to those in nonpregnant patients. In addition, pregnancy-specific causes are amniotic fluid embolism, placental abruption, eclampsia, or hemorrhage. Modifications of cardiopulmonary resuscitation in pregnancy include manual left uterine displacement to avoid aortocaval compression, anticipation of difficult airway, intravenous access above the diaphragm, administration of

100% oxygen, and a defibrillator pad placed under the breast tissue. Recommendations on chest compressions, defibrillation, and medications are the same as for nonpregnant adult resuscitation. Resuscitative hysterotomy is performed in gestational age over 20 weeks to improve the chance of maternal survival and likelihood of fetal survival. Delivery is initiated if spontaneous circulation does not return within 4 minutes of arrest, with the goal of delivering the fetus in 5 minutes. The neonatal team should be a part of the maternal resuscitation team for neonatal resuscitation.[21]

References

1. Mazze RI, Kallen B. Reproductive outcome after anesthesia and operation during pregnancy: a registry study of 5405 cases. *Am J Obstet Gynecol.* 1989;161(5):1178–1185. doi:10.1016/0002-9378(89)90659-5.

2. Brodsky JB, Cohen EN, Brown BW, Jr., Wu ML, Whitcher C. Surgery during pregnancy and fetal outcome. *Am J Obstet Gynecol.* 1980;138(8):1165–1167. doi:10.1016/s0002-9378(16)32785-5.

3. Chestnut D, Wong C, Tsen L, et al. *Chestnut's obstetric anesthesia: principles and practice.* 6th ed. Elsevier;, Philadelphia. 2019.

4. Committee on Obstetric Practice and the American Society of Anesthesiologists. Committee opinion no. 696: nonobstetric surgery during pregnancy. *Obstet Gynecol.* 2017;129(4): 777–778. doi:10.1097/AOG.0000000000002014.

5. Bouyou J, Gaujoux S, Marcellin L, et al. Abdominal emergencies during pregnancy. *J Visc Surg.* 2015;152(6 Suppl):S105–15. doi:10.1016/j.jviscsurg.2015.09.017.

6. Coleman MT, Trianfo VA, Rund DA. Nonobstetric emergencies in pregnancy: trauma and surgical conditions. *Am J Obstet Gynecol.* 1997;177(3):497–502. doi:10.1016/s0002-9378(97)70135-2.

7. Ammon Avalos L, Galindo C, Li DK. A systematic review to calculate background miscarriage rates using life table analysis. *Birth Defects Res A Clin Mol Teratol.* 2012;94(6):417–423. doi:10.1002/bdra.23014.

8. Bhavani-Shankar K, Steinbrook RA, Brooks DC, Datta S. Arterial to end-tidal carbon dioxide pressure difference during laparoscopic surgery in pregnancy. *Anesthesiology.* 2000;93(2):370–373. doi:10.1097/00000542-200008000-00014.

9. Wong CA, Loffredi M, Ganchiff JN, Zhao J, Wang Z, Avram MJ. Gastric emptying of water in term pregnancy. *Anesthesiology.* 2002;96(6):1395–1400. doi:10.1097/00000542-200206000-00019.

10. Wong CA, McCarthy RJ, Fitzgerald PC, Raikoff K, Avram MJ. Gastric emptying of water in obese pregnant women at term. *Anesth Analg.* 2007;105(3):751–755. doi:10.1213/01.ane.0000278136.98611.d6.

11. Upadya M, Saneesh PJ. Anaesthesia for non-obstetric surgery during pregnancy. *Indian J Anaesth.* 2016;60(4):234–241. doi:10.4103/0019-5049.179445.

12. D'Alton ME, Friedman AM, Smiley RM, et al. National Partnership for Maternal Safety: consensus bundle on venous thromboembolism. *Anesth Analg.* 2016;123(4):942–949. doi:10.1213/ANE.0000000000001569.

13. Reitman E, Flood P. Anaesthetic considerations for non-obstetric surgery during pregnancy. *Br J Anaesth.* 2011;107 Suppl 1:i72–i78. doi:10.1093/bja/aer343.

14. de Souza DG, Doar LH, Mehta SH, Tiouririne M. Aspiration prophylaxis and rapid sequence induction for elective cesarean delivery: time to reassess old dogma? *Anesth Analg.* 2010;110(5):1503–1505. doi:10.1213/ANE.0b013e3181d7e33c.

15. Richardson MG, Raymond BL. Sugammadex administration in pregnant women and in women of reproductive potential: a narrative review. *Anesth Analg.* 2020 Jun;130(6):1628–1637. doi:10.1213/ANE.0000000000004305.

16. ACOG Committee on Obstetric Practice. ACOG committee opinion. Nonobstetric surgery in pregnancy. Number 284, August 2003. *Int J Gynaecol Obstet.* 2003;83(1):135. doi:10.1016/s0020-7292(03)00391-6.

17. Guterman S, Mandelbrot L, Keita H, Bretagnol F, Calabrese D, Msika S. Laparoscopy in the second and third trimesters of pregnancy for abdominal surgical emergencies. *J Gynecol Obstet Hum Reprod.* 2017;46(5):417–422. doi:10.1016/j.jogoh.2017.03.008.

18. Fatum M, Rojansky N. Laparoscopic surgery during pregnancy. *Obstet Gynecol Surv.* 2001;56(1):50–59. doi:10.1097/00006254-200101000-00025.

19. Pearl JP, Price RR, Tonkin AE, Richardson WS, Stefanidis D. SAGES guidelines for the use of laparoscopy during pregnancy. *Surg Endosc.* 2017;31(10):3767–3782. doi:10.1007/s00464-017-5637-3.

20. Hans GA, Bosenge B, Bonhomme VL, Brichant JF, Venneman IM, Hans PC. Intravenous magnesium re-establishes neuromuscular block after spontaneous recovery from an intubating dose of rocuronium: a randomised controlled trial. *Eur J Anaesthesiol.* 2012;29(2):95–99. doi:10.1097/EJA.0b013e32834e13a6.

21. Jeejeebhoy FM, Zelop CM, Lipman S, et al. Cardiac arrest in pregnancy: a scientific statement from the American Heart Association. *Circulation.* 2015;132(18):1747–1773. doi:10.1161/CIR.0000000000000300.

26

Anesthesia for Fetal Surgery

Beata Evans, Kevin Quinn, Rajanya S. Petersson, Timothy Wills, and Fatoumata Kromah

Background and Overview of Fetal Surgery

Direct fetal treatment was first demonstrated by Sir William Liley, who in 1963 performed an intraperitoneal blood transfusion on a fetus suffering from erythroblastosis fetalis.[3,4] Aided by advancements in imaging, prenatal diagnostic tools, and building upon animal studies in primates and sheep, Michael Harrison performed the first fetal surgery in 1981.[1] This first fetal surgery was a vesicostomy for severe bilateral hydronephrosis secondary to lower urinary tract obstruction.[5] A year later, the International Fetal Medicine and Surgery Society (IFMSS) paved the way for the creation of a consensus statement on fetal surgery. This statement has guided case selection for fetal surgery and has remained largely unchanged.

Current guidelines for fetal surgery include:

(1) an accurate prenatal diagnosis
(2) a well-defined natural history of the congenital disorder
(3) the presence of a correctable lesion which, if untreated, will lead to fetal demise, irreversible organ dysfunction before birth, or severe postnatal morbidity
(4) the absence of severe associated anomalies
(5) an acceptable risk-to-benefit ratio for both the mother and fetus.[6]

With increasingly sophisticated prenatal diagnostic capabilities, early detection of fetal anomalies is becoming more common as early interventions and therapy may improve fetal outcomes.

Surgical and Anesthesia Management

Minimally Invasive Fetal Procedures

Minimally invasive fetal procedures (MIFP) or fetoscopic surgery are indicated for fetal conditions such as oligo- or polyhydramnios, hydrops, anemia, twin to twin transfusion syndrome, twin reversed arterial perfusion syndrome, aortic or pulmonary stenosis, congenital diaphragmatic hernia (CDH), and obstructive uropathy.[3,5] MIFP are performed either by percutaneous or laparotomy techniques under ultrasonographic and/or endoscopic guidance. During the procedure, a needle is used to puncture the abdominal wall, or a mini-laparotomy incision is made to allow a needle or fetoscope to enter the uterine cavity. Once the uterus is accessed, the needle is advanced further to contact the placenta,

Table 26.1 Anesthesia Options for MIFP

	Local infiltration (most common & well tolerated)	Neuraxial	GETA (rare)
Induction	single abdominal punctate incision	multiple abdominal wall incisions, large incision, mini laparotomy	uterine relaxation
Length of procedure	short	moderate	long
Fetal analgesia	no	no	yes
Maternal sedation needed	yes	yes	no
Postop analgesia	no	yes	no

GETA, general endotracheal anesthesia

umbilical vessels, or fetus. Compared to other types of fetal surgery, successful MIFP decrease fetal morbidity and mortality while causing fewer maternal risks due to less surgical stress, limited tissue trauma, and smaller incisions. Additionally, mothers have a faster recovery, decreased length of hospitalization, and decreased risk for perioperative blood transfusions.[7,8] However, there is still a risk of premature rupture of membranes (PROM), preterm labor, amniotic band syndrome, umbilical cord strangulation, and intrauterine fetal demise.

Before the procedure starts, a preanesthesia assessment and evaluation is required. Standard NPO guidelines and aspiration prophylaxis should be followed. A functional peripheral intravenous access, left uterine displacement, and standard ASA monitoring are recommended. It is important to obtain ultrasound imaging to identify the location of the placenta and umbilical cord. The anesthetic technique depends on the surgical approach, length of procedure, patient preference, and need for fetal analgesia and immobility (see Table 26.1).[9]

MIFP such as amniocentesis, amnioreduction, or amnioinfusion are usually well tolerated without local anesthesia or maternal sedation. Other MIFP such as percutaneous umbilical blood sampling (PUBS) and transfusion may be performed with neuraxial and/or maternal sedation. When maternal sedation alone is utilized, abdominal movement secondary to maternal respiration makes the procedure more difficult to complete. Other risks associated with maternal sedation and fetal movement should be considered (see Table 26.2).

Neuraxial anesthesia prevents maternal movement, but fetal movement also makes the surgical procedure technically challenging. MIFP do not require a surgical incision on the fetus, therefore both uterine relaxation and general anesthesia are rarely indicated. However, fetal movement may cause displacement of the needle or fetoscope, resulting in trauma or shearing of the umbilical vessels. Even though general anesthesia allows placental transfer of medication, thereby providing fetal anesthesia, fetal paralysis may still be required. If necessary, fetal immobility may be achieved by ultrasound-guided administration of a muscle relaxant, either through the umbilical vein or direct fetal intramuscular injection. A multidisciplinary contingency plan is essential for management of emergencies during the procedure. It is important to prepare for an emergency cesarean delivery under general anesthesia and to have predrawn weight-based resuscitative medications such as atropine and epinephrine readily available for the fetus. Prior to surgery, plans for fetal resuscitation should be discussed with the mother since emergency delivery of a nonviable fetus may be futile.

Table 26.2 Anesthesia Concerns with MIFP

	Concerns	Management
Maternal osedation	Respiratory depression Loss of airway reflexes Pulmonary aspiration	Titration of medications
Fetal movement	Technically difficult/impossible procedure Traumatic needle/catheter displacement Bleeding/shearing of the umbilical cord Emergency delivery	Immobility or analgesia (fetal USG IM morphine 0.3mg/kg or UVC (0.1–0.25 mg/kg), non-depolarizing neuromuscular blocker, GETA

Fetal analgesia	Needed for procedures in which the
	  needle toward the fetus or umbilical
	  vessels, i.e., shunt catheter placement/
	  septoplasty
	Fetal vagal response
	Fetal immobility
		IM/IV opioid fentanyl 10–25 mcg/kg
		  to fetus,
		Via maternal GETA placental
		  transfer

USG, ultrasound guided; UVC, umbilical venous catheter; IM, intramuscular; IV, intravenous; GETA, general endotracheal anesthesia

Open Fetal Surgical Procedures

Open fetal surgery involves an incision and procedure performed directly on the fetus. Common indications for these procedures include neural tube defect, congenital diaphragmatic hernia, congenital airway malformation, and sacrococcygeal teratoma.[10,11,12] Spina bifida is the result of an incomplete closure of the neural tube during fetal organogenesis and is the most common central nervous defect.[13,14,15] Myelomenigocele (MMC) is a subtype of spina bifida in which a multilayer defect of the vertebrae, meninges, and skin causes persistent exposure of the spinal cord to amniotic fluid, leading to possible injury and infection postdelivery (see Figure 26.1).[8,15] Fetuses diagnosed with spina bifida

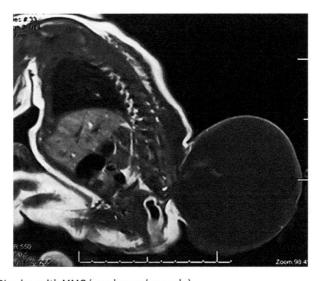

Figure 26.1 MRI spine with MMC (myelomeningocele).

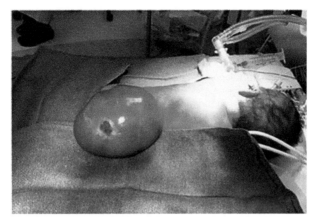

Figure 26.2 Traditional approach to MMC repair.

are at high risk for lifelong motor and sensory dysfunction, hydrocephalus, and bladder and bowel incontinence. Historically, the standard of care for spina bifida was a postnatal repair (see Figure 26.2). The prospective, randomized Management of Myelomeningocele Study (MOMS) showed that compared to the traditional approach, midgestational open fetal MMC surgery significantly decreased the neurologic dysfunction seen with spina bifida.[14,16] To qualify for open fetal surgery, both the mother and fetus must meet certain selection criteria (see Table 26.3).[15,17]

Planning for open fetal surgery involves a comprehensive multidisciplinary team collaboration from members of the maternal-fetal medicine, neurosurgery, neonatology, pediatric cardiology, and anesthesiology specialties, as well as other support staff.[11,13] The mother should be referred to a center with fetal surgery capability. The mother should undergo a thorough evaluation and assessment with baseline laboratory testing. Prior to

Table 26.3 Selection Criteria for Open Fetal Surgery

	Inclusion criteria	Possible exclusion criteria
Fetal factors	Myelomeningocele located at T1–S1 region Normal karyotype Hindbrain herniation Absent fetal malformation	Fetal kyphosis > 30 degrees Skin covered lesion
Maternal factors	Maternal age ≥ 18	BMI > 40 Maternal conditions: HTN, DM, Hep B or C, HIV, SLE, h/o preterm delivery History of incompetent cervix or shortening of cervix < 20mm Psychosocial limitations
Pregnancy factors	Gestational age < 27 wks Singleton pregnancy	Abnormal placentation, i.e., previa Uterine anomaly, i.e., septate, bicornuate uterus, fibroids

surgery, imaging is required to determine fetal and placental location.[14] Maternal blood type and crossmatch, as well as fetal O negative, CMV negative, and leukocyte-reduced blood should be readily available for emergency transfusion. The operating room must be warmed to maintain maternal and fetal temperature within normal range. Similar to a cesarean delivery, aspiration prophylaxis and multimodal pain medications should be administered. Preoperatively, catheters (arterial, large-bore intravenous, urinary, and epidural) are placed. In the operating room, the mother should be positioned in a left lateral tilt for uterine displacement and avoidance of supine hypotension syndrome, uterine hypoperfusion, and fetal anoxia. Important goals for open fetal surgery are to maintain uteroplacental circulation and prevent preterm labor until the fetus reaches term or close to term gestational age.

Open fetal surgery may be performed under neuraxial, general anesthesia, or a combination of the two anesthetic techniques.[9,17] Adequate uterine relaxation is required prior to the hysterotomy. If neuraxial anesthesia is utilized, uterine relaxation may be achieved by administration of nitroglycerine or volatile anesthetics. Uterine relaxation obtained with inhalational agents requires preoxygenation, induction of general anesthesia, and intubation with an endotracheal tube. Inhalational agents are titratable and may be used interchangeably, but desflurane has the benefit of a rapid onset and offset.[12] Although the fetus may be affected by placental passage of medication administered to the mother, intramuscular or intravenous opioids and muscle relaxant are commonly administered for fetal analgesia and immobility.[11] Fetus monitoring occurs with direct visualization, pulse oximetry, electrocardiography, ultrasonography, and/or echocardiography. Under ultrasonographic guidance, a hysterotomy is performed and amniotic membranes are fixed to the uterine wall.[7,18] Warm lactated ringer's solution is infused into the uterine cavity to prevent fetal hypothermia, cord compression, early placental separation, and preterm delivery.[7,9] When the fetal surgery is complete, amniotic fluid is replenished with additional crystalloid solution. After the procedure, the mother is monitored for preterm labor and a tocolytic agent may be administered postoperatively (see Table 26.4).[9,11,17]

Pain control is critical for prevention of preterm labor. Inadequate maternal pain management may trigger release of oxytocin, inducing uterine contraction.[9,11] In the immediate postoperative period, the mother should remain in the hospital for antenatal fetal monitoring and assessments. Hospitalization may continue until a planned term or close to term gestational cesarean delivery. However, the mother may be discharged home and undergo weekly fetal transabdominal ultrasonography.[15]

Even though open fetal surgeries may decrease neonatal morbidity and mortality, there is little to no evidence for maternal benefits. Potential maternal and fetal risks and complications associated with open fetal surgery are listed in Table 26.5.

A cesarean delivery of the fetus must be planned.[11] The mother is counseled against any future trial of labor and attempts at vaginal delivery. New developments in minimally invasive fetal surgery aim to minimize maternal risks and decrease maternal complications. MIFP for conditions that would otherwise require open fetal surgery cause less abdominal wall and uterine trauma, facilitate labor and vaginal delivery of the fetus, and decrease maternal risk of complications associated with future cesarean delivery.[13] Disadvantages of MIFP for conditions such as MMC repair are higher incidence of wound dehiscence, CSF leakage at the repair site, and possible need for postnatal revisions.[13]

Table 26.4 Tocolytic Agents

Tocolytic class	Agent	Side effect
Calcium channel blockers	Nifedipine 10–20 mg PO q 6–8 h	Vasodilation, hypotension, flushing
NSAID	Indomethacin 50–100 PR or PO (max daily dose 200 mg)	Maternal GI upset, premature closure of ductus arteriosus, fetal renal injury, intraventricular hemorrhage, necrotizing enterocolitis
Volatile anesthetic (desflurane, isoflurane, sevoflurane)	2–3 MAC	Vasodilation, hypotension
Magnesium sulfate	4–6 g loading dose over 20 min, 1–2 g/h infusion	Maternal lethargy, muscle weakness, vasodilation, cardiac arrhythmia, pulmonary edema, fetal lethargy and hypotonia
Nitroglycerine	40–100 mcg IV; 15–20 mcg/kg/min; 0.4 mg SL	Hypotension, headache
Beta agonist	Terbutaline 250 mcg SQ, IM or 5–10 mcg/min infusion	Maternal tachycardia, myocardial ischemia, pulmonary edema, hyperglycemia, hypokalemia, fetal tachycardia

Ex Utero Intrapartum Treatment Procedure

Ex utero intrapartum treatment (EXIT) procedures allow conversion of a potentially catastrophic neonatal emergency into a controlled delivery which is more likely to result in a positive outcome. EXIT procedures were initially developed for treatment of fetuses with severe congenital diaphragmatic hernia, but they are now employed for a variety of clinical indications including obstructive head, neck, and mediastinal masses, as well as tracheal and laryngeal atresia. The success of an EXIT procedure is dependent on close coordination between multiple teams including an obstetric anesthesiologist, maternal-fetal medicine specialist, radiologist, pediatric otolaryngologists and/or pediatric surgeon, neonatologist, and operating room nurses, technicians, and respiratory therapists. [19] Preprocedural preparation for every contingency of airway management is also critical for success. An EXIT procedure should be considered in cases of prenatal diagnosis of lethal or potentially lethal airway or cardiac malformations and should only be offered by institutions with appropriate

Table 26.5 Complications Associated with Open Fetal Surgery

Maternal	Fetal
Noncardiogenic pulmonary edema	Amniotic fluid leak
Uterine dehiscence	Preterm rupture of membranes
Uterine rupture	Spontaneous preterm labor
Bleeding and risk for blood transfusions	Oligohydramnios

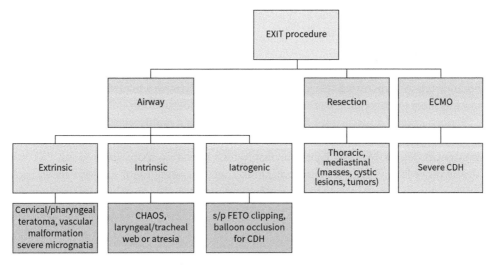

Figure 26.3 Grouped indications for EXIT procedure. EXIT, Ex utero intrapartum treatment

subspecialists available. Indications for EXIT procedures are generally divided into three subgroups (see Figure 26.3).

1. EXIT to airway: This subgroup of EXIT procedures is employed for fetuses with congenital airway compromise. The airway compromise can arise from extrinsic, intrinsic, and iatrogenic causes.
    a. Extrinsic etiologies include cervical or pharyngeal teratomas, vascular malformations, giant ranula (i.e., retention of sublingual gland), or severe micrognathia.[18,19,20] While not every fetus with a prenatally diagnosed head and neck lesion requires an EXIT procedure, head and neck lesion size greater than 5 cm, diagnosis of teratoma, evidence of airway or alimentary canal obstruction with polyhydramnios, absence of fetal gastric fluid, hyperexpanded lungs, or flattening of the diaphragm warrant close evaluation by the EXIT team.
    b. Intrinsic causes are classified as congenital high airway obstruction syndrome (CHAOS) and include laryngeal or tracheal webbing or atresia. [7,21,22]
    c. Iatrogenic airway obstruction may occur after procedures such as fetoscopic endotracheal occlusion (FETO) with tracheal clipping or balloon occlusion for treatment of congenital diaphragmatic hernia.
2. EXIT to resection: This subgroup of EXIT procedures is employed for fetuses diagnosed with thoracic or mediastinal masses including congenital cystic adenomatoid malformations (CCAM), fetal lobar interstitial tumors, and mediastinal teratomas.
3. EXIT to extracorporeal membrane oxygenation (ECMO) is employed for fetuses with severe congenital heart disease or congenital diaphragmatic hernia (CDH).[3]

Similar to other types of fetal surgery, EXIT procedures entail placing two patients at risk. It is paramount to assess individual risk factors and potential benefits for both the mother and fetus during preprocedure evaluation and discussion. While there are no absolute contraindications from the maternal standpoint, considerations such as uterine anomalies or placental position may complicate the surgical approach. From the fetal standpoint, it is important to consider viability, the degree of airway anomaly, and presence of morphological or genetic abnormalities. Maternal and fetal factors drastically impact perinatal mortality regardless of the success of the EXIT procedure. In the case of a twin or multiple gestation pregnancy, performance of an EXIT procedure on the affected fetus places the otherwise healthy, nonindex fetus at increased risk for a preterm delivery. In such situation, there should be a low threshold for involvement of an independent ethics consultation.

Performance of a successful EXIT procedure requires a multispecialty, collaborative effort and organization. Strategic location of equipment and personnel in the operating room is essential. Figure 26.4 highlights our institution's operating room setup for an EXIT to airway procedure. This arrangement maximizes our operating room area and allows each key personnel adequate access to the mother and the fetus. The anesthesiologist caring for the mother has a direct visual path of the surgical field and can anticipate next steps, while maintaining situational awareness. The pediatric anesthesiologist and ENT surgeon can work simultaneously and access critical equipment and medications from their respective trays conveniently placed nearby.

During the preoperative period, a comprehensive maternal history and physical examination, subspecialty consultations, and consents are obtained. The mother should be prepared for the extensive amount of equipment and staff members whose presence may be needed in the OR for a successful EXIT procedure (see Figure 26.5).

Preparation of equipment and medications for the fetus should include a sterile pulse oximetry probe, stethoscope, end tidal CO_2 indicator, manual resuscitation bag, supplies for intravenous catheter placement (with the Penrose drain tubes utilized as a tourniquet), saline flushes, and tape (see Figures 26.6A–C). Fetal medications should be drawn in syringes and adjusted by weight for both intravenous and intramuscular administration. Crystalloids, albumin and O negative, leukocyte reduced, and CMV negative blood product should be available in the operating room for emergency fetal resuscitation. After a proper operating room preparation a multidisciplinary pre-procedure briefing with the entire surgical team is useful to review and discuss final plans.

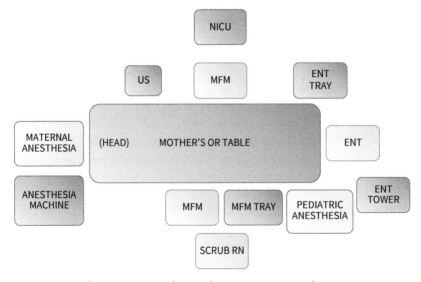

Figure 26.4 Suggested operating room layout during an EXIT procedure.

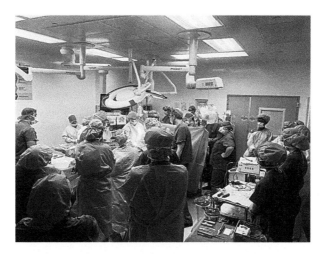

Figure 26.5 Team members and equipment during an EXIT procedure.

(A)

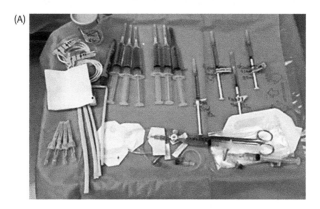

Figure 26.6A Equipment and medications prepared for the fetus.

(B)

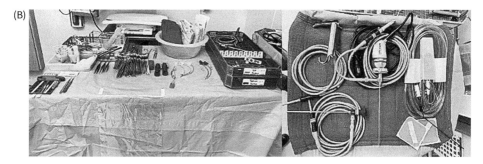

Figure 26.6B Airway equipment for the fetus.

(C)

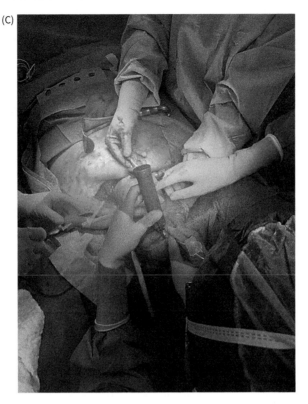

Figure 26.6C Anesthesia obtains IV access while an otolaryngologist secures the airway with intubation.

Once the mother arrives in the operating room, she is positioned in the left lateral tilt allowing for uterine displacement. Standard ASA monitors are applied. The mother's abdomen is prepped and draped as the anesthesia team ensures effective preoxygenation. Sterile ultrasonography is performed to confirm the position of the fetus and placenta and to assess for polyhydramnios before incision. Anesthesia management and considerations are discussed further in the chapter. When the uterine incision is performed, the fetus' head, a single shoulder and upper extremity are delivered. Delivery is limited in this manner to maintain thermoregulation and reduce the risk of umbilical cord and placenta compromise. A sterile pulse oximetry is applied to the delivered fetal hand or wrist; however, thick vernix often delays or makes it difficult to obtain an accurate oxygen saturation and heart rate readings. Therefore, palpation of the umbilical cord is performed for assessment of an abnormal fetal heart rate. A pediatric anesthesiologist is prepared to obtain an upper extremity intravenous or intraosseous access. Care should be taken to maintain uterine distension with amnioinfusion of warm saline and to avoid complete fetal delivery. Suppression of fetal respiratory effort and movement is achieved with intramuscular or intravenous administration of fentanyl and neuromuscular blocking agents. A definite airway, resection of a lesion or ECMO is completed while maintaining uteroplacental blood flow to the fetus.[10] At our institution, we have developed an algorithm for EXIT to airway procedures (see Figure 26.7).

The goal of airway management is to establish adequate patency or securement of the fetus's airway. Direct laryngoscopy is performed by the otolaryngologist to determine if

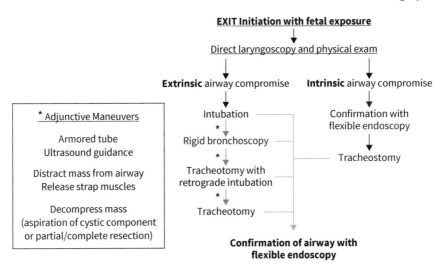

Figure 26.7 EXIT procedure algorithm.

orotracheal intubation is possible. There are many useful adjunct maneuvers that can be employed to increase the success of an orotracheal intubation (see Box 26.1). During this exam, exposure of the larynx and patency of the airway are assessed (see Figure 26.8A). A zero-degree rigid telescope may aid with visualization if necessary. If the airway is patent and larynx adequately exposed, the neonate is intubated, and placement of the endotracheal tube is confirmed (see Figure 26.8B).

If an endotracheal tube cannot be directly placed, intubation can also be performed over an airway exchange catheter. If necessary, rigid bronchoscopy may be performed to further visualize the airway. Ventilation can be carried out through the bronchoscope if the intubation was unsuccessful. An alternative to a failed endotracheal intubation is a tracheostomy with or without a bronchoscope in place or retrograde intubation. Orotracheal intubation is the preferred method of airway establishment since neonatal tracheostomy has a higher risk of complications.[21,23] While uteroplacental circulation has been maintained for up to 2.5 hours, expeditious establishment of an airway minimizes risk to both the mother and fetus, with a goal of less than 30 minutes if possible.[20] Once the airway is secured, the fetus is fully delivered and transferred to the NICU team for further management (see Figure 26.9).

Box 26.1 Adjunct Maneuvers for Successful Fetal or Neonatal Intubation During EXIT Procedures

---

Adjunct maneuvers
Armored endotracheal tube
Ultrasound guidance
Displacement or elevation of neck mass
Division of the strap muscles
Alleviation of extrinsic compression (partial/complete resection or via aspiration of cystic
    component)

(A)

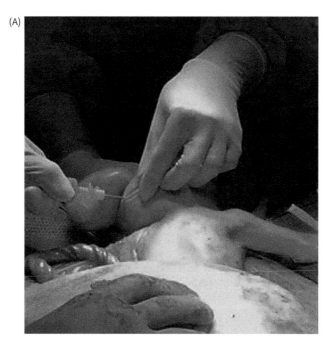

Figure 26.8A Adjunct maneuvers, such as aspiration of large cystic components, may aid in intubation.

(B)

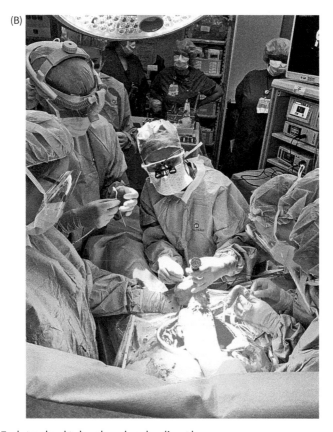

Figure 26.8B Endotracheal tube placed under direct laryngoscopy.

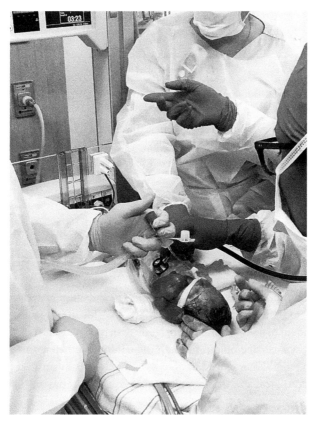

Figure 26.9 Fully-delivered neonate under NICU team care.

Anesthesia Management and Considerations for EXIT Procedures

EXIT procedures may be performed under general and/or neuraxial anesthesia. The preparation and technique for induction of general anesthesia and endotracheal intubation follow the same steps as a general anesthetic for cesarean delivery. However, there are some differences to take into considerations (see Table 26.6). An orogastric tube should be passed to decompress the mother's stomach. Anesthesia is maintained with inhalational agents at a minimum alveolar concentration of greater than 2. It is important to deeply anesthetize the mother and provide adequate uterine relaxation. Appropriate time for uteroplacental transfer of inhaled anesthetic occurs in approximately 10–15 minutes.[24] Supplemental intravenous or sublingual nitroglycerine may be utilized to enhance placental perfusion and surgical exposure. Both inhalational agents and nitroglycerine have a vasodilator effect, therefore intravenous fluid resuscitation along with vasoactive medication such as phenylephrine, ephedrine, and/or norepinephrine should be used to support maternal blood pressure. Once the fetus if fully delivered and cord clamped, reversal of uterine relaxation must promptly occur. Volatile agents should be decreased to less than 0.5 MAC and nitrous oxide may be initiated.[4,17] First-line uterotonic agents are administered and second-line uterotonics may be added as needed.

In a hemodynamically stable mother, we prefer converting to a total intravenous anesthetic technique and utilizing the epidural catheter intraoperatively. At the completion of

Table 26.6 Differences Between Cesarean Delivery and EXIT Surgery Under General Anesthesia[1,3]

EXIT procedure	Cesarean delivery
Prolonged maternal and fetal exposure to volatile agents	General anesthesia is induced after parturient is prepped and draped and surgical team ready for incision
Depressed fetus due with expected definite airway and postdelivery ventilation	Maternal medication is reduced in order to minimize anesthetic agent exposure and fetal depression
Desired uterine relaxation to preserve uteroplacental blood flow and gas exchange	Uterine relaxation increases risk of uterine atony
Increased risk for surgical site infection due to duration	Quick delivery of the fetus
Increased risk for blood loss and maternal hemorrhage	Technically common surgery

the case, extubating the mother is ideal if she meets extubation criteria. In the immediate postoperative period, the mother is frequently assessed for uterine atony and postpartum bleeding. It is prudent to use multimodal analgesia with medications such as acetaminophen, long-acting preservative-free opioid through the epidural catheter, and parenteral opioids for breakthrough pain. Other considerations for refractory post surgical pain management include a continuous local anesthetic epidural infusion, opioid based IV-PCA, and bilateral TAP blocks.

Conclusion/Summary

Fetal intervention essentially leads to the performance of two surgeries on two different patients under one operative encounter. The mother receives no immediate physical benefits from the surgical procedure but, depending on successful outcome of the surgery, fetal morbidity and mortality can be significantly reduced. Planning and execution of fetal surgeries relies on multidisciplinary expertise, teamwork, and good communication. Contingency plans and arrangements are crucial for the safety of both patients. Both patients have specific surgical and anesthetic needs that must be considered. Surgical approach to fetal surgery depends on the type of congenital anomaly requiring correction, and selection criteria. Minimally invasive techniques are reserved for procedures in which the needle enters the uterus only or advances further to contact the placenta, umbilical vessels, or fetus. In this case, the fetus requires no surgical incision, whereas in open fetal surgery, the surgical procedure is performed directly on the fetus and occurs midgestation. The fetus is not immediately delivered after the open fetal procedure is performed. Cesarean delivery of the fetus occurs at a predetermined date closer to or at term gestation. The mother is counseled against any future trial of labor and attempts at vaginal delivery. Fetuses who require an EXIT procedure are at increased risk of neonatal death at birth when separated from maternal circulation. These fetuses may undergo either an EXIT procedure to secure an airway, resect a lesion, or receive ECMO therapy. Anesthesia for fetal surgery also depends on the planned procedure, surgical needs, maternal and fetal considerations (see Table 26.7).

Table 26.7 Surgical Approach and Anesthesia Management for Fetal Procedures

Types of fetal procedures	MIS		Open	EXIT
Surgical approach	Needle entering uterus only	Needle touches the fetus or umbilical vessels	Surgical procedures directly on the fetus	Surgery/procedure directly on fetus
Examples	Amniocentesis	PUBS/TTTS/ TRAP/Paracentesis/ thoracentesis/shunts	NTD (Myelomeningocele repair)	EXIT to airway EXIT to resection EXIT to ECMO
Delivery plan	Vaginal vs. cesarean per maternal and fetal indications	Vaginal vs. cesarean per maternal and fetal indications	2 cesareans (open procedure and fetal delivery at term)	Cesarean
Anesthesia type	Not required vs. IV anxiolytic/ analgesic	MAC vs. neuraxial	GETA	GETA or/and regional
Special considerations	Minimal risks compared to open and EXIT fetal surgery	Uterine relaxation Emergent delivery of preterm fetus	Uterine relaxation Emergent delivery of preterm fetus Closure of the uterus Preterm delivery Tocolysis Postsurgical pain management	Uterine relaxation Maternal hemodynamic stability Uterine atony Postsurgical pain management

Regardless of the planned anesthetic, maternal and fetal cardiovascular stability, maintenance of placental blood flow with uterine relaxation (if required), fetal immobility and analgesia, and prompt reversal of uterine relaxation are of utmost importance. Advancements in training and experience, along with new technological innovations, hold a promise for the future of fetal interventions. As the risks to the expectant mother is reduced with newer and less invasive surgical techniques, there is potential for further growth in the field.

Abbreviations

ASA—American Society of Anesthesiologists
CCAM—congenital cystic adenomatoid malformation
CDH—congenital diaphragmatic hernia
CHAOS—congenital high airway obstruction
CMV—cytomegalo virus
DM—diabetes
ECMO—extracorporeal membrane oxygenation
ENT—ear nose and throat
ETT—endotracheal tube
EXIT—ex utero intrapartum

GA—gestational age
GETA—general endotracheal anesthesia
HIV—human immunodeficiency virus
HTN—hypertension
IM—intramuscular
IO—intraosseous
IV—intravascular
L+D—labor and delivery
LUD—left uterine displacement
MAC—minimum alveolar concentration
MFM—maternal fetal medicine
MIFS—minimally invasive fetal surgery
MIS—minimally invasive surgery
MMC—myelomeningocele
MOMS—myelomeningocele study
NDMBD—non-depolarizing muscle blockage drugs
NTD—neural tube defect
NPO—Nil per os
NSAID—nonsteroidal drug
OR—operating room
PCA—patient controlled analgesia
PO—per os
PROM— premature rupture of membranes
RN—registered nurse
SLE—systemic lupus erythromatosus
SQ—subcutaneous
TIVA—total intravenous anesthesia
US—ultrasound
USG—ultrasound guided
UVC—umbilical cord vein

References

1. Van de Velde M, De Buck F, Fetal and maternal analgesia/anesthesia for fetal procedures. *Fetal Diagnosis and Therapy*. 2012;31:201–209.
2. Spinner S, Miesnik S, Koh J, Howell L. Maternal, fetal, and neonatal care in open fetal surgery for myelomeningocele. *JCOGN*. 2012;41:447–454.
3. Bence C, Wagner A. Ex utero intrapartum treatment (EXIT) procedures. *Semin Pediatr Surg*. 2018;28:4.
4. Radic J, Illes J, McDonald P. Fetal repair of open neural tube defects: ethical, legal, and social issues. *Cambridge Quarterly of Healthcare Ethics*. 2019;28:476–487.
5. Bouchard S, Johnson M, Flake A. The EXIT procedure: experience and outcome in 31 cases. *Journal of Pediatric Surgery*. 2002;37(3):418–426.
6. Dewan M, Wellons J. Fetal surgery for spina bifida. *Journal of Neurosurgery Pediatric*. 2019;24(2):105–215.

7. Masahata K, Soh H, Tachibana K, et al. Clinical outcomes of ex utero intrapartum treatment for fetal airway obstruction. *Pediatr Surg Int.* 2019;35(8):835–843.

8. Moron AF, Barbosa MM, Milani HFJ, et al. Perinatal outcomes after open fetal surgery for myelomeningocele repair: a retrospective cohort study. *An International Journal of Obstetrics and Gynaecology.* 2018;125(10):1280–1286.

9. Cortes S, Davila I, Torres P, et al. Does fetoscopic or open repair for spina bifida affect fetal and postnatal growth? *Ultrasound Obstet Gynecol.* 2019;53(3):314–323.

10. Dinghe M, Peterson S, Dubinsky T, et al. EXIT procedure: technique and indications with prenatal imaging parameters for assessment of airway patency. *RadioGraphics.* 2011;31(2):511–526.

11. De Buck F, Deprest J, Van De Velde M. Anesthesia for fetal surgery. *Current Opinion in Anaesthesiology.* 2008;21(3):293–297.

12. Hirose S, Farmer DL, Lee H, Nobuhara KK, Harrison MR. The ex utero intrapartum treatment procedure: Looking back at the EXIT. *J Pediatr Surg.* 2004;39(3):375–380.

13. Kahr MK, Winder F, Vonzun L, et al. Risk factors for preterm birth following open fetal myelomeningocele repair: results from a prospective cohort. *Fetal Diagnosis and Therapy.* 2020;47(1):15–23.

14. Marwan A, Crombleholme TM. The EXIT procedure: principles, pitfalls, and progress. *Semin Pediatr Surg.* 2006;15(2):107–115.

15. Pucher B, Szdlowski J, Jonczyk-Potoczna K, Srocyznski J. The EXIT (ex-utero intrapartum treatment) procedure—from the paediatric ENT perspective. *Acta Otorhinolaryngol Ital.* 2018;38(5):480–484.

16. Schwarz U, Galinkin J. Anesthesia for fetal surgery. *Semin Pediatr Surg.* 2003;12(3):196–201.

17. Lapa DA. Endoscopic fetal surgery for neural tube defects. *Best Practice & Research Clinical Obstetrics and Gynaecology.* 2019;58:133–141.

18. Roby BB, Scott AR, Sidman JD, Lander TA, Tibesar RJ. Complete peripartum airway management of a large epignathus teratoma: EXIT to resection. *International Journal of Pediatric Otorhinolaryngology.* 2011;75(1):716–719.

19. Garcia P, Olutoye O, Ivey R, et al. Case scenario: anesthesia for maternal-fetal surgery: the ex-utero intrapartum therapy (EXIT) procedure. *Anesthesiology.* 2011;114(6):1446–1452.

20. Hartnick CJ, Barth WH Jr, Cote CJ, Albrecht MA, Grant PE, Geyer JT. Case records of the Massachusetts General Hospital. Case 7-2009. A pregnant woman with a large mass in the fetal oral cavity. *N Engl J Med.* 2009;360(9):913–921.

21. Walz PC, Schroeder JW. Prenatal diagnosis of obstructive head and neck masses and perinatal airway management. *Otolaryngologic Clinics of North America.* 2015;48(1):191–207.

22. Nolan HR, Gurria J, Peiro JL, et al. Congenital high airway obstruction syndrome (CHAOS): natural history, prenatal management strategies, and outcomes at a single comprehensive fetal center. *J Pediatr Surg.* 2019;54(6):1153–1158.

23. Hirose S., Sydorak R.M., Tsao K., et al. Spectrum of intrapartum management strategies for giant fetal cervical teratoma. *J Pediatr Surg.* 2003;38:446–450.

24. Bechtel A, Sheeran J. Placental transfer: anesthetic drugs [video]. *OpenAnesthesia: Keys to the Cart.* https://keywords.selfstudy.app/placental-transfer-anesth-drugs/. Accessed Nov 1, 2019.

27

Anesthesia and Assisted Reproductive Techniques

Nora Martin, Fadi Farah, and Shamantha Reddy

Background

In the United States, infertility affects 7.5 million women and 1 in 8 couples. Over 5 million children have been conceived by assisted reproductive techniques (ART), which is approximately 1.6% of children.[1] In vitro fertilization (IVF) candidates are typically women with chronic tubal disease, inadequate oocyte quality or quantity, uterine abnormalities, or other comorbidities.[2] ART may also be an avenue for men who have sperm deficiencies or genetic aberrations in couples.[2] The estimated cost is $12,500 for each IVF cycle and $41,100 for each live birth.[3] Anesthesia providers must be aware of the effects anesthetics have on gametes or embryos to optimize the outcomes.[2] ART is a four-step process (see Figure 27.1).

In Vitro Fertilization Process

Step 1: Hormonal Stimulation: A gonadotropin-releasing hormone (GnRH) agonist is administered by fertility specialists.[4] GnRH agonists bind to estrogen receptors and the body believes that the estrogen levels are low.[5] Subsequently, the body increases the levels of follicular stimulating hormone (FSH) and luteinizing hormone (LH). These hormones encourage the development of mature follicles. Human menopausal gonadotropin (hMG) is a medication composed of FSH and LH. Together, endogenous FSH and hMG are used to promote the maturity of multiple ovarian follicles. Human chorionic gonadotropin (hCG) is added to facilitate oocyte removal from the follicular wall. Usually 10–15 oocytes are generated. Due to the pituitary suppression, progesterone is used daily to build the corpus luteum.[2]

Step 2: Oocyte Retrieval (OoR): Retrieval occurs within 24–36 hours after hCG administration. Transvaginal ultrasonography is used to visualize the ovarian follicles (see Figure 27.2). A needle attached to the transvaginal ultrasound (US) is used to penetrate the vaginal fornix and aspirate the mature follicles. Laparoscopic retrieval is now reserved for oocytes that are immediately transferred to the fallopian tubes. Once the oocytes are removed, their meiotic stage is determined based upon nuclear and cytoplasmic morphology (see Figure 27.3).

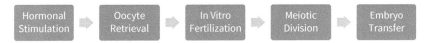

Figure 27.1 In vitro fertilization steps.

Step 3: In Vitro Fertilization and Meiotic Division: Oocytes are transferred to the spermatozoa in culture media and incubated for insemination to occur (Figure 27.2). After 16–20 hours, the oocytes are examined to see if fertilization occurred. Sometimes intracytoplasmic injection is used to assist the penetration of sperm.[2,4] The embryos divide for about 3 days and are transferred to the uterus (Figures 27.4 and 27.5). If a patient does not choose to transfer the embryos, they are frozen in 1,2 propanediol or glycerol for transfer at another time.[2,4,5]

Step 4: Embryo Transfer: The transcervical transfer (TCT) entails transferring the embryos to the uterine cavity under US guidance (Figure 27.6). This is performed without anesthesia. It is considered a standard of care for embryo transfer because it reduces the uterine contractility, which can cause embryo expulsion.[6] Potential TCT harmful adverse effects include introduction of microorganism into the uterus, prostaglandin release, and reflux of embryos.[7] TCT may not suffice for women with cervical stenosis and distortions.[6] In these cases, the transvaginal-transmyometrial embryo transfer method can be used. A needle loaded with the embryos is inserted in the middle of endometrial layer under transvaginal ultrasound guidance.[7]

Gamete or zygotic intrafallopian embryo transfers (GIFT, ZIFT): Although these methods yield higher pregnancy success, they are rarely used as they require the use of laparoscopic interventions.[6] In GIFT, mature oocytes are transferred into a catheter with sperm, then injected 3–6 cm from the fallopian tubes. Fertilization occurs in vivo and cannot be documented. In ZIFT, embryos in the pronuclear phase are transferred to the distal portion of the fallopian tube laparoscopically. ZIFT is a two-day process in which the oocytes are retrieved transvaginally, fertilized, and transferred laparoscopically the following day.

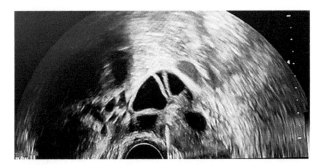

Figure 27.2 US image of the ovarian follicles.

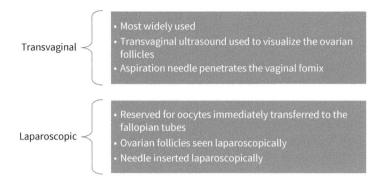

| Transvaginal | • Most widely used
• Transvaginal ultrasound used to visualize the ovarian follicles
• Aspiration needle penetrates the vaginal fornix |
| Laparoscopic | • Reserved for oocytes immediately transferred to the fallopian tubes
• Ovarian follicles seen laparoscopically
• Needle inserted laparoscopically |

Figure 27.3 Comparison between Transvaginal and Laparoscopic Approaches for Oocyte Retrieval.

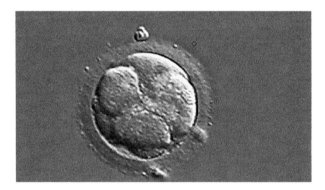

Figure 27.4 Embryonic Day 3-2.

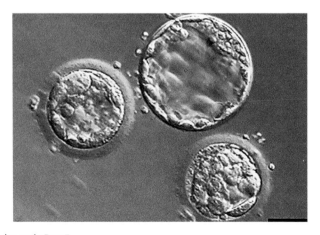

Figure 27.5 Embryonic Day 5.

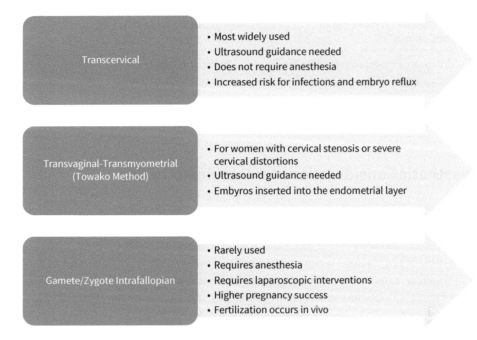

Figure 27.6 Comparison between Embryo Transfer Modalities.

Complications of Art

Ovarian Hyperstimulation Syndrome and Anesthetic Management

Ovarian hyperstimulation syndrome (OHSS) occurs when the ovaries produce prostaglandins and stimulate the renin-angiotensin system, leading to increased capillary permeability. This causes edema, ovarian enlargement, ascites, hydrothorax, anasarca, and pulmonary edema.[8] Patients afflicted with OHSS who require surgical intervention are considered full stomach due to ascites, nausea, and vomiting. Rapid-sequence induction is necessary for endotracheal intubation for airway protection. Ketamine is appropriate for induction and maintenance since these patients may be hypotensive. Monitoring of fluid status with an arterial line or central venous pressure may be indicated since these patients are intravascularly depleted.[8] Point-of-care US is helpful in determining the fluid status prior to induction. Due to increased capillary permeability, there may be altered pharmacokinetics of the anesthetics administered.[8] Paracentesis or thoracentesis for ascites before general anesthesia (GA) to optimize respiratory reserve should be considered.

Fetal Complications due to ART[1,9]	Maternal Complications due to ART[1,2,10,11]
• Low birth weight (LBW)	• Hypertensive disorders of pregnancy
• Preterm delivery	• Placental abruption/previa
• Congenital anomalies	• Cesarean deliveries
• Imprinting disorders	• Gestational diabetes (GDM)
• Neurodevelopmental disorders	• Ectopic pregnancies
	• Hypercoagulability

Transvaginal Oocyte Retrieval Complications[10, 12]	Laparoscopic Oocyte Retrieval and GIFT Complications[2]
• Hemorrhage/intraperitoneal Bleeding	• Hemoperitoneum
• Perforation	• Syncope
• Pelvic infection	• Nausea/vomiting
• Adnexal torsions	• Bowel injury

Anesthetic Considerations for Oocyte Retrieval

A safe anesthetic plan for OoR provides pain control, minimizes nausea and vomiting, facilitates quick recovery, and is nontoxic to oocytes.[13,14] Preoperatively, a review of systems to determine comorbidities and of medications including herbal medications should be completed to plan the anesthetic.[15] NPO status should be ascertained. A physical exam including cardiovascular, respiratory, neurologic, musculoskeletal, and airway exam must be documented along with baseline vital signs, pertinent labs and diagnostic tests (Figure 27.7).

Monitored Anesthesia Care

The painful and anxiety-provoking vaginal fornix penetration with the aspiration needle necessitates anesthesia. Monitored anesthesia care (MAC) is commonly used for OoR in the US and the UK.[16,17] MAC allows for faster recovery times (90 to 120 min), and is more cost effective than GA. MAC is performed with midazolam and/or propofol with fentanyl.

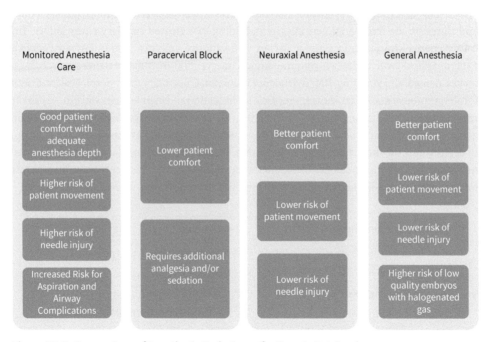

Figure 27.7 Comparison of Anesthetic Techniques for Oocyte Retrieval.

They are all considered safe for OoR (Box 27.1); however, these medications depress the respiratory drive.[13] Sedatives that do not cause respiratory depression such as ketamine and

---

Box 27.1 Common Anesthetics Used and the Effects on the In Vitro Fertilization Process

---

Local Anesthetics
- Found in fluid after PCB, but safe

Thiopental
- Safe alternative to propofol, but found in oocyte follicular fluid

Midazolam
- Found in follicular fluid, but safe and commonly used in MAC

Propofol
- Propofol found in the follicular fluid is related to the dose and the duration of administration. No differences in fertilization, cleavage, and embryo cell number

Opioids
- Fentanyl, alfentanil, remifentanil, meperidine have not been associated with fertilization or pregnancy issue for women undergoing ART
- Fentanyl and alfentanil can be found in the follicular fluid at low levels after IV administration, but no differences in fertilization or pregnancy rates were seen
- Remifentanil appeared to be superior to fentanyl in terms of pregnancy rate in MAC case

Ketamine
- Not reported to have toxic effects in the ART when used as an alternative for GA

Etomidate
- Not reported to have toxic effects in the ART when used as an alternative for GA

Dexmedetomidine
- Does not depress the respiratory drive and has analgesic properties
- Dexmedetomidine infusion provided greater patient satisfaction than midazolam for conscious sedation
- More risk of hypotension and bradycardia

Nitrous Oxide
- Nitrous oxide influences DNA synthesis in animals and humans, reducing methionine synthetase activity
- No issues were found with nitrous oxide use in ART because it has low blood solubility which allows for brief exposure and not enough time for harmful effects to take place in humans

Halogenated Volatiles
- Yields low quality oocytes
- Volatile anesthetic can increase risk of nausea, vomiting and unplanned admission
- Sevoflurane can produce compound A that is possibly genotoxic to ovarian cells
- Enflurane has been associated with increased levels of prolactin, which may suppress FSH and LH

Non-Opioid Analgesics
- Ketorolac does not affect pregnancy rates

Anti-Emetics
- Dopamine antagonists should be avoided because they are associated with hyperprolactinemia and impairment of ovarian follicle maturation and corpus luteum formation
- 5HT-3 antagonists such as granisetron or ondansetron are safe.

dexmedetomidine are also safe for OoR.[2,13,14] However, the disadvantage of using MAC is maintaining an appropriate level of anesthesia and immobility. MAC can lead to a higher hospital admission rate after OoR compared to GA due to inadvertent needle placement and intra-abdominal bleeding.[2,14] A higher number of embryos are retrieved with GA (remifentanil with propofol or isoflurane) than with MAC (midazolam, diazepam, or propofol)[14] due to increased patient comfort.

MAC with midazolam and ketamine versus GA with fentanyl, propofol, and isoflurane did not show any differences in the oocyte quality, number, or the pregnancy rate.[14] One study showed that MAC with remifentanil yielded higher pregnancy rates than with GA (alfentanil, propofol, nitrous oxide, isoflurane) and the quality of oocytes remained unchanged with remifentanil administration.[14,17] Studies have failed to consistently prove whether GA or MAC had better outcomes for pregnancy rates. A review article mentioned five studies that showed a lower pregnancy rate when ART is done under GA compared to MAC while two other studies showed no difference between GA and MAC.[14]

Paracervical Blocks

In addition to MAC, paracervical blocks (PCBs) can be utilized for OoR. Patients undergoing PCB for OoR require additional pain medication due to incomplete blockade of the vaginal and ovarian nerves. A nonrandomized prospective cohort study showed that the live births were similar between the GA versus PCB groups.[14,18] However, the vaginal pain experienced by the PCB group was greater than the GA group. Ten percent of the PCB patients required additional analgesia. Patient satisfaction and the number of mature oocytes retrieved were greater in the GA group. Smaller, immature follicles are more likely to be obtained with the use of GA.[18] Lidocaine can be found in the follicular fluid, but it is safe to use.[14] A case-controlled study looking at GA with propofol compared to PCB did not show any differences in fertilization rates, embryo cleavages, rates of development, or implantation.[19] Researchers compared the pain scores and the number of oocytes retrieved by PCB to lidocaine vaginal gel.[6] The number of oocytes retrieved was similar in both groups. However, the pain scores were higher in the vaginal lidocaine gel group.

General Anesthesia

GA is reserved for women at risk for aspiration who did not abide by the fasting guidelines. In this case, administration of a nonparticulate antacid and GA with rapid-sequence induction should be considered. Total intravenous anesthesia with propofol can be used to maintain anesthesia.[2] Volatile anesthetics increase the risk of nausea, vomiting, and unplanned hospital admission. Nausea and vomiting can be treated with 5-HT3 antagonists, but dopaminergic antagonists such as metoclopramide and droperidol should be avoided.[2] Although studies suggest that GA can yield a higher number of oocytes, the embryo quality may differ when halogenated anesthetics are used. A study showed that anesthesia with sevoflurane had lower percentage of good embryos.[14,20] Sevoflurane can produce compound A that is possibly genotoxic to ovarian cells, and isoflurane may negatively impact embryo development.[2] In other animal studies, isoflurane and nitrous oxide have toxic effects on ART.[14] Halogenated anesthetics have been shown to depress DNA synthesis and mitosis, resulting in abnormal cleavage.[2] They also reduce reproductive success.[2,4] More human studies are needed to further elucidate whether halogenated anesthetics can negatively impact the ART.

Neuraxial Anesthesia

Epidural and spinal anesthesia provide pain control with minimal oocyte exposure to anesthetic agents. Fewer complications are seen with neuraxial anesthesia (NA) compared to MAC with propofol. Spinal is preferred over epidural due to a decreased risk of anesthesia failure, lower systemic and follicular concentrations of the anesthetic agent, and faster recovery time. Using a less concentrated form of hyperbaric lidocaine leads to shorter recovery time. Incorporation of intrathecal fentanyl with hyperbaric lidocaine helps with pain control without causing urinary retention and delayed discharge time as seen with the use of bupivacaine. Although lidocaine is useful for short procedures like OoR, it is associated with transient neurologic syndrome. NA has not been found to affect fertilization rate of ART success.[14] Two studies showed that there was an advantage of increased pregnancy rates with spinal anesthesia over GA.[14,21] Vasopressor agents should be readily available if NA is utilized for evidence of a sympathectomy.

Anesthesia For Laparoscopic Art

GIFT or ZIFT is completed with laparoscopy under GA. In most cases, care is coordinated such that the patient is anesthetized once for both retrieval and transfer, if possible. Oocytes are exposed to carbon dioxide and anesthetic agents. Pelvic laparoscopy completed with GA entails the use of propofol, lidocaine, fentanyl, and muscle relaxant for induction followed by intubation and maintenance with halogenated agent or propofol/nitrous oxide. The combination of propofol/nitrous oxide for maintenance resulted in less emesis, lower pain scores, and quicker recovery compared to isoflurane/nitrous oxide for maintenance.[2] If the intraperitoneal pressures are less than 10 mm Hg, pelvic laparoscopy can also be completed with NA in nonobese patients.[2] Laparoscopy requires the Trendelenburg position, which leads to increased mean arterial pressure, increased central venous pressure, increased systemic vascular resistance, decreased stroke volume, and decreased cardiac output. To minimize the risk of brachial plexus nerve injury, it is important to keep the arms abducted less than 90 degrees and to pad all pressure points.[2]

References

1. Sullivan-Pyke CS, Senapati S, Mainigi MA, Barnhart KT. In vitro fertilization and adverse obstetric and perinatal outcomes. *Semin Perinatol.* 2017;41(6):345–353.
2. Chestnut, DH. *Chestnut's obstetric anesthesia: principles and practice.* 6th ed. Philadelphia, PA: Elsevier/Saunders, 2019.

3. Katz P, Showstack J, Smith JF. Costs of infertility treatment: results from an 18-month prospective cohort study. *Fertil Steril.* 2011;95(3):915–921.

4. Van De Velde, M. Anesthesia for in-vitro fertilization. *Current Opinion in Anesthesiology.* 2005;18(4):428–430. doi:10.1097/01.aco.0000168330.04229.c7.

5. Derksen L, Tournaye H, Stoop D, Van Vaerenbergh I, Bourgain C, Polyzos P, Haentjens P, Blockeel C. Impact of clomiphene citrate during ovarian stimulation on the luteal phase after GnRH agonist trigger. *Reproductive BioMedicine Online.* 2014;28(3):359–368.

6. Sullivan-Pyke CS, Kort DH, Sauer MV, Douglas NC. Successful pregnancy following assisted reproduction and transmyometrial embryo transfer in a patient with anatomical distortion of the cervical canal. *Systems Biology in Reproductive Medicine.* 2014;60(4):234–238. doi:10.3109/19396368.2014.917386.

7. Kato O. Transvaginal-transmyometrial embryo transfer: the Towako method; experiences of 104 cases. *Fertility and Sterility.* 1993;59(1):51–53.

8. Reed A, Tausk H, Reynolds H. Anesthetic considerations for severe ovarian hyperstimulation syndrome. *Anesthesiology.* 1990;73(6):1275–1276.

9. Wisborg K, Ingerslev HJ, Henriksen TB. In vitro fertilization and preterm delivery, low birth weight, and admission to the neonatal intensive care unit: a prospective follow-up study. *Fertility and Sterility.* 2010;94(6):2102–2106. doi.org/10.1016/j.fertnstert.2010.01.014.

10. Allahbadia G. Complications of IVF. *Journal of Obstetrics and Gynecology of India.* 2010;60:297–298. doi10.1007/s13224-010-0045-9.

11. Ashrafi M, Gosili R, Hosseini R, Arabpoor A, Ahmadi J, Chehrazi M. Risk of GDM mellitus in patients undergoing assisted reproductive techniques. *European Journal of Obstetrics and Gynecology and Reproductive Biology.* 2014;176:149–152. https://doi.org/10.1016/j.ejogrb.2014.02.009.

12. Ludwig AK, Glawatz M, Griesinger G, Ludwig M. Perioperative and post-operative complications of transvaginal ultrasound-guided OoR: prospective study of >1000 OoRs. *Human Reproduction.* 2006;21(12):3235–3240. https://doi.org/10.1093/humrep/del278.

13. Demiraran Y, Korkut E, Tamer A, et al. The comparison of dexmedetomidine and midazolam used for sedation of patients during upper endoscopy: A prospective, randomized study. *Can J Gastroenterol.* 2007;21(1):25–29. doi:10.1155/2007/350279.

14. Matsota P, Kaminioti E, Kostopanagiotou G. Anesthesia related toxic effects on in vitro fertilization outcome: burden of proof. *Biomed Res Int.* 2015;2015:475362. doi:10.1155/2015/475362.

15. Shannon J, El Saigh I, Tadrous R, Mocanu E, Loughrey J. Usage of herbal medications in patients undergoing IVF treatment in an Irish infertility treatment unit. *Irish Journal of Medical Science.* 2009;179(1):63–65. doi:10.1007/s11845-009-0378-5.

16. Ditkoff, EC, Plumb, J, Selick, A, Sauer, MV. Anesthesia practices in the United States common to in vitro fertilization (IVF) centers. *J Assist Reprod Genet.* 1997;14:145–147. doi:10.1007/bf02766130.

17. Jain D, Kohli A, Gupta L. Bhadoria P, Anand R. Anaesthesia for in vitro fertilization. *Indian journal of anaesthesia.* 2009;53(4):408–413.

18. Rolland L, Perrin J, Villes V, Pellegrin V. IVF OoR: prospective evaluation of the type of anesthesia on live birth rate, pain, and patient satisfaction. *Journal of Assisted Reproduction and Genetics.* 2017;34:1–6. doi:10.1007/s10815-017-1002-7.

19. Christiaens F, Janssenswillen C, Van Steirteghem AC, Devroey P, Verborgh C, Camu F. Comparison of assisted reproductive technology performance after OoR under general

anaesthesia (propofol) versus paracervical local anaesthetic block: a case-controlled study. *Human Reproduction.* 1998;13(9):2456–2460. https://doi.org/10.1093/humrep/13.9.2456.

20. Piroli, A, Marci R, Marinangeli F, Paladini A, Di Emidio, Artini P, Caserta D, Tatone C. Comparison of different anaesthetic methodologies for sedation during in vitro fertilization procedures: effects on patient physiology and oocyte competence. *Gynecological endocrinology: the official journal of the International Society of Gynecological Endocrinology.* 2012;28:796–799. doi:10.3109/09513590.2012.664193.

21. Azmude A, Agha'amou S, Yousefshahi F, et al. Pregnancy outcome using general anesthesia versus spinal anesthesia for in vitro fertilization. *Anesth Pain Med.* 2013;3(2):239–242.

28

Medicolegal Issues in Obstetric Anesthesia

Samuel Onyewu and Fatoumata Kromah

Introduction

James Young Simpson is considered to be the father of obstetric anesthesia. In 1847, Dr. Simpson administered chloroform for labor analgesia, and then in 1850 he utilized ether as an anesthetic for labor pain.[1] At the time the effect of ether on labor and the fetus was unknown, albeit it was proven to be effective.[1] Thus ether analgesia was met with opposition from religious proponents who had strong societal influence. Ether analgesia was believed to be an aberration to religious beliefs, but, patients, feminists, and suffragette groups campaigned for its use.[2] By the early 20th century, morphine and scopolamine were routinely combined to produce twilight sleep, which gained popularity; however, the side effect of neonatal depression led to the discontinuation of twilight sleep.[3] The mid-20th century was fraught with complications associated with cesarean delivery performed under general anesthesia. Complications such as aspiration, aspiration pneumonitis, and failed tracheal intubation led to further research and new developments. Neuraxial labor anesthesia became prominent in the 1980s[4,5] and significantly improved maternal and neonatal outcomes.

Obstetric anesthesia entails the administration and management of analgesia for labor and vaginal delivery. It also includes anesthesia for cesarean delivery, removal of retained placenta and products of conception, and other obstetric procedures. Obstetric anesthesiologists are an integral part of a multidisciplinary team comprised of obstetricians, nurses, neonatologists, and surgeons. The obstetric anesthesiologist is often involved in facilitating interdisciplinary activities aimed at improving maternal and neonatal well-being.[6] Over the years, numerous safety initiatives such as the administration of the epidural test dose, elimination of 0.75% bupivacaine for labor analgesia, and the combination of neuraxial opioids and local anesthetics have been adopted to ensure better safety while maintaining adequate sensory blockade and minimizing motor blockade.[6] Despite the advancements made, obstetric anesthesia is still laden with significant liability claims and is considered to be a high-risk practice for anesthesiologists.[7] Review of closed medicolegal claims and understanding practice guidelines in obstetric anesthesia allow anesthesiologists and team members to safely manage the peripartum care of obstetric patients.

Practice Guidelines in Obstetric Anesthesia

The American Society of Anesthesiologists Task Force on Obstetric Anesthesia and the Society for Obstetric Anesthesia and Perinatology developed recommendations to assist anesthesiologists and patients in making decisions about their health care.[8] The

Table 28.1 Summary of Preanesthetic Evaluation and Preparation

1. History	a. Prior anesthesia exposure and adverse effects
	b. Obstetric history
2. Focused examintion	a. Airway
	b. Lung
	c. Heart
	d. Neurologic
	e. Musculoskeletal—Lumbar Spine
3. Assessment	a. Baseline vital signs
4. Discussion	a. Complications
	b. Risk, benefits, and alternatives
	c. Patient preferences
	d. Anesthetic plan
	e. Consent

recommendations may be modified to address different clinical scenarios. A summary of the practice guidelines for the procedures and emergencies in anesthesia are discussed below (Table 28.1).

Preanesthetic Preparation

Before the provision of anesthesia, a preanesthetic evaluation should be performed. The preanesthesia evaluation should be focused on but should not be limited to the acquisition of the medical history, physical examination, assessment of the risk factors for poor maternal or fetal/neonatal outcome, and, if needed, discussion of concerns with the obstetrician. Possible complications involving anesthetic care and interventions should be discussed with the parturient and documented in a preoperative note and consent form.

Routine platelet count is not a requirement for the healthy parturient. For patients with a known risk factor for coagulation abnormalities, such as preeclampsia or other disease processes that may alter the platelet count or function, it is reasonable to obtain a platelet count, and further coagulation workup if needed.

A type and screen should be obtained when there is a concern for hemorrhage. Most facilities have institutional policies and guidance for ordering blood, type and screen, and crossmatch. For a healthy parturient with an uncomplicated pregnancy, cross matching of blood is not routinely recommended.

During labor, oral intake of clear liquids may be allowed for uncomplicated parturients. Pregnant patients who have risk factors for aspiration (e.g., morbid obesity, gastroparesis, diabetes mellitus, and difficult airway) should avoid oral intake of clear liquids during labor. Clear liquids should be avoided for 2 hours prior to elective cesarean delivery. Solid food should be avoided in laboring parturients. Meanwhile for pregnant patients scheduled for cesarean delivery and other operative obstetric procedures, solid food intake should be restricted for at least 6 to 8 hours. Timely administration of nonparticulate antacids, H2-receptor blockers, and/or metoclopramide should be considered for aspiration prophylaxis in pregnant patients undergoing surgical procedures such as cesarean delivery and postpartum tubal ligation.

Fetal heart rate patterns should be monitored by a qualified individual before and after administration of neuraxial analgesia for labor. Continuous monitoring may not be possible during the performance of a neuraxial procedure. However, inadequate fetal heart rate monitoring for greater than 3–5 minutes is not recommended.

Labor and Vaginal Delivery

Evidence-based research has refuted previous reports associating early neuraxial analgesia with increased duration of labor and cesarean delivery. Early neuraxial analgesia at less than 5 cm cervical dilation is advised for patients undergoing trial of labor after a cesarean delivery. For patients with twin gestation, pre-eclampsia, morbid obesity, and known difficult airway, early neuraxial placement allows the opportunity to extend the epidural analgesia into an anesthetic if an operative delivery is needed.

A single-shot spinal with administration of a combination of an opioid and local anesthetic can provide labor analgesia for the laboring patient with an imminent delivery. An epidural catheter may also be placed if there is a clinical indication that the spinal will not last as long as the surgical procedure. Pencil-point spinal needles are recommended to minimize the risk for postdural puncture headache.

Maintenance of labor analgesia with a continuous epidural infusion has proven to be effective. The addition of opioids to a low-concentration local anesthetic enhances the quality of analgesia and minimizes motor blockade. Patient-controlled epidural analgesia (PCEA) is an effective and flexible technique for maintenance of labor analgesia. A PCEA technique reduces the local anesthetic requirement and is useful with and without a background continuous infusion.

Delivery of retained products of conception (e.g., placenta) can be undertaken with an epidural or other neuraxial anesthetic technique if the parturient is hemodynamically stable. The use of sedation and other analgesic medications may increase the risk for respiratory depression and aspiration. If hemorrhage occurs with hemodynamic instability, general anesthesia is preferred. Nitroglycerin can be administered in incremental doses intravenously or sublingually to help with uterine relaxation. Terbutaline and general anesthesia with halogenated agents are also alternatives. However, careful monitoring and management of the patient's blood pressure is required to maintain appropriate end-organ perfusion assessed by the patient's level of consciousness, urine output, or laboratory findings.

Cesarean Delivery and Other Obstetric Procedures

Cesarean delivery can be performed under either neuraxial or general anesthesia. The decision of neuraxial versus general anesthesia depends on patient risk factors, clinical scenario, allotted time, urgency, and preference. There should be equipment both in the labor and delivery area and operating room to manage possible difficulties, such as failed intubation, hypotension, aspiration or hemorrhage. The anesthetic plan must be one that is tailored to facilitate prompt and safe delivery of the fetus.

Postpartum tubal ligation should follow cesarean delivery guidelines because recommendations for oral intake, timing, patient characteristics, and anesthetic preference are similar. Postpartum tubal ligation may be performed either with neuraxial or general anesthesia, but neuraxial is preferred.

Anesthesia Management of Obstetric Emergencies

Anesthesia management for obstetric emergencies is saddled with peculiarities. The anesthesiologist is tasked with providing quality and safe care for both mother and the fetus/neonate, with the focus on maternal care. Recent data from US Maternal Mortality Review Committees indicate that a majority of maternal deaths are due to preventable causes, such as cardiovascular diseases, infection/sepsis, hemorrhage, cardiomyopathy, thrombotic pulmonary embolism, cerebral vascular accidents, hypertension disease of pregnancy, amniotic fluid embolism/anaphylactoid syndrome of pregnancy, and anesthesia. Obstetric emergencies involving maternal hemorrhage are a preventable cause of severe morbidity and mortality. A process for massive transfusion of blood products should be readily available, and intraoperative cell salvage is a safe and useful modality for autologous blood transfusion. The staff should be trained and prepared to implement standard resuscitative measures for maternal cardiac arrest, which involves immediate cesarean delivery if return of spontaneous circulation does not occur in 4 minutes. Basic and advanced life support equipment availability are required in the labor and delivery and the operating room areas along with medications for emergency airway management. These equipment and medication are laryngoscopes, video-laryngoscopes, smaller-size endotracheal tubes, laryngeal mask airways, ambu bags, an oxygen source, a difficult airway cart, and medications for induction of anesthesia and muscle relaxants. There should be an individual skilled at surgical airway management available for airway emergencies.

Liability Trends Over the Years

Over the years, the practice of obstetrics and gynecology has been associated with increasing malpractice claims, and obstetric anesthesiologists have been listed as defendants in lawsuits even though the anesthesiologists are consultants managing maternal and fetal/neonatal care. The manifestation of complications related to obstetric care may be lifelong and present years after the initial event. For example, neonatal asphyxia manifests as cerebral palsy and other neurological deficits years after the initial injury. Therefore, higher payments may be awarded to plaintiffs of malpractice. The frequency of malpractice liability claims has gradually declined over the past three decades. However, the proportion of the claims have changed. In the 1980s the most common malpractice liability claim was for maternal/neonatal death and brain damage (Table 28.2).[9] Maternal and neonatal death or brain damage comprise approximately 20% of all obstetric liability claims. Maternal deaths and brain damage were commonly due to hemorrhage, embolic events, and anesthesia-related complications (Table 28.3). [9] Neonatal death and brain damage were often attributed to delay in delivery following a nonreassuring fetal monitoring pattern, poor communication between

Table 28.2 Frequency of Liability Claims and Proportion Trends Over the Past Three Decades

	1980s (N=407) N (%)	1990s (N=481)	2000s (N=263) N (%)	2005–2015 (N=107) N (%)
Maternal death and severe brain damage	89 (21)	91 (19)	89 (34)	16 (15)
Neonatal death and severe brain damage	125 (31)	115 (23)	76 (19)	10 (9)
Maternal nerve damage	51 (12)	114 (23)	51 (19)	58 (54.2)
Maternal major and minor injuries	112 (32)	121 (30)	47 (20)	23 (21.5)

Data from:

Davies JM, Stephens LS. Obstetric anesthesia liability concerns. *Clin Obstet Gynecol*. 2017;60:431-446.

Kovacheva VP, Brovman EY, Greenberg P, Song E, Palanisamy A, Urman RD. A Contemporary Analysis of Medicolegal Issues in Obstetric Anesthesia Between 2005 and 2015. *Anesth Analg*. 2019;128(6):1199-1207.

care team members, and inappropriate resuscitation of the neonate by an anesthesia provider following delivery.[9,10,11]

In the 1990s and 2000s, maternal nerve injury and minor injuries made up most obstetrics litigations (see Table 28.2).[9] Maternal nerve injury claims have increased over the past two decades with greater than 50% of the claims due to maternal nerve injury (see Table 28.2).[12] Common anesthesia-related complications were epidural hematoma (only one patient had a known coagulopathy), epidural abscess, inadequate or lack of appropriate documentation, and poor communication during procedure.[10] Claims for neurological injury mainly involved nerve root, spinal cord injury, and permanent neurological deficits. Other maternal malpractice claims described retention of objects in the lumbar spine (e.g., epidural catheter tip), inadequate analgesia during surgical delivery, delay in providing pain management during labor, and lack of compassionate care during labor.[13]

Table 28.3 Most Common Causes for Maternal Deaths and Severe Brain Damage Over the Past Three Decades

	1980s N (%)	1990s N (%)	2000s N (%)	2005–2015 N (%)
Excessive blood loss	4 (4.5)	15 (16.5)	31 (34.8)	2 (12.5)
High/total neuraxial block/arrest	10 (11.2)	22 (24.1)	14 (15.7)	5 (31.2)
Embolic events	5 (5.6)	13 (14.3)	16 (18)	4 (25)
Failed intubation or airway issues	37 (41.6)	14 (15.3)	4 (4.5)	3 (18.8)

Data from:

Davies JM, Stephens LS. Obstetric anesthesia liability concerns. *Clin Obstet Gynecol*. 2017;60:431-446. Kovacheva VP, Brovman EY, Greenberg P, Song E, Palanisamy A, Urman RD. A Contemporary Analysis of Medicolegal Issues in Obstetric Anesthesia Between 2005 and 2015. *Anesth Analg*. 2019;128(6):1199-1207.

Pitfalls Associated With Liability

Although anesthesiologists have been named in many obstetric-related malpractice claims, liability claim payments made on behalf of anesthesiologists have been secondary to issues in which the availability of a qualified anesthesia provider has been reported. Payments have also been made when poor communication with other obstetric team members was determined, anesthetic care plan for parturients were deemed inappropriate, and inadequate documentation of records were noted.

Availability of Qualified Personnel

Over the past three decades, the issue of availability of a qualified anesthesia provider during critical periods of the peripartum period account for 5–50% of claims settlements made on behalf of anesthesiologists.[7,12] A high proportion of these claims were associated with maternal and neonatal death and permanent brain damage where prompt intervention from an anesthesia provider may have impacted the outcome.[7,9,12] A practice model in which the obstetric anesthesiologist is assigned home call may be counterproductive especially when the decision-to-skin incision time of approximately 30 minutes is the goal. Designated high-risk centers should always have an anesthesiologist readily available to provide timely and emergent obstetric care. According to the American College of Obstetrics and Gynecology and the Society for Maternal Fetal Medicine, facilities with a designated maternal care level II or greater must have a board certified anesthesiologist physically present at all times to manage the care of pregnant patients with complex maternal conditions, obstetric complications, and fetal conditions.[14] Also, prioritization of nonobstetric patient care by the obstetric anesthesiologist may be a challenge for anesthesiologists who are assigned to cover general or specialty call while covering obstetric patient care. Recently, the Society of Obstetric Anesthesia and Perinatology awarded Centers for Excellence (COE) in obstetric anesthesia care. Anesthesiologists at designated Centers of Excellence are required to cover the obstetric service without the additional responsibilities of caring for nonobstetric patients.[15]

Communication

There should be clear communication between obstetric anesthesiologists and other members of the patient care team. This fosters a collegial environment and may avoid an impending catastrophe. For example, in the case of uterine atony and hemorrhage, early awareness of bleeding may result in early recognition and transfusion of blood products and resuscitation. Closed claim studies have shown that 10–26% of obstetric malpractice payments were due to lack of communication or miscommunication.[12,16] Clear communications between the obstetric anesthesiologist and the patient is important. Risks associated with epidural placement, such as postdural puncture headache, hypotension, and its impact on the fetus should be discussed with the patient during the informed consent.[12]

Anesthetic Care Plan

An appropriate anesthetic plan should be made based on the patient's preanesthetic evaluation and assessment, clinical scenario, available resources, and preferences. The decision for neuraxial versus general anesthesia should not significantly impede the obstetric plan. Inappropriate anesthetic plan and poor care plans for anticipated complications were associated with approximately 10% of obstetric malpractice claim payments.[12] The availability of airway equipment and emergency medications is key to managing obstetric emergencies and anesthesia-related complications. Early recognition of maternal and fetal risk factors for poor outcomes, along with routine assessments of parturient and fetal monitoring during the peripartum period, cannot be overemphasized.

Documentation

Poor or inaccurate documentation accounts for 4–8% of obstetric malpractice claim payments.[12]

Medical documentation is crucial for recall of events. Proper documentation facilitates acquisition of information and data collection for research purposes, outcome studies, and chart review, and it enhances patient safety and quality care initiatives. Although it is important to record preanesthetic evaluation, assessments, and anesthetic plans, patient consents and other additional discussions should also be documented. Medications administered must be documented appropriately. Procedure notes should describe the equipment/instrument and technique used and mention the safety measures followed. Complications should be noted along with precautionary steps taken to address or mitigate further decompensation. Medical records captured electronically or on paper must be legible.

Finally, in this era of technology and social media, the use of smart phones poses a significant risk for health care information and privacy violations. It is important to protect patient information from data breach and properly discard medical records. Cyber attacks have not been named in obstetric malpractice claims but it is important to recognize this new threat to medicine and to understand that obstetric anesthesia records are no different.

Summary

As medical therapies and technology advances, more women with complex medical conditions present with risk factors for increased maternal and fetal morbidity and mortality during pregnancy, labor and delivery. Therefore, the anesthesia management of obstetric patients often involves greater risk for malpractice claims. The additional involvement of the fetus/neonate increases the likelihood for litigations. Currently, maternal nerve injury constitutes a large proportion of obstetric malpractice claims in the United States. For a developed county, maternal and neonatal deaths and brain damage claims remain high, and this continues to result in significant settlement and plaintiff compensation. Practice Guidelines in obstetric anesthesia provide useful recommendations for quality obstetric care during the peripartum period. Appropriate communication, availability of qualified personnel, planning, and management of obstetric emergencies enhances maternal and fetal care and may impact outcomes as well as prevent litigations.

References

1. Caton D. John Snow's practice of obstetric anesthesia. *Anesthesiology*. 2000;92:247–252.
2. Caton D. The influence of social values on obstetric anesthesia. *AMA J Ethics*. 2015;17:253–257.
3. Lim G, Facco FL, Nathan N, Waters JH, Wong CA, Eltzschig HK. A review of the impact of obstetric anesthesia on maternal and neonatal outcomes. *Anesthesiology*. 2018;129(1):192–215.
4. Mendelson CL. The aspiration of stomach contents into the lungs during obstetric anesthesia. *Am J Obstetric Gynecology*. 1946;52:191–205.
5. Thorp JA, Hu DH, Albin RM, McNitt J, Meyer BA, Cohen GR, et. al. The effect of intrapartum epidural analgesia on nulliparous labor: a randomized, controlled, prospective trial. *Am J Obstetric Gynecology*. 1993;169:851–858.
6. Hawkins JL, Chang J, Palmer SK, Gibbs CP, Callaghan WM. Anesthesia related maternal mortality in the United States: 1979-2002. *Am J Obstetric Gynecology*. 2011;117:69–74.
7. Chadwick HS, Posner K, Caplan RA, Ward RJ, Cheney FW. A comparison of obstetric and non-obstetric anesthesia malpractice claims. *Anesthesiology*. 1991;74:242–249.
8. Practice guidelines for obstetric anesthesia: an updated report by the American Society of Anesthesiologists Task Force on Obstetric Anesthesia and Society for Obstetric Anesthesia and Perinatology. *Anesthesiology*. 2016; 124: 270–300.
9. Davies JM, Stephens LS. Obstetric anesthesia liability concerns. *Clin Obstet Gynecol*. 2017;60:431–446.
10. Jordan LM, Quraishi JA. The AANA Foundation malpractice closed claims study: a descriptive analysis. *AANA J*. 2015;83:318–323.
11. Crawford K. The AANA Foundation closed malpractice claims study: obstetric anesthesia. AANA J. 2002;70:97–104.
12. Kovacheva VP, Brovman EY, Greenberg P, Song E, Palanisamy A, Urman RD. A contemporary analysis of medicolegal issues in obstetric anesthesia between 2005 and 2015. *Anesth Analg*. 2019;128(6):1199–1207.
13. Davies JM, Posner KL, Lee LA, Cheney FW, Domino KB. Liability associated with obstetric anesthesia: a closed claims analysis. *Anesthesiology*. 2009;110: 131–139.
14. American College of Obstetricians and Gynecologists, Society for Maternal-Fetal Medicine. *Obstetric Care Consensus*. Obstet Gynecol. 2014 Mar;123(3):693–711.
15. Carvalho B, Mhyre JM. Centers of Excellence for anesthesia care of obstetric patients. *Anesthesia Analgesia*. 2019;128(5):844–846.
16. Domino KB, Davies JM. Neonatal injury and resuscitation: a liability for anesthesiologists? An update from the Anesthesia Closed Claims Project. *ASA Monitor 02*. 2017;81:16–17.

Index

Tables, figures and boxes are indicated by *t*, *f* and *b* following the page number